Nerve Growth Factor and its Antiserum

Edited by
ELEANOR ZAIMIS
and
Julie Knight

AF797826

Papers presented at the Symposium entitled *Nerve Growth Factor and its Antiserum*, held at University College London, 15–16 April 1971

THE ATHLONE PRESS *of the University of London*
1972

Published by
THE ATHLONE PRESS
UNIVERSITY OF LONDON
at 4 *Gower Street, London* WC1

Distributed by Tiptree Book Services Ltd
Tiptree, Essex.

© *University of London* 1972

0 485 11132 2

Printed in Great Britain by
WESTERN PRINTING SERVICES LTD
BRISTOL

luction

very, about 20 years ago, that 'more than 90 per cent of
ation of sympathetic nerve cells can be increased up to
, conversely wiped out, by supplying a protein or its
to newborn animals', was so extraordinary that for
s it was viewed by a great number of scientists, at least
Britain, with some disbelief. In 1964, however, we were
Professor Levi-Montalcini's advice and using her anti-
demonstrate to the Physiological Society the first
ympathectomized rats produced in this country. A few
ter she visited us at the invitation of London University.
of her lectures I received a letter from Sir Henry Dale,
doubting Thomases, thanking me for the opportunity
ng from Professor Levi-Montalcini of the stages by
has been able to open so fascinating and important a
pter in developmental physiology'. He subsequently
ne of the most ardent supporters of her work.
sts all over the world have not only confirmed the
Professor Levi-Montalcini and those of her colleagues
also produced a number of additional and striking
ons on the nerve growth factor (NGF) and its anti-
ecause of this, the time seemed ripe to bring together
orking on the different aspects of this problem in order
s freely their more recent results. This took the form of
ational Symposium held 15–16 April 1971 at University
ondon. The papers presented at the symposium provide
ance of this volume.
ubject of NGF and its antiserum, as will become
, is still full of intriguing uncertainties. For example,
at total purification of NGF from various sources have
ghly conflicting reports. Professor Levi-Montalcini and
agues consider the problem of the chemical nature of
settled; moreover they stress the similarity of NGF's

Contents

NGF–Antiserum

Problems in the Assay

Introc

The disco
the popul
sixfold, o
antiserum
many yea
in Great I
able, with
serum, t
immunos
months la
After one
one of th
'of heari
which sh
new cha
became c
Scienti
results o
but have
observati
serum. B
people w
to discus
an Intern
College I
the subs
The s
apparent
attempts
led to hi
her colle
NGF as

isolated from mouse salivary glands and snake venom. In contrast, Professor Vernon and his group, conclude that proteins with NGF activity, from different sources, differ considerably in gross chemical properties although, as they point out, their biological effects are highly specific and apparently indistinguishable. To make things even more perplexing, the antigenic properties may be quite distinct. For example, the antiserum to the mouse NGF has little effect on the activity of the snake venom NGF in tissue culture, while the antiserum to NGF from the venom of *Vipera russelli*, fails to block the effects in tissue culture of the mouse NGF. Professor Larrabee also believes that we are dealing with a variety of proteins and because of this he objects to the abbreviation 'NGF', used in this volume. However, I feel that as long as we are aware of these uncertainties and until all the questions are answered, we can go on using, for brevity's sake, the presently popular abbreviation.

There are many other questions which still await an answer: What is the primary source of production of NGF? What is the physiological role of NGF? Are there similar factors for other types of cells? No one will deny that a great deal remains to be learned about nerve growth factor and its mechanism of action but the discussion of what is so far known, and a great deal of what we know, is included in the present volume, makes a very exciting scientific story.

I am sure that my colleagues on the Organizing Committee, Professor C. A. Vernon and Dr D. C. Edwards, wish to join me in acknowledging the essential and notable parts played by Dr E. D. Bueker, Dr S. Cohen—two of the pioneers in the field—Dr M. Abercrombie, FRS and Dr Marthe Vogt, FRS, who chaired the four sessions of the symposium. Their presence was of the greatest value to the success of the meeting. Finally, this symposium could not be arranged without the generous financial support of the Wellcome Trust and the International Union of Biochemistry. We are most grateful to them.

March 1972 E. Z.

List of Participants

P. U. ANGELETTI *Laboratorio di Biologia Cellulare, C.N.R., Rome, Italy and Department of Biology, Washington University, St Louis, Mo., USA*

BARBARA E. C. BANKS *Department of Physiology, University College London, UK*

M. J. BRODY *Department of Pharmacology, College of Medicine, University of Iowa, Iowa City, USA*

KATHERINE A. CHARLWOOD *Department of Chemistry, University College London, UK*

D. C. EDWARDS *Department of Biological Chemistry, Wellcome Research Laboratories, Beckenham, Kent, UK*

I. A. HENDRY *Department of Pharmacology, University of Cambridge, Cambridge, UK*

RUTH HOGUE ANGELETTI *Department of Biology, Washington University, St Louis, Mo., USA and Laboratorio di Biologia Cellulare, C.N.R., Rome, Italy*

G. I. KLINGMAN *School of Medicine, State University of New York at Buffalo, Buffalo, New York 14214, USA*

M. G. LARRABEE *Thomas C. Jenkins Department of Biophysics, Johns Hopkins University, Baltimore, Maryland, USA*

RITA LEVI-MONTALCINI *Laboratorio di Biologia Cellulare, C.N.R., Rome, Italy and Department of Biology, Washington University, St Louis, Mo., USA*

A. LIUZZI *Laboratorio di Biologia Cellulare, C.N.R., Rome, Italy and Department of Biology, Washington University, St Louis, Mo., USA*

ELENA NICOLESCU *Department of Physiology, Faculty of Medicine, Bucharest, Rumania*

LUCIENNE PAPADAKI *The School of Pathology, Middlesex Hospital Medical School, London, UK*

F. L. PEARCE *Department of Chemistry, University College London, UK*

M. SANDLER *Institute of Obstetrics and Gynaecology, Queen Charlotte's Maternity Hospital, Goldhawk Rd, London, UK*

N. R. SAUNDERS *Department of Physiology, University College London, UK*

E. M. SHOOTER *Department of Biochemistry, Stanford University Medical School, Stanford, California, USA*

G. STEINER *Department of Medicine, University of Toronto, Canada*

C. VAN-TOLLER *Department of Psychology, University of Durham, UK*

C. A. VERNON *Department of Chemistry, University College London, UK*

BERNICE WENZEL *Department of Physiology and Brain Research Institute, University College of Los Angeles School of Medicine, Los Angeles, California, USA*

ELEANOR ZAIMIS *Department of Pharmacology, Royal Free Hospital School of Medicine, Hunter St, London, UK*

SECTION I

Nerve Growth Factor

The Isolation and Characterization of Nerve Growth Factor from the Venom of *Vipera russelli*

F. L. PEARCE, BARBARA E. C. BANKS,* D. V. BANTHORPE, A. R. BERRY, H. ff. S. DAVIES and C. A. VERNON

Departments of Chemistry and Physiology, University College London, UK*

The effects of implants of mouse sarcoma 180 in chick embryos were discovered by Bueker (1948) and were further investigated by Levi-Montalcini & Hamburger (1951, 1953). The hypothesis that the effects arise from some diffusible chemical agent released by the sarcoma was advanced by Levi-Montalcini in 1952 and has since been amply confirmed. The development of a simple tissue culture technique (Levi-Montalcini, Meyer & Hamburger, 1954) for the detection of similar agents led to the discovery that snake venoms and the submaxillary gland of the male mouse are potent sources (Cohen & Levi-Montalcini, 1956; Cohen, 1958). Since the primary effect of the agents, *in vitro*, is to promote the growth of fibres from explants of chick embryonic dorsal root and sympathetic ganglia, they were given the name nerve growth factor (NGF). It must be emphasized that the name refers to a group of substances and not to a unique chemical species.

The first attempt to purify NGF used mouse sarcoma 180 as source and led to the view that activity is associated with a specific protein (Cohen & Levi-Montalcini, 1957). All subsequent work has confirmed this view and it is now firmly established that NGF refers to a group of proteins with very similar or, perhaps, identical effects on embryonic dorsal root and sympathetic ganglia.

It is somewhat surprising that the complete chemical characterization of NGF has proceeded rather slowly. All attempts at total purification have been made with mouse submaxillary gland or snake venoms as the source and have led to highly conflicting reports. The first purification from mouse submaxillary glands was that reported by Cohen (1960). He isolated a protein, active in tissue culture at a concentration of 10^{-8} g/ml, that was homogeneous to sedimentation analysis: no other criteria of homogeneity were used. On the basis of the value of the sedimentation coefficient ($s_{20} = 4.33S$), Cohen estimated the molecular weight to be about 40 000. This preparation, although highly active, was obtained by using somewhat unorthodox chromatographic procedures, and was almost certainly heterogeneous. The reported value of the sedimentation coefficient has not been confirmed by other workers.

Schenkein, Levy, Bueker & Tokarsky (1968), using a rather different purification procedure, isolated a protein fraction which, they claimed, was active at a concentration of 10^{-16} g/ml. Electrophoresis on acrylamide gel showed that the active fraction was not homogeneous and it was suggested that it contained two forms of NGF, one active at high concentration and the other at low concentration. This finding has not been confirmed by other workers. The remarkably high level of activity reported may be an artefact, generated as described by one of us (F. L. Pearce) elsewhere in this volume (pp. 253–61).

However, multiple forms of NGF from mouse submaxillary gland have also been reported by Zanini, Angeletti & Levi-Montalcini (1968). These workers used a modification of Cohen's procedure and reported that 'under appropriate conditions' NGF could be separated into molecular forms which were multiples of a basic unit having a molecular weight of about 14 000. It is difficult to assess this work since it appears to have been ignored in a later publication (Bocchini & Angeletti, 1969). In this paper, standard chromatographic methods were used to isolate a protein that was homogeneous to sedimentation analysis and to electrophoresis. The molecular weight, calculated from the sedimentation and diffusion coefficients ($s_{20} = 2.43S$, $D_{20} = 7.30 \times 10^{-7}$ cm^2 s^{-1}) was given as 32 000. The substance was active in tissue culture at about the same concentration as Cohen's preparation (10^{-8} g/ml).

Shooter and his co-workers (Varon, Nomura & Shooter, 1967*a*, *b*; 1968; Smith, Varon & Shooter, 1968) have isolated NGF from mouse submaxillary glands as a high molecular weight aggregate (s_{20} = 7.1S, estimated molecular weight 140 000). This preparation, which is active in tissue culture at a concentration of about 10^{-8} g/ml, has also been obtained in several other laboratories and is certainly reproducible. The aggregate is stable only within the range pH 5–8; outside these limits it reversibly dissociates into a mixture of acid, neutral and basic subunits each having a molecular weight of about 30 000. The subunits can easily be separated by ion-exchange chromatography and NGF activity is found to be associated only with the basic component. This subunit, which was shown to be homogeneous to electrophoresis in acrylamide gel, is clearly similar to or identical with the preparation produced by the procedure described by Bocchini & Angeletti (1969). It represents the only well-characterized form of NGF from submaxillary glands that has so far been described.

A high molecular weight aggregate showing NGF activity from mouse submaxillary glands has also been described by Levi-Montalcini, Angeletti and their co-workers (Levi-Montalcini, Tentori, Vivaldi, Angeletti & Marini-Bettolo, 1965; Salvi, Angeletti & Frati, 1965). This aggregate, like that described by Shooter and his colleagues, could be dissociated into subunits, only one of which was active. However, Levi-Montalcini and her co-workers consider that the aggregate has no functional significance, whereas Shooter and his colleagues disagree. They suggest that the presence of inactive subunits might be relevant in permitting 'the control of biological activity through allosteric effects' (Varon *et al.*, 1967*b*).

The purification of NGF from snake venoms has progressed less far. The first preparation, using the venom of *Angkistrodon piscivorus*, was also made by Cohen (1959). His purification procedure, although somewhat ill-defined, led to a protein which gave a single peak on sedimentation analysis (s_{20} = 2.2S). A more conventional procedure (Banks *et al.*, 1968) gave a protein of similar biological activity and with a similar value of the sedimentation coefficient to that reported by Cohen. However, it proved to be heterogeneous on starch gel electrophoresis. Angeletti (1970), using standard chromatographic methods, purified NGF from the venom of *Naja naja*. The final product was claimed to be homogeneous to sedimentation analysis (s_{20} = 2.37S) and to electrophoresis in acrylamide gel. Gel filtration gave a molecular weight of approximately 25 000.

Gel filtration has been used to study the behaviour of a number of crude snake venoms and it has been concluded (Angeletti, Calissano, Chen & Levi-Montalcini, 1967; Angeletti, 1968*a*) that NGF is present in various molecular forms corresponding to different degrees of aggregation of some fundamental subunit. Angeletti and co-workers (1967) considered the molecular weight of the subunit to be approximately 20 000. However, Angeletti (1968*b*), working with the venoms of *Crotalus admanteus* and *Bothrops jararaca*, has claimed that the monomeric species has a molecular weight of only 5000. In evaluating this work it must be remembered that gel filtration can be a highly misleading technique. Later in this paper we offer evidence to suggest that this is especially true with NGF from snake venoms.

Our own work has been largely concerned with NGF from the venom of *Vipera russelli*. The procedures described below are elaborations of those briefly reported earlier (Banks *et al.*, 1968; Vernon *et al.*, 1969).

The purification of NGF from the venom of '*Vipera russelli*'

The venom of *Vipera russelli* was purchased from the Haffkine Institute, Bombay, India. The procedure which leads to a homogeneous product is as follows:

Step 1 Lyophilized whole venom (2.5 g) was dissolved in sodium chloride solution (0.5 M, 20 ml), centrifuged to remove insoluble material and applied to a column of Sephadex G-150 that had been equilibrated with the solvent. The NGF was eluted in the apparent molecular weight range 20 000–60 000. Yield 17.4 per cent; active* at 1.5×10^{-7} g/ml.

* Yields are percentages of the dry weight of the whole venom. The concentrations quoted are those required to produce a standard response of 2.5 on an arbitrary scale of 0–5 in tissue culture, using dorsal root ganglia from eight-day chick embryos cultured in liquid medium on collagen.

Step 2 The previous step was repeated, using Sephadex G-75. The NGF was eluted in the apparent molecular weight range 25 000–55 000. Yield 7.4 per cent; active at 10^{-7} to 5×10^{-8} g/ml.
Step 3 The active material from Step 2 was dissolved in sodium carbonate-bicarbonate buffer (0.05 M, pH 10.6) and dialysed against this buffer for 36 hours. It was then applied to a column of QAE A-25 Sephadex equilibrated at the same pH. The NGF was not adsorbed on to the resin and was eluted with the starting buffer. The remaining components were eluted by application of a salt gradient of parabolic form. Yield 0.39 per cent, active at 10^{-8}–10^{-9} g/ml.
Step 4 The active fraction from Step 3 was dissolved in acetate buffer (0.05 M, pH 5.0) and dialysed against this buffer for 36 hours. It was then applied to a column of SP C-25 Sephadex equilibrated at the same pH. The NGF was bound to the resin and was eluted by application of a linear salt gradient. Yield 0.29 per cent; active at 10^{-8}–10^{-9} g/ml.
Step 5 The material was finally passed through a column of Sephadex G-100 that had been equilibrated with sodium choride solution (0.1 M) and was calibrated by measuring the elution volumes of proteins of known molecular weight over the range 10 000–70 000. Two peaks were obtained: the first, with an apparent molecular weight of 54 000, contained no NGF activity. The second peak, corresponding to an apparent molecular weight of 34 000, showed NGF activity at a concentration of 10^{-8}–10^{-9} g/ml. Yield 0.15 per cent.

As described below, this final material was homogeneous to all criteria available to us.

Some comment on the purification procedure is required, since it presents some unusual features. Step 4 removed a number of contaminating proteins. In many preparations it proved to be unnecessary, since the contaminants were removed by the QAE-Sephadex. In these cases, and in other preparations after Step 4, the active material was found to be homogeneous both to sedimentation and to diffusion analysis in the ultracentrifuge, and its behaviour was indistinguishable by these methods from that of the active material from Step 5. It follows that the two proteins finally separated by the Sephadex G-100 column must have the same molecular weight. The separation depends, therefore, on a factor other than size. The explanation of this anomalous behaviour is probably to be found in the fact that both proteins contain large amounts of carbohydrate; 26 per cent for the inactive component and 20 per cent for the NGF. Glycoproteins are normally eluted from calibrated Sephadex columns with apparent molecular weights which are too large (Andrews, 1965); and this is presumably because hydration of the carbohydrate residues increases the effective Stokes radius. The inactive component of the mixture from Step 4 is, therefore, showing expected behaviour; but the NGF is heavily retarded. The obvious interpretation of this is that the molecule interacts with the matrix of the resin, which thus slows its passage through the column. As described below, we have found that the material is strongly adsorbed on to a number of surfaces, both polar and nonpolar. Its behaviour on a Sephadex column is consistent with this; but, whatever the explanation of the results obtained with the Sephadex G-100 column, the dangers inherent in inferring molecular sizes of snake venom components from this type of result, particularly when using crude venom mixtures, are clearly illustrated.

It is perhaps surprising that the two components separated in the final step should have failed to separate in the four earlier ones. This, and the fact that both molecules have the same molecular size and similar carbohydrate contents, suggests that they may be closely related. However, all attempts to generate NGF activity from the inactive component by chemical treatments have so far failed.

Electrophoretic properties

There is no doubt that electrophoresis in a supporting medium is the most sensitive method for detecting heterogeneity in a protein preparation. However, the number of buffer systems suitable for examining the NGF from the venom of *Vipera russelli* is rather limited. The discontinuous buffer system using β-alanine/acetic acid described by Reisfeld, Lewis & Williams (1962) showed that at pH 3.8 the active material migrated towards the cathode as a slightly diffuse band. No contaminants were observed. Electrophoresis, using a continuous buffer system at pH 2.9, was carried out by a modification of the method described by Jordan &

Raymond (1969). As before, the active material migrated towards the cathode as a slightly diffuse single band. Electrophoresis at pH 5.2 was carried out, using a buffer system developed by two of us (Berry & Davies, unpublished work). This buffer system contains 6-amino-*N*-hexanoic acid/cacodylic acid and provides considerable resolving power. Again, no contaminants were detected.

Isoelectric focusing in acrylamide gels is another technique used to examine the heterogeneity of protein samples; it depends upon the migration of proteins under the influence of an electric field to regions of their isoelectric pH values in a stable pH gradient. The protein zones then become stationary and are further sharpened as electrophoresis proceeds. The method used in the present work has been described by Pearce (1971). The result was clear-cut: the active material showed a single sharp band at the bottom of the gel. No trace of contaminant was found. From the results obtained the isoelectric point of NGF (pI) was estimated to be 10.5 ± 1.0. However, since the NGF migrated to the end of the gel, it was still possible that two highly basic proteins might not have been resolved. To exclude this possibility, the technique of dynamic gel electrofocusing was applied (Wrigley, 1968). In this procedure, electrophoresis is stopped before equilibrium is attained. The method showed that NGF migrated through the gel as a single diffuse band which sharpened as equilibrium was approached. Again, no contaminant was detected. Staining with periodate Schiff's reagent, which detects the presence of carbohydrates associated with proteins (Clarke, 1964), gave bands in the same position as those developed by the protein-detecting stains.

There is no doubt that as far as the techniques of electrophoresis in acrylamide gel are concerned, the NGF prepared by the method described above consists of a single, unique chemical species.

The molecular weight of NGF

The molecular weight of NGF was calculated from values of the sedimentation and diffusion coefficients measured by standard procedures using an analytical ultracentrifuge. The experimental and computational methods were as described by Banks,

Doonan, Lawrence & Vernon (1968). In each sedimentation run the material showed a single, symmetrical peak. In the diffusion runs the area under the curve given by the Schlieren optical system was constant with time to within 2 per cent. The partial specific volume ($\bar{v}$) was calculated from the amino acid and carbohydrate content as 0.710. The data obtained are shown in Table 1. Since there is no obvious change of estimated molecular

Table 1 The molecular weight of NGF from the venom of *Vipera russelli* determined by ultracentrifugation analysis

Protein concentration (% *w/v*)	*pH*	s_{20}	D_{20}	*Molecular weight*
0.3	10.5	2.92	6.48	38 000
0.7	7.4	3.07	6.67	39 000
0.8	10.5	2.83	6.86	35 000
0.8	10.5	2.86	6.72	36 000
0.9	10.5	2.63	5.50	40 000
1.0	10.5	2.70	6.15	37 000
1.0	10.5	2.65	5.65	39 000
1.2	10.5	2.88	7.12	34 000

s_{20}, sedimentation coefficient ($\times 10^{-13}$ s^{-1}).
D_{20}, diffusion coefficient ($\times 10^{-7}$ cm^2 s^{-1}).
pH 10.5 was obtained using carbonate-bicarbonate buffer (0.1 M).
pH 7.4 was obtained using phosphate buffer (0.1 M).

weight with concentration or with pH the mean value has been taken as 37 000. The data provide no evidence for dissociation into subunits, since the concentration of protein decreases in this admittedly limited range. However, it is not possible to work with dilute solutions in the ultracentrifuge and, for this reason, the behaviour of NGF on a calibrated Sephadex column was examined as a function of concentration. As mentioned above, this method does not give the correct value of the molecular weight with this particular protein; but it should nevertheless provide evidence for a change in molecular weight; that is, for dissociation at high dilution. The data, given in Table 2, are not very precise because of the difficulty of estimating the activity maxima with dilute solutions of NGF. However, it is clear that even at low concentrations (10^{-8}–10^{-9} M) there is no evidence for the dissociation of the molecule into subunits.

The values of the sedimentation and diffusion coefficients can also be used to calculate the frictional ratio which can then be used, given certain assumptions, to provide information about the shape of the molecule. The frictional ratio for NGF is found to be 1.54 and, assuming that the value normally cited (30 per cent) for the degree of hydration of unconjugated proteins (Alexander & Johnson, 1949) also applies to glycoproteins, this means that the molecule can be represented by a prolate ellipsoid of axial ratio 7:1. Consequently, the molecule, unlike most globular proteins, more closely resembles a rod than a sphere.

Table 2 The elution volumes from G-100 Sephadex of samples of NGF at different concentrations

Sample applied	*Maximum protein concentration in eluate* (M)	*Elution volume (ml)*	*Apparent molecular weight*
30 000 μg 0.86×10^{-3} M	1.4×10^{-5}	266	34 000
500 μg 1.4×10^{-5} M	2.3×10^{-7}	260–285	31 000–35 000
50 μg 1.4×10^{-6} M	2.3×10^{-8}	260–295	29 000–35 000
10 μg 2.8×10^{-7} M	4.6×10^{-9}	260–300	28 000–35 000

Chemical composition of NGF

The amino acid composition of NGF was determined by conventional methods. Tryptophan was estimated by the spectrophotometric method of Bencze & Schmid (1957). The carbohydrate content was analysed by the very convenient method developed by Bolton, Clamp & Hough (1965), in which a known amount of salt-free protein is hydrolysed with hydrochloric acid in methanol. The carbohydrates are then converted into the corresponding trimethyl silyl ethers, which are analysed by gas-liquid chromatography. The peaks obtained are identified by comparison with standards. The results of both the amino acid and the carbohydrate analyses are summarized in Table 3—the number of residues being calculated for a molecular weight of 37 000. These results show a number of features of interest. The carbohydrate content is high (19.3 per cent). The number of acidic amino acid residues (59) greatly exceeds the number of basic ones (29). Since the molecule is highly basic most of the acidic residues must be present in the amide form and may possibly be points of attachment for *N*-acetyl glucosamine. The number of residues of threonine and serine is also relatively high (38); some of these no doubt also serve as points of attachment of the carbohydrate residues.

Table 3 The chemical composition of NGF

Amino acid	*Number of residues*	*Carbohydrate*	*Number of residues*
Aspartic acid	44	Fucose	4
Glutamic acid	15	Mannose	8
Threonine	22	Galactose	9
Serine	16	*N*-acetyl glucosamine	14
Proline	14	*N*-acetyl neuraminic acid	2
Glycine	13		
Alanine	14	Total	37
Valine	33		
Isoleucine	12		
Leucine	7		
Half-cystine	12		
Methionine	6		
Tyrosine	7		
Phenylalanine	12		
Tryptophan	12		
Histidine	6		
Lysine	14		
Arginine	15		
Total	274		

Stability

The NGF from the venom of *Vipera russelli* is a very stable molecule. It retains its biological activity after being subjected to extremes of pH, and after treatment with trypsin and chymotrypsin. The details of the effects of the various treatments are given in Table 4.

It can be seen that rapid loss of activity occurs only on heating to high temperature or on treatment with pepsin. The extreme stability of the protein suggests that the half-cystine residues may be present in the form of six disulphide bridges. The polypeptide chain may also be protected by the carbohydrate content of the molecule.

Table 4 Effects of various treatments on the biological activity of NGF

Treatment	*Effect on biological activity*
0.1 N-HCl, 37°C	None
0.1 N-NaOH, 37°C	None
Trypsin (5–100 μg), 37°C, pH 7.2	None
Chymotrypsin (5–100 μg), 37°C, pH 7.2	None
DNase (5–100 μg), 37°C, pH 7.2	None
RNase (5–100 μg), 37°C, pH 7.2	None
Dialysis against EDTA (10^{-2} M), 4°C, 72 hours	None
Dialysis against urea (6 M), 4°C, 72 hours	Partial loss (90%)
Pronase (5–100 μg), 37°C, pH 7.2	Partial loss (50%)
Pepsin (5 μg), 37°C, pH 2.0	Total loss
Heating to 90°C, 15 minutes	Total loss

Time of treatment 4 hours unless otherwise stated

Other properties of NGF

The ultraviolet absorption spectrum is typical of a protein, the ratio of the absorbance at 280 nm to that at 260 nm being 1.68. The optical density at 280 nm of a solution of 1 mg/ml is 1.10 and this value is also within the normal range.

Perhaps the most interesting property of the NGF from the venom of *Vipera russelli* is its ready adsorption onto a variety of surfaces. This phenomenon led us to underestimate the concentration required for biological activity by several orders of magnitude (Banks *et al.*, 1968; Pearce, this volume pp. 253–61). One might suppose that the adsorption arises from interaction between the positively charged protein and the negatively charged glass surface, but this cannot be the correct explanation since equally strong adsorption occurs on polypropylene and on a number of other non-polar surfaces. Since the molecule has a rod-like shape, it may be that London forces are sufficiently strong to account for the observed effect. Although the phenomenon is interesting from the physico-chemical viewpoint it presumably has nothing to do with the general biological action of NGF, since the high molecular weight material from mouse submaxillary gland prepared by the method of Varon and coworkers (1967*a*, 1968) does not show this property (Helen Davies, unpublished experiments).

Comparison with NGF from other sources

Comparison of the properties of NGF from the venom of *Vipera russelli* with those of NGF from other sources is not easy, since the published literature contains few of the necessary data. However, the NGF from mouse submaxillary gland as prepared by Bocchini & Angeletti (1969) has been well characterized (Bocchini, 1970) and the NGF from the venom of *Naja naja* as prepared by Angeletti (1970) has been partially characterized. Some comparison is therefore possible. The relevant data are collected in Table 5. It would appear that the three molecules differ considerably both in size and in charge. An important difference occurs between the NGF from the two snake venoms: one is highly basic whereas the other is not. This is particularly surprising since other snake venoms examined by us (for example, the venom of *Vipera ammodytes ammodytes*) were also found to contain highly basic NGF.

Table 5 Properties of NGF from different sources

	Venom of Naja naja	*Venom of* Vipera russelli	*Mouse submaxillary gland*
Sedimentation coefficient (s_{20}, 10^{-13} s^{-1})	2.37	2.82	2.43
Diffusion coefficient (D_{20}, 10^{-7} cm^2 s^{-1})	—	6.39	7.30
Partial specific volume	—	0.710	0.716
Molecular weight (ultracentrifuge)	—	37 000	32 000
Molecular weight (gel filtration)	25 000–28 000	34 000	30 000
Frictional ratio	—	1.54	1.40
Isoelectric point	6.75	10.5	9.3
OD_{280} of 1 mg/ml	1.27	1.10	1.39
OD_{280}/OD_{260}	1.4	1.68	1.54

The amino acid compositions of all three forms of NGF may also be compared. The data are given in Table 6: the number of residues of each amino acid is expressed as an approximate percentage of the total number of residues. No very obvious similarities are revealed by this comparison.

Table 6 Percentage amino acid composition of NGF from different sources

Residue	*Naja naja*[1]	*Vipera russelli*	*Mouse submaxillary gland*[2]
Aspartic acid	14.8	16.1	9.4
Glutamic acid	8.7	5.5	7.6
Threonine	11.3	8.0	11.3
Serine	7.0	5.8	8.7
Proline	4.3	5.1	1.9
Glycine	7.0	4.7	4.9
Alanine	5.2	5.1	7.2
Valine	7.7	12.0	10.9
Isoleucine	5.2	4.4	4.5
Leucine	3.5	2.2	3.0
Half-cystine	3.5	4.4	3.9
Methionine	0.9	2.2	0.8
Tyrosine	1.8	2.6	1.5
Phenylalanine	3.5	4.4	6.0
Tryptophan	1.8	4.4	2.3
Histidine	3.5	2.2	3.0
Lysine	7.7	5.1	7.2
Arginine	2.6	5.5	6.0

1 From Angeletti, 1970.
2 From Bocchini & Angeletti, 1969; Bocchini, 1970.

Discussion

The purification procedure described here leads to a product which is homogeneous both to ultracentrifugation analysis and to a variety of electrophoretic techniques of high resolution. However, the method is time-consuming if used on more than a small scale since the initial gel filtration step cannot be conveniently carried out with more than about 2 g of material. The venom of *Vipera russelli* is a rather poor source of NGF and is, in any case, not available in large amount. We have found that the largest practicable amount of starting material is 50 g of lyophilized crude venom, which yields about 75 mg of final material. Large quantities of NGF cannot, therefore, be made by this method. We have tried a number of variations in the procedure, including isoelectric focusing, but these have generally proved unsuccessful.

The product finally obtained was found to be a highly basic, stable glycoprotein of molecular weight 37 000 and containing approximately 20 per cent carbohydrate. The molecule is rod-shaped and this probably helps to explain its ready adsorption on to a variety of surfaces both polar and non-polar. It is probable that the carbohydrate component has no functional significance since the NGF of low molecular weight from mouse submaxillary gland appears to contain little, if any, carbohydrate. In tissue culture the NGF from the venom of *Vipera russelli* is active towards chick embryonic dorsal root ganglia at a concentration of 10^{-8}–10^{-9} g/ml (i.e. 3×10^{-10} to 3×10^{-11} M) and the response obtained is indistinguishable from that produced by NGF from other sources.

The substance has been shown to be active in neonatal mice and it produces the characteristic hypertrophy and hyperplasia of the superior cervical ganglia (Charlwood & Edwards, unpublished experiments). Perhaps not surprisingly, however, it is less active in this species, by about one order of magnitude, than is the NGF from mouse submaxillary gland. It is also active in kittens, but the effects may not be precisely identical with those produced by NGF from mouse submaxillary gland (Zaimis, personal communication).

A potent antiserum was prepared in rabbit by Dr D. C. Edwards of the Wellcome Research Laboratories. This antiserum, however, did not produce immunosympathectomy in neonatal rats and failed to block the effects in tissue culture of the NGF from mouse submaxillary gland except when it was used at a concentration a thousand-fold higher than that required to abolish the *in vitro* effects of the NGF from the venom of *Vipera russelli*. The reverse procedure gave consistent results: antiserum to the mouse NGF had little effect on the activity of the snake venom NGF in tissue culture. The antigenic properties of these two forms of NGF are therefore quite distinct; but the extent to which this behaviour is due to differences in their polypeptide chains, or to differences in their carbohydrate contents, is not known.

The results presented here show that proteins with NGF activity from different sources appear to differ considerably in gross chemical properties. This is in some ways surprising, since the biological effects are highly specific and, apparently, indistinguishable. One might argue, by analogy with enzymes, that only the active sites need to be the same; and that this would permit large variations in gross chemical properties. However, enzymes which differ, other than in the active site, are always distinguishable by stability, substrate specificity and so on. For example, trypsin and chymotrypsin have the same active site in the sense that both depend on a serine residue which is activated by the aspartate-histidine-serine relay system. The mechanism of catalysis is essentially the same in both cases; but nevertheless, the two enzymes are easily distinguishable. Furthermore, it is by no means obvious that the notion of the active site can be carried over to molecules with activities of the kind shown by NGF. Clearly much more comparative work is necessary in this field.

Acknowledgements

The authors wish to thank the Whitehall Foundation, New York for generous financial support. Thanks are also due to the University of London, the Medical Research Council and the Science Research Council for financial support (to F.L.P. and A.R.B.).

References

Alexander, A. E. & Johnson, P. (1949). *Colloid Science*, p. 148. Oxford: Clarendon Press.

Andrews, P. (1965). *Biochem. J.* **96**, 595.

Angeletti, P., Calissano, P., Chen, J. S. & Levi-Montalcini, R. (1967). *Biochim. biophys. Acta* **147**, 180.

Angeletti, R. H. (1968*a*). *J. Chromat.* **36**, 535.

Angeletti, R. H. (1968*b*). *J. Chromat.* **37**, 62.

Angeletti, R. H. (1970). *Proc. natn. Acad. Sci. U.S.A.* **65**, 668.

Banks, B. E. C., Banthorpe, D. V., Berry, A. R., Davies, H. ff. S., Doonan, S., Lamont, D. M., Shipolini, R. & Vernon, C. A. (1968). *Biochem. J.* **108**, 157.

Banks, B. E. C., Doonan, S., Lawrence, A. J. & Vernon, C. A. (1968). *Eur. J. Biochem.* **5**, 528.

Bencze, W. L. & Schmid, K. (1957). *Analyt. Chem.* **29**, 1193.

Bocchini, V. (1970). *Eur. J. Biochem.* **15**, 127.

Bocchini, V. & Angeletti, P. U. (1969). *Proc. natn. Acad. Sci. U.S.A* **64**, 787.

Bolton, C. H., Clamp, J. R. & Hough, L. (1965). *Biochem. J.* **96**, 5C.
Bueker, E. D. (1948). *Anat. Rec.* **102**, 369.
Clarke, J. T. (1964). *Ann. N.Y. Acad. Sci.* **121**, 428.
Cohen, S. (1958). In *The Chemical Basis of Development*, p. 665. Ed. by B. McElroy and W. D. Glass. Baltimore: Johns Hopkins Press.
Cohen, S. (1959). *J. biol. Chem.* **234**, 1129.
Cohen, S. (1960), *Proc. natn. Acad. Sci. U.S.A.* **46**, 302.
Cohen, S. & Levi-Montalcini, R. (1956). *Proc. natn. Acad. Sci. U.S.A.* **40**, 1014.
Cohen, S. & Levi-Montalcini, R. (1957). *Cancer Res.* **17**, 15.
Jordan, E. M. & Raymond, S. (1969). *Analyt. Biochem.* **27**, 205.
Levi-Montalcini, R. (1952). *Ann. N.Y. Acad. Sci.* **55**, 330.
Levi-Montalcini, R. & Hamburger, V. (1951). *J. exp. Zool.* **116**, 321.
Levi-Montalcini, R. & Hamburger, V. (1953). *J. exp. Zool.* **123**, 233.
Levi-Montalcini, R., Meyer, H. & Hamburger, V. (1954). *Cancer Res.* **14**, 49.
Levi-Montalcini, R., Tentori, L., Vivaldi, G., Angeletti, P. U. & Marini-Bettolo, G. B. (1965). *Gazz. chim. ital.* **95**, 333.
Pearce, F. L. (1971). Ph.D. Thesis, University of London, p. 46.
Reisfeld, R. A., Lewis, U. J. & Williams, D. E. (1962). *Nature, Lond.* **195**, 281.
Salvi, M. L., Angeletti, P. U. & Frati, L. (1965). *Farmaco* **20**, 12.
Schenkein, I., Levy, M., Bueker, E. D. & Tokarsky, E. (1968). *Science* **159**, 640.
Smith, A. P., Varon, S. & Shooter, E. M. (1968). *Biochemistry, N.Y.* **7**, 3259.
Varon, S., Nomura, J. & Shooter, E. M. (1967*a*). *Biochemistry, N.Y.* **6**, 2202.
Varon, S., Nomura, J. & Shooter, E. M. (1967*b*). *Proc. natn. Acad. Sci. U.S.A.* **57**, 1782.
Varon, S., Nomura, J. & Shooter, E. M. (1968). *Biochemistry, N.Y.* **7**, 1296.
Vernon, C. A., Banks, B. E. C., Banthorpe, D. V., Berry, A. R., Davies, H. ff. S., Lamont, D. M., Pearce, F. L. and Redding, K. A. (1969). In *Ciba Foundation Symposium on Homeostatic Regulators*, p. 57. Ed. by G. E. W. Wolstenholme and J. Knight. London: J. & A. Churchill.
Wrigley, C. (1968). *Science Tools* **15**, 17.
Zanini, A., Angeletti, P. & Levi-Montalcini, R. (1968). *Proc. natn. Acad. Sci. U.S.A.* **61**, 835.

Nerve Growth Factors of the Mouse Submaxillary Gland

J. R. PÉREZ-POLO,* JAMES R. BAMBURG,* W. W. W. DE JONG,† DANIEL STRAUS, MICHAEL BAKER and E. M. SHOOTER

Departments of Genetics and Biochemistry, and Lt. Joseph P. Kennedy, Jr Laboratories for Molecular Medicine, Stanford University School of Medicine, Stanford, California, USA

The submaxillary gland of the adult male mouse is a principal source of nerve growth factor (NGF) proteins and a number of laboratories have been concerned over the past few years with their isolation and characterization. It was already apparent from the early work of Cohen (1960), and it has become increasingly apparent in later studies, that NGF activity is not uniquely associated with a single protein species. However, the molecular heterogeneity of NGF activity can now be explained in terms of the properties of a number of well-defined proteins and of the relationships between them. The two major protein classes which elicit NGF activity are the high molecular weight forms, which exist in neutral pH homogenates of the gland, and the smaller, basic proteins, which can be isolated from the high molecular weight species after exposure to mild acid or alkaline pH. This review will be primarily concerned with the properties and relationships of these two classes.

The two classes of NGF proteins

It is generally agreed that NGF activity in the initial homogenates of the gland is found with a relatively high molecular weight,

* Postdoctoral Fellow, National Multiple Sclerosis Society.
† Fellow, UNESCO International Brain Research Organization.

complex protein which readily undergoes dissociation (Varon, Nomura & Shooter, 1967*a*, *b*; Angeletti, Calissano, Chen & Levi-Montalcini, 1967; Bocchini & Angeletti, 1969). This form has been isolated and characterized by its electrophoretic and sedimentation properties, the latter, together with its biological activity, giving rise to the designation 7S NGF (Varon *et al.*, 1967*b*; Smith, Varon & Shooter, 1968). Its molecular weight has not yet been accurately determined. The value of 140 000 (Varon *et al.*, 1967*b*) is an estimate based on its sedimentation coefficient, assuming the molecule to be spherical. The values of 80 000–90 000 are those obtained on calibrated Sephadex G-100 columns (Varon & Shooter, 1966; Bocchini & Angeletti, 1969) and as such are subject to the usual errors of the method, particularly in so far as they relate to elution of glycoproteins and of proteins in equilibrium with their subunits, both of which apply to 7S NGF. These problems are illustrated by the fact that, on a calibrated Sephadex G-200 column, the higher value of 130 000 is obtained (Angeletti *et al.*, 1967). Irrespective of the actual molecular weight, the current methods for isolating either the high or low molecular weight forms all use gel filtration as a first step and consistently isolate a fraction containing 7S NGF. Probably because of the removal of substances which interfere in the bioassay, the recovery of NGF activity at this stage often exceeds 100 per cent of the activity applied to the column (Varon *et al.*, 1967*b*; Bocchini & Angeletti, 1969). The question of whether all the NGF activity of the gland homogenate can be accounted for as 7S NGF, has not yet been satisfactorily answered. It is true that essentially all the assayable NGF activity in a gland homogenate or supernatant analysed by gel filtration or sucrose-gradient sedimentation coincides with 7S NGF (Varon *et al.*, 1967*a*, *b*; Bocchini & Angeletti, 1969). However, the recovery of the low molecular weight form, the β-subunit, in these analyses is very low (Greene, Varon, Piltch & Shooter, 1971) and a sizeable fraction of these species could be present in the homogenate and yet remain undetected.

Provided that the pH is kept near neutrality and certain other precautions are observed, the high molecular weight 7S NGF species can be isolated as stable reproducible proteins accounting for some 60 per cent of the NGF activity and 2 per cent of the total protein in the gland homogenate. Their properties have recently been described in detail (Varon & Shooter, 1970). If, on the other hand, at any stage of the isolation procedure the pH is brought below 5 or above 8, all the NGF activity is recovered in smaller, basic proteins whose size, and possibly also specific NGF activity, is dependent on the method of isolation (Varon, Nomura & Shooter, 1968; Zanini, Angeletti & Levi-Montalcini, 1968; Bocchini & Angeletti, 1969). One of these proteins is the subunit of 7S NGF, a protein of molecular weight 23 000 and isoelectric point of pH 9.2. The specific NGF activity of this protein is altered by its interaction with the other two subunit types in 7S NGF. Another is the basic protein isolated by Bocchini & Angeletti (1969) and further studied by Angeletti, Bradshaw and Wade (1971), the molecular weight of which is closer to 30 000 and which accounts for a higher proportion of the initial NGF activity of the gland than does the β-subunit.

The high molecular weight form 7S NGF

Composition. Electrophoresis of 7S NGF in acrylamide gel systems near neutrality gives rise to a single broad band of protein (Varon *et al.*, 1967*b*; Varon *et al.*, 1968; Smith *et al.*, 1968; Smith, Greene, Fisk, Varon & Shooter, 1969). When 7S NGF is subjected to isoelectric focusing in an acrylamide gel containing ampholine (pH 3–10) such that it is never exposed to a pH outside the range of 5 to 8, it again forms a broad band when it reaches its equilibrium position near pH 5.1 (Varon & Shooter, 1970). However, prolonged exposure of the 7S NGF to this pH in the gel causes the complex to dissociate into three types of subunit which give rise to additional bands at quite acidic (α-subunits) slightly acidic (γ-subunits) and very alkaline (β-subunits) regions of the gel. If 7S NGF is applied to these same isoelectric focusing gels from either the acidic or alkaline end, only the subunit components appear, since the complex has completely dissociated (Varon & Shooter, 1970). The subunits of 7S NGF can be separated on a cation-exchange column (Smith *et al.*, 1968) and it has been found that the ratio of subunits isolated from many different 7S NGF preparations remains constant. The purified α- and γ-subunits each migrate as multiple bands on acrylamide gels (Smith *et al.*, 1968) and it is this microheterogeneity in the subunits which accounts for the broadness of the migrating 7S NGF band on acrylamide gels. Any one of the α-subunits will recombine with any individual γ-subunit in the presence of β at neutral pH to re-form as 7S NGF (Smith *et al.*, 1968). The recombination always occurs in a fixed proportion of the subunits which is similar to the ratios of the subunits isolated from a typical 7S NGF preparation (Shooter & Varon, 1970). The net charge of the 7S NGF species which is formed upon recombination of subunits depends only on the nature of the species of α-subunit used, those 7S NGF molecules containing the most acidic α-subunit having the highest mobility on acrylamide gels (Varon & Shooter, 1970).

The individual species of 7S NGF cannot be resolved by ion-exchange chromatography or by electrophoresis, because of a mobile equilibrium between the 7S NGF complex and the subunits which exists at all pH values, even those where 7S NGF appears quite stable (Smith *et al.*, 1969). Species of 7S NGF made by specific recombination of a single type of α-subunit with β- and γ-subunits show exchange of their α-subunit with added α-subunit of a different type. Additionally, iodination of α-subunits with ^{125}I and incubation of the labelled α with intact unlabelled 7S NGF results in the incorporation of α-subunits into the complex with a half-time of about 30 minutes at 27°C. Labelled γ- and β-subunits have also been prepared but exchange is much slower than for the α-subunits, which probably indicates that around neutral pH the 7S NGF species consists mainly of α-subunits associated with a more tightly bound β-γ complex (Smith *et al.*, 1969). A consequence of this subunit equilibrium is that in the chromatography of the 7S NGF complex on anion-exchange resins, the α-subunits will be selectively removed unless the column is run at a rate which is considerably shorter than the half-life of the exchange process (300 minutes at 4°C). The diethylaminoethyl cellulose (DEAE-cellulose) column procedure used in the isolation of 7S NGF is an example of such a column (Varon *et al.*, 1967*b*) and must be operated at the high flow rates suggested by the authors, if the purification of the 7S NGF complex is to succeed.

Biological properties. Using the plasma clot assay of Levi-Montalcini, Meyer and Hamburger (1954), 7S NGF, at a concentration of 10–20 ng/ml, causes a typical halo of neurite fibres to appear around embryonic sensory and sympathetic ganglia (Varon *et al.*, 1967*b*). *In vivo* 7S NGF injected into newborn mice caused a four- to six-fold increase in the size of the superior cervical ganglia (Varon *et al.*, 1968). The nerve growth factor activity of 7S NGF resides in only the β-subunit, which by itself will give similar responses at identical concentration to those of 7S NGF. Since the β-subunit accounts for only about 20 per cent of the protein in the 7S NGF complex, its activity is increased about five-fold when it is in the complex (Varon & Shooter, 1970).

The other known biological activity of 7S NGF is that of an esteropeptidase enzyme which is capable of hydrolysing esters and, to a lesser extent, amides of free or substituted amino acids, especially arginine, which however has very low activity toward protein substrates (Greene, Shooter & Varon, 1968, 1969). This enzymic activity appears only to be associated with the γ-subunits of 7S NGF; in solution at neutral pH the complex has very little initial esterase activity and there is a long time-lag until a maximum rate is obtained. The free γ-subunit, on the other hand, demonstrates maximum activity with no lag period. One interpretation of these results is that the 7S NGF complex probably has no esterase activity but depends on dissociation to a different form (either free subunits or a different complex) for the esteropeptidase activity to be expressed (Greene *et al.*, 1969). This is further evidence that a specific interaction between the subunits of 7S NGF exists.

Is 7S NGF a naturally occurring protein?

The evidence that 7S NGF is a specific multisubunit protein may be summarized as follows:

(*a*) the sedimentation behaviour of 7S NGF as judged by NGF activity remains constant throughout the various steps of the isolation procedure (Varon *et al.*, 1967*b*);

(*b*) the final product, 7S NGF, is the same from preparation to preparation in terms of its sedimentation and electrophoretic properties, as well as in terms of specific NGF and enzymic activities, with the latter always showing an atypical time-course of the hydrolysis of substrate (Greene *et al.*, 1968; 1969);

(*c*) the amounts of the three subunit types obtained by pH

dissociation of a variety of 7S NGF preparations are constant, and

(*d*) the distribution of individual subunits within the α- and γ-subunit groups also remains reasonably constant between preparations.

Two additional lines of evidence also support this conclusion. Previous studies (Varon, Nomura & Raiborn, unpublished results) have shown that 7S NGF is present in salivary glands of female mice. It has now also been found in salivary glands from males of other inbred strains of mice.

NGF was isolated from the submaxillary glands of five strains of inbred mice (Table 1), using the procedures of Varon and co-workers (1967*b*) and Pérez-Polo & Shooter (1971*a*). The NGF activity from all strains of mice was found in a high molecular weight fraction which chromatographed identically to 7S NGF on a Sephadex G-150 column (Bamburg, Derby & Shooter, 1971). Assay of the purified NGF in plasma clots with eight-day embryonic sensory ganglia (Levi-Montalcini *et al.*, 1954) showed an identical biological activity of all samples with a maximum response at 20 ng/ml, also identical with a control of 7S NGF. The esterase activities of the NGF's of the inbred mice were

Table 1 Yield and biological activity of 7S NGF from submaxillary glands of inbred mice

Strain	*Yield (mg NGF/ g fresh glands)*	*NGF activity (ng/BU)*	*Enzymic activity*[3] (*μmoles/min/mg*) *pH* 7.4	*pH* 9.0
Random bred[1]	2.5	20	24.1	42.0
C57/BL/6[2]	0.4	20	23.7	44.5
SWR[2]	0.9	20	25.9	48.8
C57/BL/10[2]	0.3	20	23.7	37.9
DBA/2[2]	0.75	20	18.5	51.4
Balb/C[1]	1.5	20	14.7	51.0

[1] From Simonsen Laboratory, Gilroy, California.

[2] From Jackson Laboratory, Bar Harbor, Maine.

[3] Assayed by the method of Hummel (1959). Solutions of 7S NGF of 1–2 μg/ml were preincubated in 3 ml phosphate buffer, pH 7.4, I = 0.2 for 3½ hours, or in tris chloride buffer, pH 9.0, I = 0.05 for 15 min. The substrate was *p*-toluene sulphonyl-L-arginine methyl ester at 5×10^{-4}M and temperature 23° C.

compared with those of a standard 7S NGF using the assay system of Hummel (1959) after a preincubation of the diluted enzyme in buffer for 3½ hours at 23°C. The results (Table 1) show that the specific activities of the NGF isolated from three of the five strains of mice were identical with the control 7S NGF and that the NGF isolated from the remaining two strains of mice which had a low specific activity in the assay at pH 7.4 had a higher activity than the control at pH 9.0, perhaps indicating some differences in their degree of dissociation at different pH values. Isoelectric focusing of NGF from inbred mice in acrylamide gels containing ampholine (pH 3–10) allowed their subunit content to be estimated. Results of scanning the trichloroacetic acid precipitated protein in the gel at 280 nm (Table 2) show that

Table 2 7S NGF from inbred strains of mice: percentages of subunits as measured from areas of isoelectric focusing acrylamide gel scans

Strain	*Relative area of each subunit*		
	α	γ	β
Randomly bred	34	50	16
C57BL/6	42	42	15
SWR	33	52	15
C57BL/10	40	46	14
DBA/2	37	47	16
Balb/C	41	46	13

a fairly constant ratio of α:β:γ was maintained from one strain to another. Analysis of these gel scans, however, showed that the inbred strains each had slightly different proportions of the individual α- and γ-subunits, the differences being independent of the method of isolation (Bamburg *et al.*, 1971). Therefore, these heterogeneous subunits probably exist in the animal and are not an artefact of the isolation procedure.

Another critical test relates to the affinity of the 7S NGF subunits for each other. If these proteins are subunits of a specific protein, rather than simple aggregates of indifferent proteins, then their affinity for one another should lead to the re-formation of 7S NGF even in the presence of a large excess of inert protein.

This type of experiment can be done by dissociating the 7S NGF complex in the original homogenate and asking if substantial amounts of 7S NGF re-form under appropriate conditions. The recombined material can also be compared to the 7S NGF isolated in the standard way (Varon *et al.*, 1967*b*) and both the affinity of the subunits for each other, as well as the uniqueness of the subunit composition of the 7S form, can be tested. To determine the affinity of the α-, β-, and γ-subunits for each other in the presence of a 20–30-fold excess of inert protein, native to the mouse submaxillary gland, 7S NGF was made to dissociate reversibly into its component subunits by shifting the pH of the supernatant outside the 5–8 (pH) range and then allowing the subunits to recombine by adjusting the pH of the supernatant back to neutrality (Pérez-Polo & Shooter, 1972). The amount of 7S NGF isolated from the supernatant after this treatment is an indication of the relative affinities of the subunits for one another. The control for this type of experiment is the amount of 7S NGF isolated from gland supernatant stored at pH 6.8 for the length of time required to go through the dissociation and recombination process. At this pH the supernatant is an unstable medium for 7S NGF; and after 36 hours of incubation, only about half the original 7S NGF remains (Table 3). The low recovery is probably

Table 3 Recovery of 7S NGF due to recombination of subunits in gland supernatant

Supernatant treatment (24–36 h)	*mg protein/50 gland pairs*	*Percentage recovery*
None	19.0	100
(1) pH 6.8→6.8	11.0	58
(2) pH 10.3→6.8	12.4	65
(3) pH 4.0→6.8	3.6	19

(1) Phosphate buffer, I = 0.05, pH 6.8 at 25°C.
(2) Carbonate buffer, I = 0.2, pH 10.3 at 25°C.
(3) Acetate buffer, I = 0.05, pH 4 at 25°C.

a result of the proteolytic activity present in the gland supernatant. After dissociation at alkaline pH, the recovery of 7S NGF was about 10 per cent higher than the control; while the yield of 7S NGF from recombination following acid dissociation was only about 20 per cent of control (Table 3).

The experiment at alkaline pH shows clearly that the subunits of 7S NGF do have a high affinity for each other and recombine specifically in the presence of inert protein. The increased yield, compared with the control at pH 6.8, could be due to a decrease in proteolytic activity and thus less degradation of 7S NGF or its subunits at the high pH. Correspondingly, acid pH may enhance proteolytic activity, although the low recovery at this pH may be primarily due to the appearance of a copious precipitate and adsorption of the subunits to it. The differences in recovery are not dependent on the pathway of dissociation, since 7S NGF dissociated at either pH 10.3 or 4.0 recombined completely at neutral pH (Varon *et al.*, 1968).

In order to check that the partial recoveries of 7S NGF in the experimental and control situations were due to enzymic degradation rather than incomplete recombination, the recombined supernatants were divided by molecular sieving into high and low molecular weight fractions; and the NGF activity was measured in each. In each instance the major fraction of the NGF activity was recovered in the high molecular weight, 7S NGF fraction (Table 4). Little, if any, was found in the low molecular weight fraction which would contain free β-subunits. The total recovery of NGF activity in these experiments paralleled the recoveries of 7S NGF in the preparative experiment, being about 50 per cent of the original for the control maintained at neutral pH; greater than 50 per cent for the supernatant incubated at high pH; and significantly lower for the acid incubation (Table 4). That the recombined product is 7S NGF was shown by the identity of the enzymic and NGF activities of this product with those of authentic 7S NGF (Table 5), as well as the identity of sedimentation and electrophoretic properties and subunit composition. Although proteolytic activity in the gland supernatant makes it impossible in this type of experiment to recover by recombination all the 7S NGF subunits originally present, the recovery is high enough to support the hypothesis that 7S NGF is a naturally occurring protein in the mouse submaxillary gland with both a high affinity among subunits and a uniquely determined subunit composition.

Table 4 Recovery of 7S NGF by recombination of subunits in gland supernatant after ultrafiltration through XM–100 membrane

Supernatant treatment (24–36 h)	*Retained by XM-100* $BU \times 10^{-3}$	*Percentage of biological activity recovered*	*Overall biological activity recovered (per cent)*
None	216	90	80
(1) pH 6.8→6.8	91	80	38
(2) pH 10.2→6.8	174	100	58
(3) pH 4.0→6.8	33	100	11

(1) Phosphate buffer, I = 0.05, pH 6.8 at 25°C.
(2) Carbonate buffer, I = 0.2, pH 10.2 at 25°C.
(3) Acetate buffer, I = 0.05, pH 4.0 at 25°C.

Table 5 Comparison of the two 7S NGF preparations by biological and enzymic assay

	NGF activity ng/BU	*Enzymic activity poly-L-arg*[3]	*(μmol/min/mg) TAME*[4]
7S NGF	16[1]	8.3	38.0
Amicon 7S NGF	17[2]	8.5	37.6

[1] Average of 2 preparations.
[2] Average of 5 preparations.
[3] Assayed in phosphate buffer, pH 6.8, I = 0.05, substrate concentration 5×10^{-4}M and 7S NGF concentration of 1–5 μg/ml. Hydrolysis followed at 238 nm in Carey 14.
[4] Assayed by method of Hummel (1959) using 5×10^{-4}M TAME in phosphate buffer, pH 7.0, I = 0.2 at 25°C using 1–5 μg/ml 7S NGF.

The low molecular weight class of NGF proteins

The β-subunit of 7S NGF. The basic β-subunit of 7S NGF, when isolated by chromatography on CM-cellulose at acid pH, is eluted from the column as the last protein. It shows a major component of isoelectric point 9.2 and a minor component (about 5 per cent) of lower isoelectric point and it accounts for approximately 20 per cent of the 7S NGF protein. It produces optimum fibre outgrowth in the *in vitro* assay at the same protein concentrations as 7S NGF and, therefore, is less active than is the β-subunit in 7S NGF. The significance of this difference is not easy to evaluate. In spite of the relative inaccuracy of the bioassay, the difference is consistently found in replicate analyses of 7S NGF and β-subunit done under identical conditions. However, the β-subunit is known to bind more readily to surfaces than does 7S NGF, as is shown by the very poor recovery of the β-subunit from Sephadex or Biogel (Greene *et al.*, 1971) and the protective action of serum albumin (Zanini *et al.*, 1968); and it is possible that significant amounts of the β-subunit are lost by adsorption during the serial dilutions. An argument against this point of view is that Bocchini & Angeletti (1969) report such high recoveries of NGF activity in a fraction similar to, if not identical with the β-subunit that it is unlikely that any of this fraction failed to be assayed because of adsorption losses.

Alternative methods of isolating the β-subunit have been developed, and in both instances the product has been found to have the same nerve growth and physical properties as the original preparation. In one method (Pérez-Polo & Shooter, 1972) 7S NGF was dissociated at pH 11 and the β-subunit isolated on QAE-Sephadex at the same pH. Under these conditions, little or none of the subunit binds to the column matrix. In the second method, 7S NGF was separated into its subunit components by isoelectric focusing on acrylamide gel and the β-subunit fraction was eluted from the gel. In both procedures the recovered β-subunit comprised approximately 20 per cent of the 7S NGF protein, displayed the same electrophoretic mobility or isoelectric point as the β-subunit prepared by chromatography at acid pH; and elicited optimum fibre outgrowth at the same concentration as 7S NGF (Table 6). These results suggest that, if no problems remain with the bioassay, the lower nerve growth activity of the free β-subunit is an intrinsic property of the subunit which is independent of the method of isolation.

Table 6 Comparison of β-subunit in 7S complex and isolated at both acid and alkaline pH

Species	*Percentage β recovered*	*Specific activity ng/BU*	*Specific activity*[1] *ngβ/BU*
7S NGF	—	14	3
βAcid (3)	20	26	26
βAlkaline(5)	23	16	16

[1] Assuming β constitutes 21.5 per cent of 7S NGF.

Structure of the β-subunit. A variety of methods indicate that the β-subunit consists of two identical peptide chains associated by non-covalent forces. The molecular weight of the β-subunit, determined by the meniscus depletion method of sedimentation equilibrium (Yphantis, 1964), is 23 000 (Table 7). Good agree-

Table 7 Molecular weight of β-subunit, determined by sedimentation equilibrium using the meniscus depletion method

Conditions	ω	M_n	M_w
0.1M-acetate, pH 4.0 + 0.1M-NaCl	44 067	21 000	21 500
	36 050	22 000	22 000
	32 050	23 000	23 500
	30 037	21 700	22 000
0.1M-carbonate, pH 10.0	44 033	22 500	23 000
	36 000	22 000	23 500
	30 000	23 500	24 500

ment was obtained between M_n and M_w values after equilibrium was reached at three different speeds in acetate buffer at pH 4. The linearity of the plot of log C against r^2 at this pH suggested that little, if any, self-aggregation of the β-subunit occurred. In contrast, at pH 10.0, close to the isoelectric point of the subunit, and especially at neutral pH, considerable aggregation of the native subunit was noted. The extrapolated values of M_n and M_w, however, even under these conditions, were close to 23 000 (Table 7). Under strong denaturing conditions, such as 8M-urea or 6M-guanidine-HCl, the molecular weight, as measured by gel filtration, fell to about 12 000 (Greene *et al.*, 1971). This result was also obtained on electrophoresis in sodium dodecyl sulphate, the conversion of the native subunit to the 12 000 unit having a half-time of 2 hours at 37°C. Since none of these conditions caused reduction of disulphide bonds, it is apparent that the two chains in the subunit are not held together by this type of covalent link. Reduction and carboxymethylation by itself did not result in dissociation into peptide chains; this was only achieved after adding urea, guanidine-HCl or sodium dodecyl sulphate. The fact that only one major protein component was observed in the analysis of untreated or reduced and carboxymethylated β-subunit in isoelectric focusing gels containing 8M-urea, suggests that the two chains are identical, a conclusion so far sustained by amino acid sequence data.

On the basis of a molecular weight of 24 000, the β-subunit contains 16 lysine and 14 arginine residues (these numbers will have to be rounded up or down to even values to accommodate identical chains). Thirteen soluble peptides were isolated and characterized in tryptic digests of reduced and carboxymethylated β-subunit. These 13 peptides contained 5 carboxymethylcystine residues, just under half of the 12 half-cystine residues present in the protein. Such data are highly suggestive of the presence of two identical chains, each of which contains six half-cystine residues in the form of three disulphide bridges. The *N*-terminal sequence of the β-subunit was present as one of the insoluble tryptic peptides. Its sequence determined by the automatic Edman procedure is given in Fig 1. The first lysine residue occurs at position 25 and the second at position 32, while the

1 10
SER-SER-THR-HIS-PRO-VAL-PHE-HIS-MET-GLY-GLU-PHE-

20
SER-VAL-CYS-ASN-SER-VAL-SER-VAL-TRY-VAL-GLY-ASP-
←——AE Tp1——

30
LYS-THR-THR-ALA-THR-ASP-ILE-LYS-
→ ←——AE Tp4——→

AE Tp1 and AE Tp4 are sequences of two soluble tryptic peptides from the digest of the aminoethylated β-subunit.

Fig. 1 Amino-terminal sequence of β-subunit.

first half-cystine residue is at position 15. One additional tryptic peptide (AE Tpl) resulted from cleavage at this modified cysteine residue in the aminoethylated β-subunit. Three additional soluble peptides were also found in the digest of aminoethylated β-subunit: they result from cleavage at three of the other modified cysteine residues. Although the sequence given in Fig. 1 was predominant, the sequence data showed the presence, in small quantities, of a second chain, having the methionine residue of position 9 as its *N*-terminal, and proceeding thereafter in identical fashion. These results suggest that a small fraction of the chains have lost the octopeptide SER-SER-THR-HIS-PRO-VAL-PHE-HIS from their *N*-terminus. At what stage this occurs is not yet known.

The 2.5S NGF species isolated by Bocchini & Angeletti

Bocchini & Angeletti (1969) described the isolation of a basic protein similar to the β-subunit. This 2.5S species was separated directly from the NGF-containing Sephadex G-100 fraction (i.e. from 7S NGF) by chromatography on CM-cellulose at pH 5. The isoelectric point and amino acid composition of this protein are close to those of the β-subunit (Bocchini & Angeletti, 1969; Bocchini, 1970; Varon & Shooter, 1970; Angeletti *et al.*, 1971). The recovery of NGF activity was much higher for the 2.5S species than for the β-subunit, approaching that of 7S NGF. The reported molecular weights of 30 000 (Bocchini & Angeletti, 1969) and 29 000 (Angeletti *et al.*, 1971) are also higher than those of the β-subunit, although the sedimentation coefficients are more nearly identical. Angeletti and co-workers (1971) found 15 soluble peptides in the tryptic digest of the S-^{14}C carboxymethyl derivative of the 2.5S species, which included five residues of *S*-carboxymethylcysteine. A sixth residue was located in a thermolysin digest of the insoluble tryptic peptides. The *N*-terminal residue was found to be serine. Angeletti and co-workers (1971) and Angeletti & Bradshaw (this volume, pp. 35–8) concluded from these data that the 2.5S species contained two similar chains, each with three intrachain disulphide bridges. This preparation is clearly similar to the β-subunit in many respects; and a detailed comparison of the two preparations will be of considerable interest.

Acknowledgements

Research described in this paper was supported by research grants from the National Institutes of Health (NS 04270) and the National Science Foundation (GB 14458). We are indebted to Dr Charles Yanofsky for the use of the Beckman Sequenator.

References

Angeletti, R. H., Bradshaw, R. A. & Wade, R. D. (1971). *Biochemistry, N.Y.* **10**, 463.
Angeletti, P., Calissano, P., Chen, J. S. & Levi-Montalcini, R. (1967). *Biochim. biophys. Acta* **147**, 180.
Bamburg, J. R., Derby, M. A. & Shooter, E. M. (1971). *Neurobiology* **1**, 115.
Bocchini, V. (1970). *Eur. J. Biochem.* **15**, 127.
Bocchini, V. & Angeletti, P. U. (1969). *Proc. natn. Acad. Sci. U.S.A.* **64**, 787.
Cohen, S. (1960). *Proc. natn. Acad. Sci. U.S.A.* **46**, 302.
Greene, L. A., Shooter, E. M. & Varon, S. (1968). *Proc. natn. Acad. Sci. U.S.A.* **60**, 1383.
Greene, L. A., Shooter, E. M. & Varon, S. (1969). *Biochemistry. N.Y.* **8**, 3735.
Greene, L. A., Varon, S., Piltch, A. & Shooter, E. M. (1971). *Neurobiology* **1**, 37.
Hummel, B. C. W. (1959). *Canadian J. Biochem. Physiol.* **37**, 1393.
Levi-Montalcini, R., Meyer, H. & Hamburger, V. (1954). *Cancer Res.* **14**, 49.
Pérez-Polo, J. R. & Shooter, E. M. (1972). Manuscript in preparation.
Pérez-Polo, J. R. & Shooter, E. M. (1972). Manuscript in preparation.
Shooter, E. M. & Varon, S. (1970). In *Protein Metabolism of the Nervous System*, p. 419. Ed. by Lajtha, A. New York: Plenum Press.
Smith, A. P., Greene, L. A., Fisk, H. R., Varon, S. & Shooter, E. M. (1969). *Biochemistry, N.Y.* **8**, 4918.
Smith, A. P., Varon, S. & Shooter, E. M. (1968). *Biochemistry, N.Y.* **7**, 3259.
Varon, S., Nomura, J. & Shooter, E. M. (1967*a*). *Proc. natn. Acad. Sci. U.S.A.* **57**, 1782.
Varon, S., Nomura, J. & Shooter, E. M. (1967*b*). *Biochemistry, N.Y.* **6**, 2202.
Varon, S., Nomura, J. & Shooter, E. M. (1968). *Biochemistry, N.Y.* **7**, 1296.
Varon, S. & Shooter, E. M. (1966). In *Variations in the Chemical Composition of the Nervous System*, p. 108. Ed. by Ansell, G. B. Oxford: Pergamon Press.

Varon, S. & Shooter, E. M. (1970). In *Biochemistry of Brain and Behavior*, p. 41. Ed. by Bowman, R. E. & Datta, S. P. New York: Plenum Press.
Yphantis, D. A. (1964). *Biochemistry, N.Y.* 3, 297.
Zanini, A., Angeletti, P. & Levi-Montalcini, R. (1968). *Proc. natn. Acad. Sci. U.S.A.* **61**, 835.

The Amino Acid Sequence of 2.5S Nerve Growth Factor from the Mouse Submaxillary Gland

RUTH HOGUE ANGELETTI* and
RALPH A. BRADSHAW

Departments of Biology and Biochemistry, Washington University, St Louis, Missouri, USA

In view of the considerable interest in the biological, immunochemical and metabolic phenomena elicited by the nerve growth factor (NGF), we have begun detailed studies designed to relate the structural properties of this factor to its functional role in neural tissue. Specifically, 2.5S NGF from mouse submaxillary glands, selected for its relative abundance and ease of purification (Levi-Montalcini & Angeletti, 1968), has been examined and the complete amino acid sequence determined. This form of the factor (Bocchini & Angeletti, 1969), which is somewhat smaller than that isolated by Varon, Nomura & Shooter (1967), possesses the only nerve growth-promoting activity present in the gland and, as such, represents the fundamental unit of biological activity.

Previous studies (Hogue Angeletti, Bradshaw & Wade, 1971), using sedimentation equilibrium, amino end-group analyses and tryptic peptide mapping, indicated that 2.5S NGF was composed of two identical or very similar subunits of about 14 500 molecular weight. A similar conclusion has been reached by Greene, Varon, Piltch & Shooter (1971) regarding the quaternary structure of the β-subunit of 7S NGF, which corresponds very closely to 2.5S NGF.

The primary structure has been elucidated by classical methods

* Present address: Laboratorio di Biologia Cellulare, C.N.R., Rome, Italy.

in which tryptic, chymotryptic, thermolytic and peptic peptides were prepared and isolated by means of ion-exchange chromatography. After sequence analysis of the purified peptides by Edman degradation and digestion by carboxypeptidase A and/or B, an entirely self-consistent overlapping structure was assembled. The sequence is shown in Fig. 1. The 33 amino-

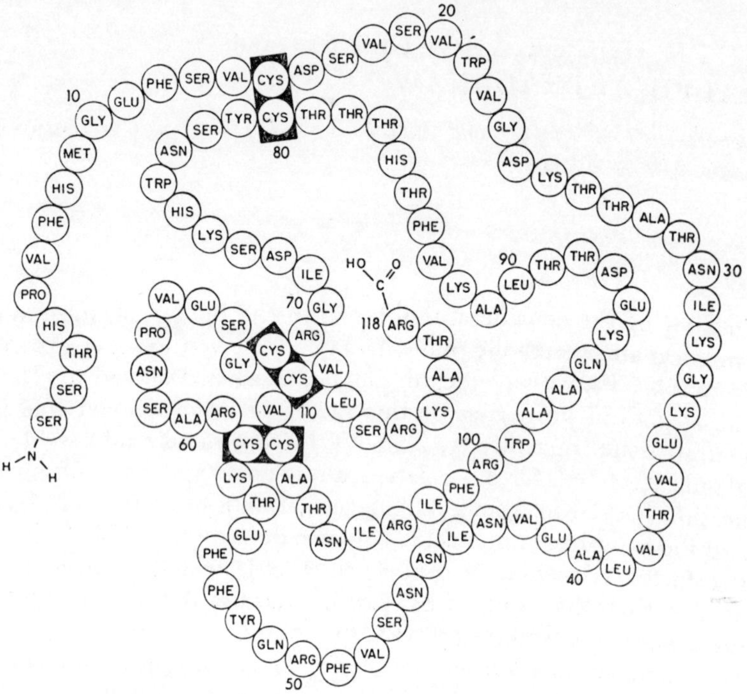

Fig. 1

terminal amino acids were confirmed using the Beckman Amino Acid Sequenator, in collaboration with Dr Mark Hermodsen, University of Washington, Seattle.

These data also indicated that one of the two chains composing the native dimer was shorter by eight amino acids (Hermodsen, Hogue Angeletti, Frazier & Bradshaw; in preparation). Thus, depending on the method of preparation, 2.5S NGF may be isolated as a dimer containing two identical chains (denoted as A chains); or as a heterogeneous dimer containing one long chain and one short chain (denoted as the B chain). The relation of A/A and A/B dimers to the physiological activity is now being investigated.

The correct pairing of the disulphide bonds was determined from peptic digests of native NGF. However, all the disulphides were located in one large peptide and a second digestion of this fragment by thermolysin was necessary to release the individual bridges. The component half-cystinyl peptides of each disulphide-containing fragment were subsequently identified by means of performic acid oxidation and ion-exchange chromatography.

The complete primary and secondary structure of the fundamental subunit (A chain) of 2.5S mouse NGF (shown in Fig. 1) contains 118 amino acids with amino-terminal serine and carboxyl-terminal arginine, and has a molecular weight of 13 259. Consequently, the homogeneous A/A dimers have a molecular weight of 26 518 while the A/B dimers are lower by about 900 daltons. These values may be compared with the determined molecular weight of 29 000 $\pm$ 1000 (Bocchini, 1970). The amino acid composition, as determined from the sequence, is in excellent agreement with those previously reported (Bocchini, 1970; Hogue Angeletti *et al.*, 1971), when those results are corrected to the proper molecular weight. It should also be noted that the amide content determined from the primary structure (seven out of eleven aspartic acids and two out of eight glutamic acids), is in excellent agreement with the observed isoelectric point of 9.3 determined by isoelectric focusing (Bocchini, 1970).

The completion of the primary structure of mouse 2.5S NGF provides an excellent basis for probing the structure-function relationships of this factor. In turn, it is hoped that these data will provide an insight into the means by which NGF plays its central role in promoting the growth and differentiation of neural tissue.

Acknowledgements

We should like to express our appreciation to Mr Delio Mercanti for his assistance in this work and to Mr Charles Yates and Mr Robert Sherman for their assistance with the amino acid analyses. We should also like to record our gratitude to Dr Levi-Montalcini for her financial and intellectual support of this project, and to Mr William Frazier for many helpful discussions.

This investigation has been supported by grants from the National Institutes of Health, AM-13362 and NS-03777. R.A.B. is a Research career development awardee of the National Institutes of Health, AM-23968.

References

Bocchini, V. (1970). *Eur. J. Biochem.* **15**, 127.

Bocchini, V. & Angeletti, P. U. (1969). *Proc. natn. Acad. Sci. U.S.A.* **69**, 787.

Greene, L. A., Varon, S., Piltch, A. & Shooter, E. M. (1971). *Neurobiology* **1**, 1.

Hermodsen, M., Hogue Angeletti, R., Frazier, W. A. & Bradshaw, R. A. Manuscript in preparation.

Hogue Angeletti, R., Bradshaw, R. A. & Wade, R. D. (1971). *Biochemistry* **10**, 463.

Levi-Montalcini, R. & Angeletti, P. U. (1968). *Physiol. Rev.* **48**, 534.

Varon, S., Nomura, J. & Shooter, E. M. (1967). *Biochemistry, N.Y.* **6**, 222.

Localization of the Nerve Growth Factor in Subcellular Fractions of Peripheral Tissues

P. U. ANGELETTI, R. LEVI-MONTALCINI and E. VIGNETI

Laboratorio di Biologia Cellulare, C.N.R., Rome, Italy

Before the physiological significance of nerve growth factor (NGF) can be understood we need to know its localization at cellular level. The recognition and characterization of the receptor sites at which this unique molecule binds would be of the utmost importance in clarifying its mechanism of action.

It has long been known that, aside from its two richest natural sources, mouse submaxillary glands and snake venoms, NGF activity is displayed *in vitro* by several other tissue extracts and body fluids (Bueker, Schenkein & Bane, 1960; Levi-Montalcini, 1966; Levi-Montalcini & Angeletti, 1960).

The NGF molecule has recently been completely purified and chemically characterized (Bocchini & Angeletti, 1969; Hogue Angeletti, Bradshaw & Frazier, 1971; Hogue Angeletti, Bradshaw & Wade, 1971), and a specific, monovalent antiserum to this protein has been used in our laboratory for quantitative and qualitative studies using micro-complement fixation (Zanini & Angeletti, 1971; Zanini, Angeletti & Levi-Montalcini, 1968). In the experiments here reported the concentration of NGF in several peripheral tissues from different animal species has been measured by this immunochemical technique. Evidence will be presented that in peripheral tissues NGF is present in a particulate form, associated with the microsomal fraction.

Materials and methods

Hearts, kidneys and spleen from mice and rats were used to

prepare tissue homogenates. Calf heart and swine heart taken from the slaughterhouse were also used. Tissue homogenates were made in isotonic sucrose containing 1mM-Mg^{2+} and sodium phosphate buffer, pH 7.4. The homogenates were subjected to differential centrifugation according to the scheme shown in Fig. 1. The pellet recovered after centrifugation at 105 000 ***g*** was resuspended in sucrose and was then centrifuged again.

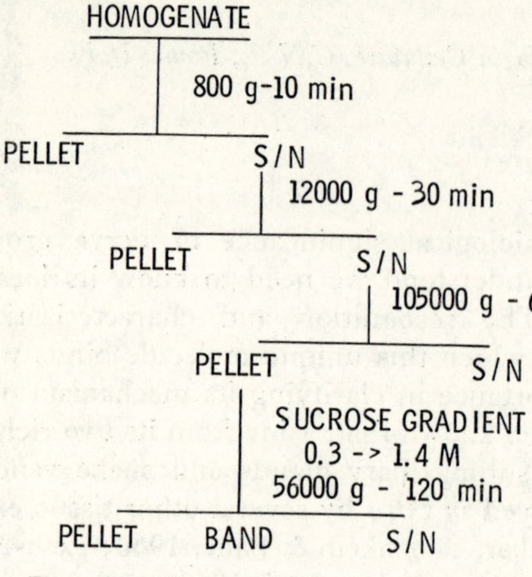

Fig. 1 Procedure for centrifugation of tissue homogenates.

In most experiments this microsomal fraction, after the second centrifugation, was dissolved in 0.01M-phosphate buffer, dialysed overnight against the same buffer, and then used for complement fixation.

In some experiments, the microsomal pellet was further fractionated by centrifugation on a sucrose gradient from 0.3 to 1.4 M-sucrose. These fractions were then collected, as shown in Fig. 1.

Proteins were measured by the Lowry method, using bovine albumin as a standard. Complement fixation was carried out by the micro-method of Wasserman and Levine (1961), with some modifications according to Moore and Peréz (1966).

The biological activity of various samples was also assessed *in vitro* by the tissue culture method of Levi-Montalcini (1966).

Results

The sensitivity of the micro-complement fixation in our system allowed a reliable assay of NGF in the range 2–10 ng. This sensitivity could be further increased almost ten times (from 0.2 to 1 ng) using the modifications suggested by Moore and Pérez (1966). This, however, proved unnecessary in the present experiments. Fig. 2 shows a micro-complement fixation curve obtained with a purified mouse NGF and its own antiserum.

As can be seen from the first part of the curve (zone of antibody excess), the percentage of complement fixation increases almost linearly with increasing antigen concentration.

When crude extracts of peripheral organs such as heart, kidney and spleen from mice and rats were used, it was not possible to determine the presence or the concentration of NGF by complement fixation, because of the haemolytic or anti-complementary effect of the extracts. A completely different picture was obtained when NGF was assayed in the microsomal pellets from different peripheral tissues. In all instances, with mouse tissues, clear-cut complement fixation curves were obtained with fixation reaching a maximum of 85 to 95 per cent, as occurs using the pure NGF antigen (Fig. 2). A semiquantitative assay of NGF in the various microsomal preparations was then possible by calculating the amount of protein required to obtain 50 per cent complement fixation, both with the microsomal fraction and with the pure NGF. The results are shown in Table 1.

NGF was present in the microsomal fraction of all mouse tissues examined in relatively high concentrations, ranging from 0.1 to 0.5 per cent of the total proteins. When the preparations were assayed in tissue culture, NGF activity was also clearly observed. The activity displayed in tissue culture, however, was from 10 to 100 times less than that expected from the NGF concentration in the microsomal samples as measured by complement fixation. NGF was also detected in the microsomal fractions from rat tissues. Complement fixation curves were run with the antiserum to mouse NGF; complement fixation never reached values higher than 60 to 65 per cent.

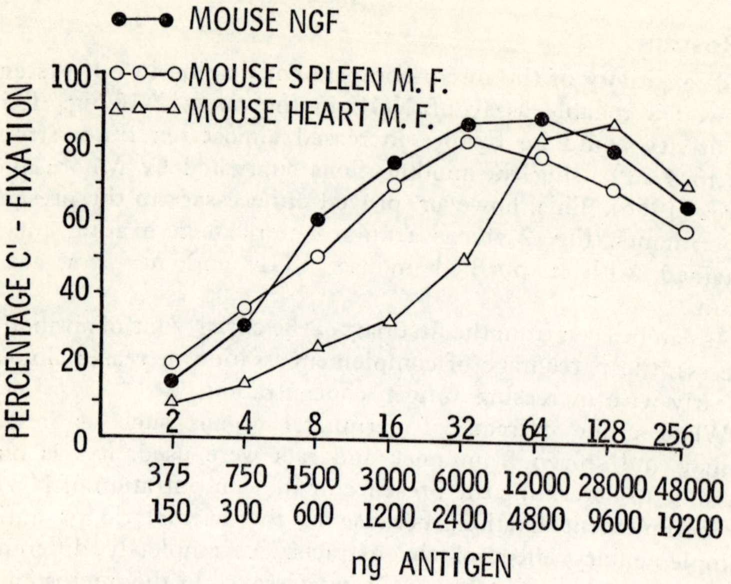

Fig. 2 Complement fixation curves with mouse NGF-antiserum and purified NGF, mouse heart microsomal fraction (M.F.) and mouse spleen microsomal fraction (M.F.).

Table 1 Relative concentration of NGF in microsomal fractions from mouse tissues calculated from the amount of protein required to give a 50 per cent complement-fixation with purified NGF and with the microsomal fraction

Tissue	*Experiment*	*NGF ng*	*Microsomal fraction ng*	*NGF concentration mg per cent*
Heart	1	6.0	2400	0.25
	2	4.5	3300	0.14
	3	7.0	1400	0.50
	4	5.4	3200	0.17
Spleen	1	7.0	3500	0.20
	2	4.5	3200	0.14
	3	5.4	1800	0.30
Kidney	1	4.5	3800	0.12
	2	5.4	2200	0.24
	3	6.4	4500	0.14

This vertical shift in the complement fixation curve indicates a cross-reaction between two similar but not identical NGF molecules in mouse and rat tissues (Fig. 3). Table 2 shows the relative concentration of NGF in rat kidney, heart and spleen in

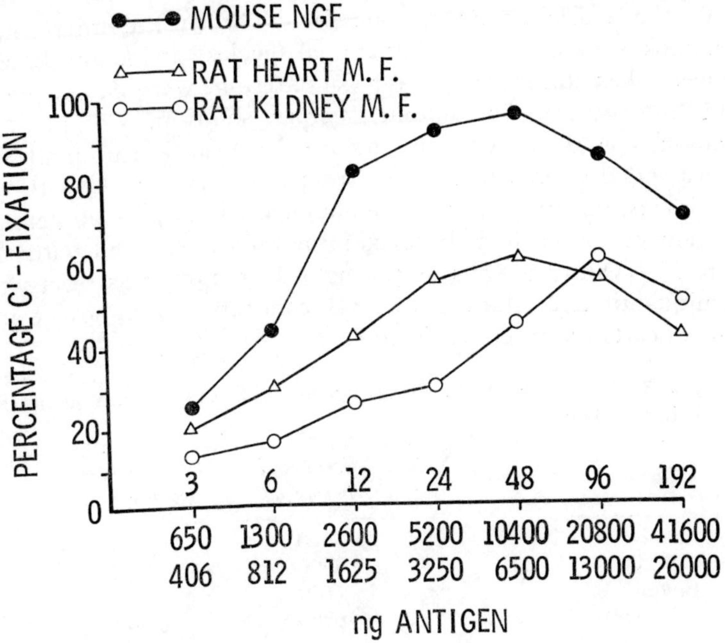

Fig. 3 Complement fixation curves with mouse NGF-antiserum and purified mouse NGF, rat heart microsomal fraction (M.F.) and rat kidney microsomal fraction (M.F.).

Table 2 NGF concentration in the microsomal fractions from rat tissues, determined as in Table 1

Tissue	*Experiment*	*NGF ng*	*Microsomal fraction ng*	*NGF concentration mg per cent*
Heart	1	7.0	4600	0.15
	2	4.5	6200	0.075
Kidney	1	7.0	9500	0.08
	2	4.5	5200	0.08
Spleen	1	7.0	6400	0.10
	2	4.5	7300	0.06

microsomal fractions. The presence of NGF activity in this preparation was confirmed by tissue culture and again it was found that, at corresponding NGF concentrations, the activity of the rat extracts was about 100 times less than the purified NGF from mouse submaxillary gland.

We have also begun to look for NGF in the microsomal fractions of tissues from other animal species. Swine and bovine hearts, taken immediately after slaughtering, were cut in pieces and homogenized in isotonic sucrose solution. Complement fixation was done with the mouse NGF-antiserum and the resuspended microsomal pellets from these tissues. As with the rat tissues, positive results were obtained, although complement fixation never reached the maximum values obtained with the pure NGF antigen, thus indicating a degree of cross-reactivity. Semiquantitative values of the NGF concentration in bovine and swine hearts are given in Table 3.

Table 3 NGF concentration in microsomal fractions from swine and bovine heart

Tissue	*Experiment*	*NGF ng*	*Microsomal fraction ng*	*NGF concentration mg per cent*
Swine	1	6	5600	0.100
heart	2	6	8200	0.073
Bovine	1	6	7500	0.080
heart	2	6	6500	0.092

Further attempts were made to fractionate the microsomal pellet by sucrose-density centrifugation and to localize the NGF in the various fractions. Preliminary results indicate that most of the NGF can be localized in the second of three fractions obtained after centrifugation in a gradient from 0.3 to 1.4 M-sucrose. Experiments along this line are still in progress.

Conclusions

The results of these experiments confirm the widespread presence of NGF in several peripheral mammalian tissues. The immunochemical evidence presented proves that the biological activity displayed by these tissues *in vitro* is indeed due to the same molecule as that purified from the submaxillary glands.

Furthermore, the protein appears to be mostly present in a membrane-bound form, associated with the microsomal fraction. The apparent discrepancy between the concentration of NGF in this fraction as measured by immunochemical methods, and that calculated by the tissue culture method, could be explained in several ways. In its membrane-bound form the NGF could be less active, or it could be associated with other regulatory proteins which limit its activity in the *in vitro* test, or its activity could be inhibited by extraneous molecules present in the microsomal fraction.

The isolation of NGF in particulate form from the microsomal pellet is now in progress. The identification of the receptor will be a significant step forward in elucidating the physiological role played by NGF in its peripheral localization.

References

Bocchini, V. & Angeletti, P. U. (1969). *Proc. natn. Acad. Sci. U.S.A.* **64**, 787.

Bueker, E. D., Schenkein, I. & Bane, J. L. (1960). *Cancer Res.* **20**, 1220.

Hogue Angeletti, R., Bradshaw, R. A. & Frazier, W. A. (1971). In *Third Int. Congress of Neurochemistry. Abstracts of Communications*, Budapest.

Hogue Angeletti, R., Bradshaw, R. A. & Wade, R. C. (1971). *Biochemistry* **10**, 463.

Levi-Montalcini, R. (1966). *Harvey Lectures, Ser.* **60**, 217.

Levi-Montalcini, R. & Angeletti, P. U. (1960). In *Regional Neurochemistry, Proc. Fourth Int. Neurochemical Symp.*, p. 362. Ed. by Kety, S. S. & Elkes, J. New York: Pergamon Press.

Moore, B. W. & Perez, V. J. (1966). *J. Immun.* **96**, 1000.

Wasserman, E. & Levine, L. (1961). *J. Immun.* **87**, 290.

Zanini, A. & Angeletti, P. U. (1971). *Biochim. biophys. Acta* **229**, 724.

Zanini, A., Angeletti, P. U. & Levi-Montalcini, R. (1968). *Proc. natn. Acad. Sci. U.S.A.* **61**, 835.

Nerve Growth Factor: Evaluation and Perspectives

R. LEVI-MONTALCINI and P. U. ANGELETTI

Laboratorio di Biologia Cellulare, C.N.R., Rome, Italy, and Department of Biology, Washington University, St Louis, Missouri, USA

Twenty years after the discovery that some mouse sarcomas release a diffusible agent which selectively enhances the growth and differentiation of sensory and sympathetic nerve cells, the time seems ripe for an evaluation of the phenomenon and of the perspectives opened up in this area of research.

The various aspects of this investigation, which from the beginning departed from the beaten track of experimental neuroembryology and opened up new vistas on the growth control mechanisms in the nervous system, have been reviewed frequently and extensively in recent years. We shall therefore recall only that the first experiment was performed by E. D. Bueker in 1948 and consisted in implanting a fragment of mouse sarcoma 180 into the body wall of a three-day chick embryo. The finding that sensory nerve fibres from adjacent spinal ganglia of the host innervated the explant and that the ganglia considerably increased in size led to new investigations, which resulted in the discovery that this tumour and other similar sarcomas release a diffusible nerve growth factor responsible for the growth response of the sensory and sympathetic ganglia of the host (Bueker & Hilderman, 1953; Levi-Montalcini, 1952; Levi-Montalcini & Hamburger, 1951; 1953).

This same factor, which in 1954 became known as the nerve growth factor (Cohen, Levi-Montalcini & Hamburger, 1954), was found in much larger quantities in snake venom and in mouse salivary glands in 1956 and 1958 respectively (Cohen,

1958; Cohen & Levi-Montalcini, 1956; Levi-Montalcini, 1958; Levi-Montalcini & Cohen, 1956).

In this paper we shall consider the main facets of the phenomenon which are at present under investigation. They are:

(1) the chemical nature of the nerve growth factor (NGF);
(2) the target cells;
(3) characteristics of the growth response; and
(4) site of production and physiological role of NGF.

Chemical nature of NGF

The protein nature of NGF was demonstrated by Cohen in 1956 for the snake venom NGF (Cohen & Levi-Montalcini, 1956), and in 1958 for the salivary gland NGF (Cohen, 1958).

During the last decade our efforts have been directed to characterizing this molecule, isolated from both sources (Angeletti, Calissano, Chen & Levi-Montalcini, 1967; Bocchini & Angeletti, 1969; Cohen, 1959, 1960; Hogue Angeletti, Bradshaw & Wade, 1971). The primary and secondary structure of the salivary gland NGF have now been elucidated. These results have been discussed in this volume by Drs Hogue Angeletti and Bradshaw (see p. 35), and it will suffice to mention here that the active NGF molecule is a dimer of molecular weight 26 518, composed of two identical subunits of molecular weight 13 259. Three intrachain disulphide bridges are present. The terminal residues in each polypeptide chain are serine and arginine. These findings settle the long-debated question of the molecular weight of NGF, and open up the possibility of a systematic investigation of the structure-function relationship of this unique protein: a prerequisite to understanding its mechanisms of action. Hence, from a chemical viewpoint, remarkable progress has been made in the knowledge of this growth-promoting factor which stands comparison with the best-known biologically active proteins, such as insulin, growth hormone, or ACTH.

Although the elucidation of the nature of the NGF has rewarded twenty years of efforts directed to this end, some points remain to be clarified. One of these, to be considered in more detail elsewhere in this volume (Pérez-Polo *et al.*, p. 19) concerns the association of the native NGF with other proteins present in the homogenate of mouse salivary glands. This high molecular weight aggregate, known as 7S NGF, has been extensively investigated by Shooter and Varon (Greene, Shooter & Varon, 1968; Varon, Nomura & Shooter, 1967*a*, *b*), and an elaborate theory has been proposed in which the association of the NGF molecule or β-subunit, as it has been named by these authors, with other proteins referred to as α- and γ-subunits, results in the enhancement of the NGF activity of the β-subunit *in vitro*. Neither the α- nor the γ-subunit display NGF activity when assayed alone. Using our purification procedures and *in vitro* techniques, we were unable to confirm the hypothesis that the α- and γ-molecules activate the NGF protein molecule (Zanini, Angeletti & Levi-Montalcini, 1968).

Another aspect of the chemical nature of NGF requires comment. According to some authors, the snake venom and the salivary gland NGF differ from each other to a considerable extent; and the concept has thus been developed that different molecules are endowed with NGF activity (Banks *et al.*, 1968; Pearce *et al.*, p. 3; Varon, 1968). However, extensive comparative studies, carried out in our laboratory with the snake venom and salivary gland NGF's, do not substantiate this hypothesis. On the contrary, immunochemical and chemical studies stress the remarkable similarity of NGF's from these two sources (Zanini *et al.*, 1968; Hogue Angeletti, 1970*a*, *b*; 1971). These findings seem all the more impressive in view of the phylogenetic separation of the two groups—reptiles and mammals—which supply the native NGF. Analytical studies aimed at determining the primary structure of cobra venom NGF are now in progress in our laboratory (R. Hogue Angeletti, unpublished results).

The target cells

NGF elicits the growth response from two nerve cell types: embryonic sensory nerve cells during a restricted period of their development; and sympathetic nerve cells throughout their life cycle, from early differentiation to maturity (Levi-Montalcini, 1966; Levi-Montalcini & Angeletti, 1968*a*).

In our early studies of the growth effects of mouse sarcomas 180 and 37 on the sensory ganglia of the chick embryo, we reported that of the two morphologically and topographically distinct cell populations, designated as medio-dorsal (M-D) and ventrolateral (V-L) cells on account of their position in cephalic and spinal ganglia, only the M-D cells are receptive to the action of the NGF (Levi-Montalcini, 1962; Levi-Montalcini & Angeletti, 1968*a*). These results were recently confirmed by Weis (1970). The growth response, to be considered in the next section, is first apparent in six-day chick embryos; it increases between the seventh and the ninth day of incubation and decreases thereafter. It is no longer apparent in three-week-old chick embryos nor in ganglia from hatched chicks. A similar pattern of response occurs in ganglia of mammals, but neither the first appearance nor the extinction of the growth response has been accurately analysed. Experiments *in vitro*, however, have shown that sensory ganglia dissected out from a large number of mammalian foetuses (ganglia from human foetuses available through surgical abortion were also assayed) respond to NGF *in vitro* in the same way as do avian embryonic ganglia (Levi-Montalcini & Angeletti, 1961). During postnatal life, mammalian spinal ganglia show no growth response when treated either *in vivo* or *in vitro* with NGF (Levi-Montalcini, 1966).

Sympathetic nerve cells from the para- and prevertebral chain ganglia are receptive to the effects of the NGF from their early inception to maturity. One exception to the rule that adrenergic nerve cells increase in size and number in NGF-treated birds and mammals is the ganglionic complexes which innervate the gonads in both sexes. Cell counts and volume determinations made in mice showed comparable values in experimental and control ganglia (Levi-Montalcini, 1966; Levi-Montalcini & Angeletti, 1968*a*).

A third cell type, the medullary adrenergic cell, was examined as a possible target of NGF in chick embryos bearing transplants of mouse sarcomas, and in newborn and adult mice injected with the salivary gland NGF. Histological studies in the chick embryos gave ambiguous results: at times an increase in this cell population was apparent in 10–15-day embryos with large transplants of mouse sarcomas (Levi-Montalcini & Hamburger, 1951; 1953), while in other instances no increase was noticeable. Subsequent studies of embryos injected with the venom or salivary gland NGF did not provide decisive evidence for or against the hypothesis that medullary adrenergic cells are a target of NGF (unpublished results). Likewise, histological studies in newborn and infant mice injected with salivary gland NGF failed to show clear-cut effects of NGF on this cell population; and we concluded that only sensory and sympathetic nerve cells respond to this factor (Levi-Montalcini, 1966; Levi-Montalcini & Angeletti, 1968*a*). Markedly different results were obtained by Professor E. Zaimis, whose findings are presented elsewhere in this volume (pp. 59–70).

Characteristics of the growth response at structural, ultrastructural and metabolic levels

The growth response elicited by NGF has been studied extensively at structural, ultrastructural and metabolic levels. Only the most relevant data will be summarized here, as they have been reported in detail in recent original and review articles (Angeletti, Levi-Montalcini & Calissano, 1968; Angeletti, Liuzzi & Levi-Montalcini 1964*a*; Angeletti, Liuzzi, Levi-Montalcini & Gandini-Attardi, 1964*b*; Levi-Montalcini, 1952; Levi-Montalcini & Angeletti, 1968*a*).

Structural and ultrastructural changes elicited by the NGF in embryonic sensory and sympathetic nerve cells

The growth effects elicited by NGF on embryonic sensory and sympathetic nerve cells are so very similar that they can be considered together. They were investigated both in the developing organism and after dissection of the ganglia and their explantation *in vitro* in a semi-solid medium, consisting of rooster plasma and basal amino acid solution; or in fluid medium, consisting of the same amino acid solution. The animal chosen for these experiments was the chick embyro. Since the same effects were obtained with fragments of mouse sarcomas, venom or salivary gland NGF, we shall summarize the results obtained with the salivary gland NGF which was obtained in a highly purified form, and therefore enabled a more rigorous analysis to be made *in vivo* and *in vitro*.

Injections of salivary gland NGF into the yolk of 7–10-day chick embryos resulted in marked hypertrophic and hyperplastic changes in sensory and sympathetic ganglia. Sympathetic nerve fibres appeared in excessive numbers, branched in large numbers into the viscera of the host and entered the lumen of blood vessels obliterating small veins and capillaries (Levi-Montalcini, 1964; 1966).

In vitro, the NGF elicits a fibrillar halo around both types of ganglia in a 6–10-hour period. This growth response occurs with 0.01 μg of NGF per ml of culture medium. The effects of NGF excess have been described previously (Levi-Montalcini & Angeletti, 1968*b*). It will suffice to mention here that the growth effect keeps pace with the amount of the growth factor added to the culture medium.

Of particular interest, and even more revealing than the effect of NGF on whole ganglia explanted *in vitro* in a semi-solid medium, is the effect of the same factor on dissociated embryonic nerve cells cultured in basal amino acid solution. In the absence of NGF, sensory and sympathetic nerve cells attach to the glass surface in the culture vessel but deteriorate progressively, and all but a few cells disintegrate in the first two days of culture. In the presence of the NGF, nerve cells survive for as long as one month, and produce a dense fibrillar network. These results suggest that the NGF not only enhances the production of neurofibrillar material in the target cells and causes marked hyperplastic and hypertrophic effects, but also plays a key role in the life of these cells (Levi-Montalcini & Angeletti, 1963; 1968*a*).

The main feature of the growth response of both sensory and sympathetic cell types at the ultrastructural level is the massive production of neurofibrillar material in the cell perikaryon. This is already apparent two hours after the start of incubation, and is, in fact, so extensive as to overshadow other less prominent ultrastructural changes, such as an increase in the Golgi complex and a disarray of the endoplasmic reticulum. Prominent changes are also apparent in the nucleus. The nucleoplasm is denser than it is in controls and aggregates of more electron-dense chromatin are irregularly dispersed throughout the nucleus (Levi-Montalcini, Caramia, Luse & Angeletti, 1968).

Structural and ultrastructural changes elicited by NGF in sympathetic nerve cells of newborn and adult mice

Newborn mice injected daily with the salivary gland NGF for periods ranging between three days and one month show a progressive size increase of sympathetic ganglia and no other apparent effects. Volume measurements of the superior cervical ganglia in mice injected daily with the NGF from birth to the tenth day and of littermates, showed that ganglia of experimental mice are six-to-ten-fold larger than are controls (Levi-Montalcini, 1966; Levi-Montalcini & Booker, 1960).

Ganglia of experimental and control mice were studied by light and electron microscopy. Cytological examination showed that the hypertrophic neurones differ from controls not only in their larger size but also in the more intense basophilia and in the size of the nucleoli, which are much larger than in controls (Levi-Montalcini, 1964; 1966). A parallel increase in neurofibrillar material is apparent in silver-stained ganglia. A study of the peripheral distribution of sympathetic nerve fibres in NGF-treated mice showed a markedly increased innervation of the viscera, the tunica of blood vessels and the hair bulbs. A detailed analysis, made by Olson (1967) using the histochemical technique of Falck and Hillarp, impressively demonstrated increased density of the adrenergic ground plexus in the iris, the submaxillary and parotid glands, and of the intramural ganglionic plexuses of the intestinal tract in NGF-treated mice. Varicose adrenergic terminals were also detected in areas normally deprived of adrenergic innervation. The previous finding, that the NGF does not affect the adrenergic ganglionic complex innervating the vas deferens, was confirmed by these studies of Olson. The fluorescent histochemical technique showed no increase in the adrenergic ground plexus around this organ. Increased catecholamine content in ganglia and several peripheral organs in mice, rats and kittens injected with NGF has been demonstrated with quantitative fluorometric techniques by other authors (Olson, 1967).

The life-long responsiveness of sympathetic neurones to NGF raised the question of whether the growth effects obtained *in vivo* compare at the ultrastructural level with those observed *in vitro* in embryonic sensory nerve cells. The results indicated a remarkable similarity between the *in vitro* and *in vivo* effects when explored at the ultrastructural level. Newborn and adult mice were injected for five days with NGF. The treatment resulted in a five-fold increase of sympathetic chain ganglia in newborn mice; and in a two-fold increase of the same ganglia in adult specimens. When examined in the electron microscope, sympathetic neurones of newborn and adult NGF-treated mice differed from those of controls due to a massive increase of neurofibrillar material; an increase in the endoplasmic reticulum; a dilatation of the Golgi complex, and a change in the cellular contour from ovoid in controls to polyhedral in NGF-treated neurones (Angeletti, Levi-Montalcini & Caramia, 1971).

While these studies re-emphasize the extraordinary effect of NGF on the production of neurofibrils in its target cells, it is conceivable that the primary site of action of this growth factor is not at the level of neurofibrillar formation. Their striking increase may well be caused by the stimulation of some more basic and highly specific processes in the sequence of events which result in growth and differentiation of the receptive nerve cells. The massive production of neurofibrils should therefore be regarded as a consequence of the enhancement of all anabolic processes in the cells triggered by NGF. Supporting this view are the results of some metabolic studies which will be considered briefly in the next section.

NGF-induced metabolic changes in sensory and sympathetic ganglia

The growth response elicited by NGF is accompanied by several metabolic changes, such as increases in RNA, protein and lipid synthesis and carbohydrate utilization. The latter occurs through activation of the pentose-phosphate pathway (Angeletti, Gandini-Attardi, Toschi, Salvi & Levi-Montalcini, 1965; Angeletti *et al.*, 1964*a*, *b*; 1968; Angeletti, Liuzzi & Pocchiari, 1967). A specific induction of enzymes related to the synthesis of the noradrenergic neurotransmitter has recently been demonstrated (Thoenen, Angeletti & Levi-Montalcini, 1971). The primary site of action of NGF is, however, not yet identified. The hypothesis first suggested—that it could be at the level of DNA transcription (Levi-Montalcini, 1966; Levi-Montalcini & Angeletti, 1968*a*)—was not supported by subsequent investigations with actinomycin D. The addition of this inhibitor to the culture medium at doses which block RNA synthesis does not completely prevent the production of a neurofibrillar halo around ganglia cultured in the presence of NGF (Larrabee, 1969; Levi-Montalcini &

Angeletti, 1971). The possibility that NGF might be endowed with enzymic activity has been considered, but extensive screening of possible substrates does not reveal any specific catalytic property which could account for the biological effect of this molecule. A new lead, which may eventually provide the answer to this question, came with the discovery that NGF is present in considerable amounts in peripheral tissues such as heart, spleen, and kidney of several animal species; in these tissues NGF is membrane-bound and comes down in the microsomal pellet. The results of these investigations are presented elsewhere in this volume (Angeletti, Levi-Montalcini & Vigneti, 1972).

Site of production and physiological role of the NGF

Twenty years after the discovery of the NGF in some mouse sarcomas, and 15 and 13 years, respectively, since the discovery of the same molecule in snake venom and mouse salivary glands, we still have no explanation nor, for that matter, any clue as to why this molecule, which is endowed with such a potent and specific nerve growth-promoting activity, should be released by some neoplastic cells, snake venom and salivary glands. The screening of other tissues and body fluids for the same agent showed that it is widespread (Bueker, Schenkein & Bane, 1960; Levi-Montalcini, 1966) and can in fact be detected in trace amounts in the blood of several mammals, man included; and also in extracts of a number of organs and tissues. Granuloma tissue, experimentally produced in mice, rats, cats and monkeys by local implantation of carrageenin, elicits the same nerve growth-promoting effect *in vitro* as do fragments of mouse sarcomas (Levi-Montalcini & Angeletti, 1961).

The occurrence of this protein in so many different organs and animal fluids, while attesting to its functional value, leaves us with an embarrassing wealth of potential sources of this potent factor, and also a distressing awareness of our inability to solve the apparently simple problem of detecting its primary source of production.

We have previously presented the reasons why we reject the most simple and appealing explanation, which would identify the salivary glands as the source of this factor (Levi-Montalcini,

1965; 1966). At present, although we have by no means proved it, we favour the hypothesis that this protein is produced, not in a specific organ, but everywhere in animal tissues. Its presence in such a large quantity in snake venom and mouse salivary glands, where the NGF is synthesized *in situ* (Burdman & Goldstein, 1965; Goldstein & Burdman, 1965; Levi-Montalcini & Angeletti, 1968*a*, *b*), suggests that this molecule might be endowed with another activity related to one of the two main functions of this gland in reptiles and rodents: the production of toxic factors or of hydrolytic enzymes.

Another equally powerful protein with the property of enhancing growth of epithelial cells was discovered by Cohen in mouse salivary glands (Cohen, 1964; 1965*a*, *b*). The remarkable potency and specificity of action of these two proteins, nerve growth factor and epidermal growth factor, and their presence in large quantities in the tubular portion of the mouse salivary glands, underline at once their similarity and their difference from other agents, such as hormones.

It is tempting to think that each cell type might depend upon a similar specific factor for its growth. The identification of such factors would greatly add to our knowledge of growth regulatory mechanisms, which remain among the most challenging and unsolved problems in biology.

Conclusions

While a great deal remains to be learned about nerve growth factor and its mechanism of action on sensory and sympathetic nerve cells, one can feel optimistic about the future of this field, which began in the area of classical neuroembryology and has progressed increasingly rapidly toward the identification of the NGF molecule, to the structural, ultrastructural and metabolic effects of the growth factor, and to its physiological role in the life of its target cells. Perhaps in no other area of neuroembryology, nor indeed in the more general field of growth control mechanisms in the nervous system, has progress been so fast, and has the information gathered in two decades of intensive efforts so much exceeded expectation.

With the identification of NGF as a protein molecule and the elucidation of its primary and secondary structure one can predict that we shall soon be able to identify the biologically active group of this small protein molecule and its mechanism of action at the molecular level. The NGF compares favourably with hormones such as insulin and the growth hormone in one important respect; its field of action is much more specific and its target sensory and sympathetic nerve cells (leaving aside the adrenal medullary cells) have distinct and unique differentiative characteristics which enable us to detect the successive morphological stages of the growth response. It is also of considerable significance that the time between stimulus and response is remarkably short, thus narrowing down the search for the earliest changes subsequent to the action of this factor. Experiments with ferritin-labelled NGF, delayed until now because of lack of evidence on the purity of the NGF, are at present in progress to identify the site of action of this factor.

In another way the identification of the receptor site or sites of this unique protein seems now to be within reach. With the discovery that this molecule is present in fairly large amounts in membrane-bound particles isolated from a microsomal fraction of peripheral tissues, its physiological role is ascertained and its localization in the target system is a definite possibility. Since the achievements of the past two decades have far exceeded expectation and the phenomenon of NGF is so much more sharply in focus now than at the time of its discovery, we feel justified in anticipating further progress which may open up new perspectives in the field of neurobiology.

References

Angeletti, P. U., Calissano, P., Chen, J. S. & Levi-Montalcini, R. (1967). *Biochim. biophys. Acta* **147**, 180.

Angeletti, P. U., Gandini-Attardi, D., Toschi, G., Salvi, M. L. & Levi-Montalcini, R. (1965). *Biochim. biophys. Acta* **95**, 111.

Angeletti, P. U., Levi-Montalcini, R. & Calissano, P. (1968). *Advn. Enzymol.* **31**, 51.

Angeletti, P. U., Levi-Montalcini, R. & Caramia, F. (1971). *J. Ultrastruct. Res.* **36**, 24.

Angeletti, P. U., Levi-Montalcini, R. & Vigneti, E. (1972). These proceedings, p. 39.

Angeletti, P. U., Liuzzi, A. & Levi-Montalcini, R. (1964*a*). *Biochim. biophys. Acta* **84**, 778.

Angeletti, P. U., Liuzzi, A., Levi-Montalcini, R. & Gandini-Attardi, D. (1964*b*). *Biochim. biophys. Acta* **90**, 445.
Angeletti, P. U., Liuzzi, A. & Pocchiari, F. (1967). In *First Int. Meeting of Neurochemistry. Abstracts of Communications*, Strasbourg, France. p. 6.
Banks, B. E. C., Banthorpe, D. V., Berry, A. R., Davies, H. ff. S., Doonan, S., Lamont, D. M., Shipolini, R. & Vernon, C. A. (1968). *Biochem. J.* **108**, 157.
Bocchini, V. & Angeletti, P. U. (1969). *Proc. natn. Acad. Sci. U.S.A.* **64**, 787.
Bueker, E. D. (1948). *Anat. Rec.* **102**, 369.
Bueker, E. D. & Hilderman, H. L. (1953). *Cancer* **6**, 397.
Bueker, E. D., Schenkein, I. & Bane, J. L. (1960). *Cancer Res.* **20**, 1220.
Burdman, J. A. & Goldstein, M. N. (1965). *J. exp. Zool.* **160**, 183.
Cohen, S. (1958). In *Chemical Basis of Development*, p. 665. Ed. by McElroy, W. D. & Glass, B. Baltimore: Johns Hopkins Press.
Cohen, S. (1959). *J. biol. Chem.* **234**, 1129.
Cohen, S. (1960). *Proc. natn. Acad. Sci. U.S.A.* **46**, 302.
Cohen, S. (1964). In *Metabolic Control Mechanisms in Animal Cells*, p. 14. Ed. by Rutter, W. J. Washington, D.C.: Natl. Cancer Inst. Monograph 13.
Cohen, S. (1965*a*). *Develop. Biol.* **12**, 394.
Cohen, S. (1965*b*). In *Developmental and Metabolic Control Mechanisms and Neoplasia*. A Collection of Papers Presented at the Nineteenth Annual Symposium on Fundamental Cancer Research, p. 251. Baltimore: Williams & Wilkins.
Cohen, S. & Levi-Montalcini, R. (1956). *Proc. natn. Acad. Sci. U.S.A.* **42**, 571.
Cohen, S., Levi-Montalcini, R. & Hamburger, V. (1954). *Proc. natn. Acad. Sci. U.S.A.* **40**, 1014.
Goldstein, M. N. & Burdman, J. A. (1965). *Anat. Rec.* **151**, 199.
Greene, L. A., Shooter, E. M. & Varon, S. (1968). *Proc. natn. Acad. Sci. U.S.A.* **60**, 1383.
Hogue Angeletti, R. (1970*a*). *Proc. natn. Acad. Sci. U.S.A.* **65**, 668.
Hogue Angeletti, R. (1970*b*). *Biochim. biophys. Acta* **214**, 478.
Hogue Angeletti, R. (1971). *Brain Res.* **25**, 4244.
Hogue Angeletti, R. & Bradshaw, R. A. (1972). These proceedings, p. 35.
Hogue Angeletti, R., Bradshaw, R. A. & Wade, R. C. (1971). *Biochemistry* **10**, 463.
Larrabee, M. G. (1969). *Progr. Brain Res.* **31**, 95.
Levi-Montalcini, R. (1952). *Ann. N.Y. Acad. Sci.* **55**, 330.
Levi-Montalcini, R. (1958). In *Chemical Basis of Development*, p. 646. Ed. by McElroy, W. D. & Glass, B. Baltimore: Johns Hopkins Press.
Levi-Montalcini, R. (1962). *Sci. Repts. 1st Super. Sanità* **2**, 345.
Levi-Montalcini, R. (1964). *Ann. N.Y. Acad. Sci.* **118**, 149.
Levi-Montalcini, R. (1965). *Proc. R. Soc. Med.* **58**, 357.
Levi-Montalcini, R. (1966). *Harvey Lectures Ser.* **60**, 217.

Levi-Montalcini, R. & Angeletti, P. U. (1961). In *Regional Neurochemistry Proc. Fourth Int. Neurochemical Symp.* p. 362. Ed. by Kety, S. S. & Elkes, J. New York: Pergamon Press.

Levi-Montalcini, R. & Angeletti, P. U. (1963). *Devl. Biol.* **7**, 653.

Levi-Montalcini, R. & Angeletti, P. U. (1968*a*). *Physiol. Rev.* **48**, 534.

Levi-Montalcini, R. & Angeletti, P. U. (1968*b*). In *Ciba Found. Symp. on Growth of the Nervous System*, p. 126. Ed. by Wolstenholme, G. E. W. & O'Connor, M. London: Churchill.

Levi-Montalcini, R. & Angeletti, P. U. (1971). In *Hormone Regulation*, p. 719. Ed. by Hamburgh, M. & Barrington, E. J. W. New York: Appleton Century Crofts.

Levi-Montalcini, R. & Booker, B. (1960). *Proc. natn. Acad. Sci. U.S.A.* **46**, 373.

Levi-Montalcini, R., Caramia, F., Luse, S. A. & Angeletti, P. U. (1968). *Brain Res.* **8**, 347.

Levi-Montalcini, R. & Cohen, S. (1956). *Proc. natn. Acad. Sci. U.S.A.* **42**, 695.

Levi-Montalcini, R. & Hamburger, V. (1951). *J. exp. Zool.* **116**, 321.

Levi-Montalcini, R. & Hamburger, V. (1953). *J. exp. Zool.* **123**, 233.

Olson, L. (1967). *Z. Zellforsch. mikrosk. Anat.* **81**, 155.

Pearce, F. L., Banks, B. E. C., Banthorpe, D. V., Berry, A. R., Davies, H. ff. S. & Vernon, C. A. (1972). These proceedings, p. 3.

Pérez-Polo, J. R., Bamburg, J. R., de Jong, W. W. W., Straus, D., Baker, M. & Shooter, E. M. (1972). These proceedings, p. 19.

Thoenen, H., Angeletti, P. U. & Levi-Montalcini, R. (1971). *Proc. natn. Acad. Sci. U.S.A.* In press.

Varon, S. (1968). *J. Pediatric Surgery: Conference on the Biology of Neuroblastoma* **3**, 120.

Varon, S., Nomura, J. & Shooter, E. M. (1967*a*). *Proc. natn. Acad. Sci. U.S.A.* **57**, 1782.

Varon, S., Nomura, J. & Shooter, E. M. (1967*b*). *Biochemistry* **6**, 2202.

Weis, P. (1970). *J. Embryol. Exptl. Morphol.* **24**, 381.

Zaimis, E. (1972). These proceedings, p. 59.

Zanini, A., Angeletti, P. U. & Levi-Montalcini, R. (1968). *Proc. natn. Acad. Sci. U.S.A.* **61**, 835.

Nerve Growth Factor: The Target Cells

ELEANOR ZAIMIS

Department of Pharmacology, Royal Free Hospital School of Medicine, University of London, UK

Levi-Montalcini & Booker (1960) demonstrated that the daily administration of nerve growth factor (NGF) to newborn mice produces a hypertrophy of the sympathetic ganglia. Histological investigations showed an increase in both the nerve-cell population and the size of each nerve cell. By injecting purified NGF into rabbits, Stanley Cohen (1960) prepared an antiserum to it. Together with Professor Levi-Montalcini (Levi-Montalcini & Cohen, 1960) he demonstrated that the administration of this antiserum to newborn mice resulted in a rapid and extensive destruction of the nerve cells of the sympathetic ganglia.

Animals with either hypertrophied or atrophied sympathetic ganglia provide ideal material on which to test current theories concerning the role of the sympathetic system and the way in which structures innervated by it can be affected by drugs. Because of this and because the cat and the rat are very convenient animals for cardiovascular studies, it was decided to investigate the effect of NGF on newborn kittens and rats.

Immediately after birth the animals were treated for several days with NGF prepared either from submaxillary glands of adult male mice or from Russell's viper venom, generously provided by Dr D. C. Edwards and Professor C. A. Vernon, respectively. Table 1 shows the number of animals used, the duration of treatment, and the amount of NGF administered. Daily subcutaneous injections of NGF resulted, in both kittens and rats, in an increase in the size of the sympathetic ganglia and of the adrenal medulla.*

Table 1

	Treatment	*Number of animals*	*Duration of treatment (days)*	*NGF units (total)*
RATS	Mouse salivary gland NGF	55	9–14	440 000–550 000
	Russell's viper venom NGF	5	9–14	60 000–110 000
	Saline	62	9–14	
KITTENS	Mouse salivary gland NGF	11	8	90 000
	Russell's viper venom NGF	6	8	9 000–14 000
	Saline	16	8	

The existing methods for assaying NGF (Levi-Montalcini, Meyer & Hamburger, 1954; Cohen, 1959; Fenton, 1970) are based on subjective estimates of the outgrowth of nerve fibres from sensory ganglia of chick embryos in tissue cultures containing serial dilutions of NGF. The concentration which produces a maximum fibre outgrowth (the 4+ response) is defined as one Biological Unit/ml. However, the correlation between the *in vitro* and the *in vivo* potencies is not always good (Edwards, Fenton & Hendry, this volume, p. 237). Moreover, differences also exist among the NGF's isolated from various sources. For example, in one experiment Dr Edwards and his colleagues have compared the effects of mouse salivary gland NGF with those of NGF isolated from snake venom. The specific activities of the two samples *in vitro* were 600 000 units/mg for the mouse salivary gland NGF and 300 000 for the Russell's viper venom NGF. Their potency *in vivo*, however, differed by a much larger factor,

* Some of the results I shall describe come from the Ph.D. theses of my students, Drs Lucienne Papadaki (1969) and Bryan Large (1969). Accounts and demonstrations of the preliminary findings have been given to the Physiological Society (Edwards, Fenton, Kakari, Large, Papadaki & Zaimis, 1966; Zaimis, 1971).

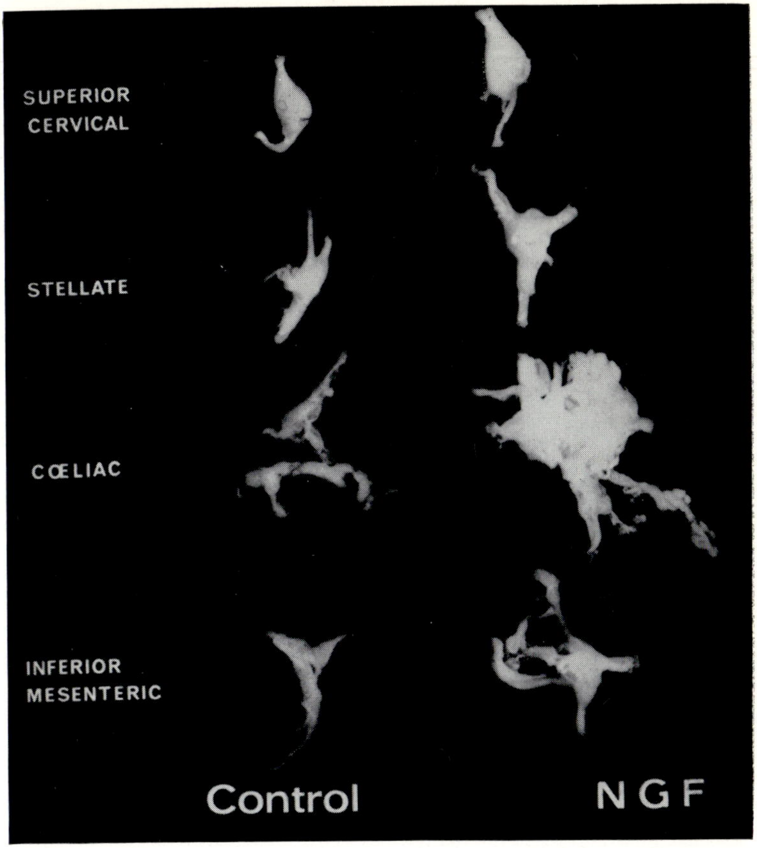

Fig. 2 Sympathetic ganglia removed from two nine-day-old kittens, one treated with saline (control), the other with mouse salivary gland NGF.

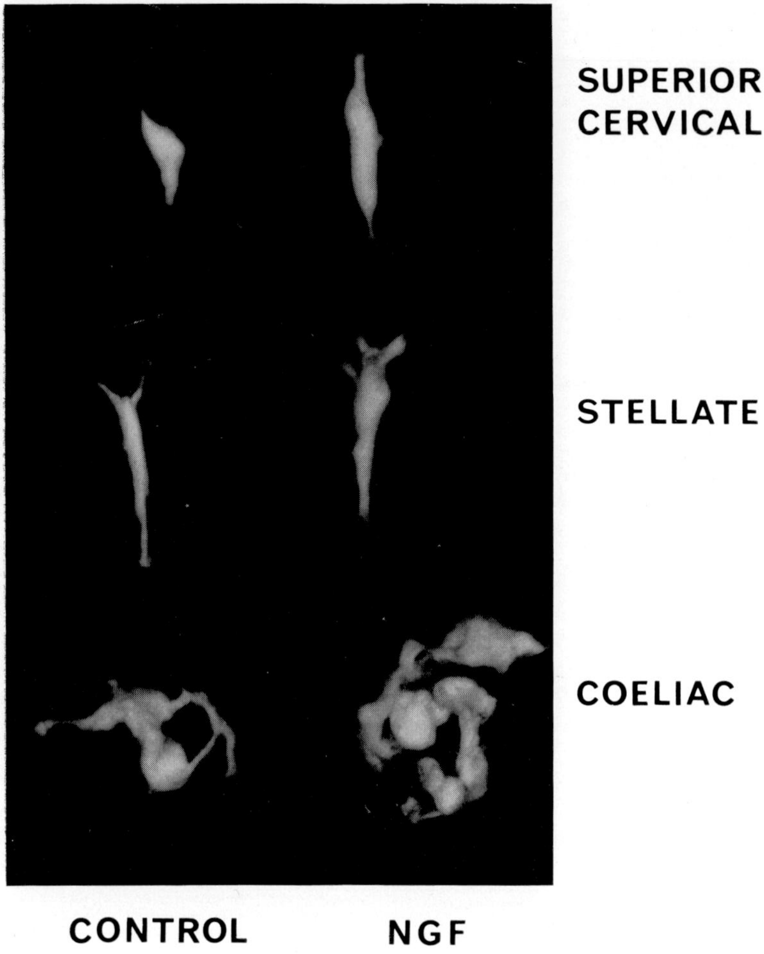

Fig. 3 Sympathetic ganglia removed from two 14-day-old rats, one treated with saline (control), the other with mouse salivary gland NGF.

PLATE III

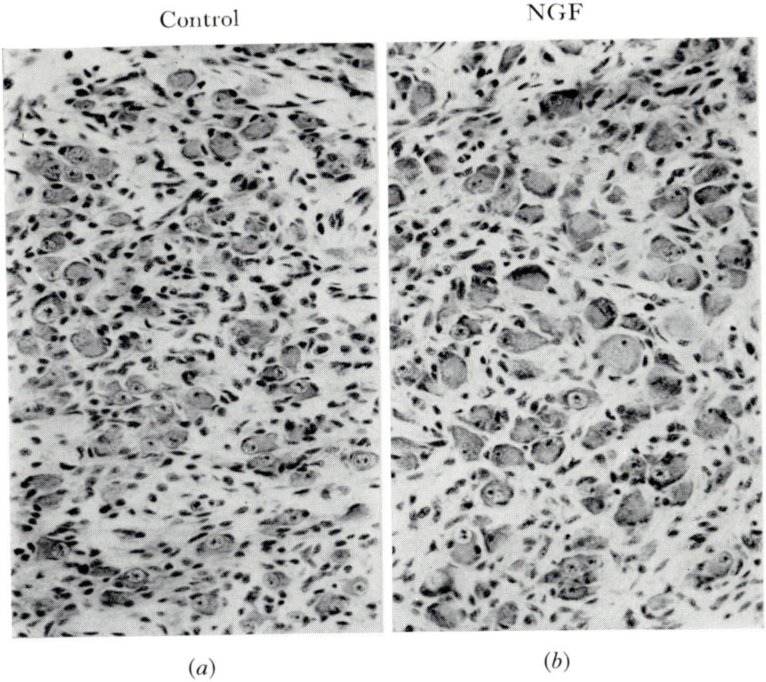

Fig. 4 Nine-day-old kittens: (*a*) control; (*b*) treated with mouse salivary gland NGF. Micrographs of sections through the superior cervical ganglion. Haematoxylin-eosin. (×185)

PLATE IV

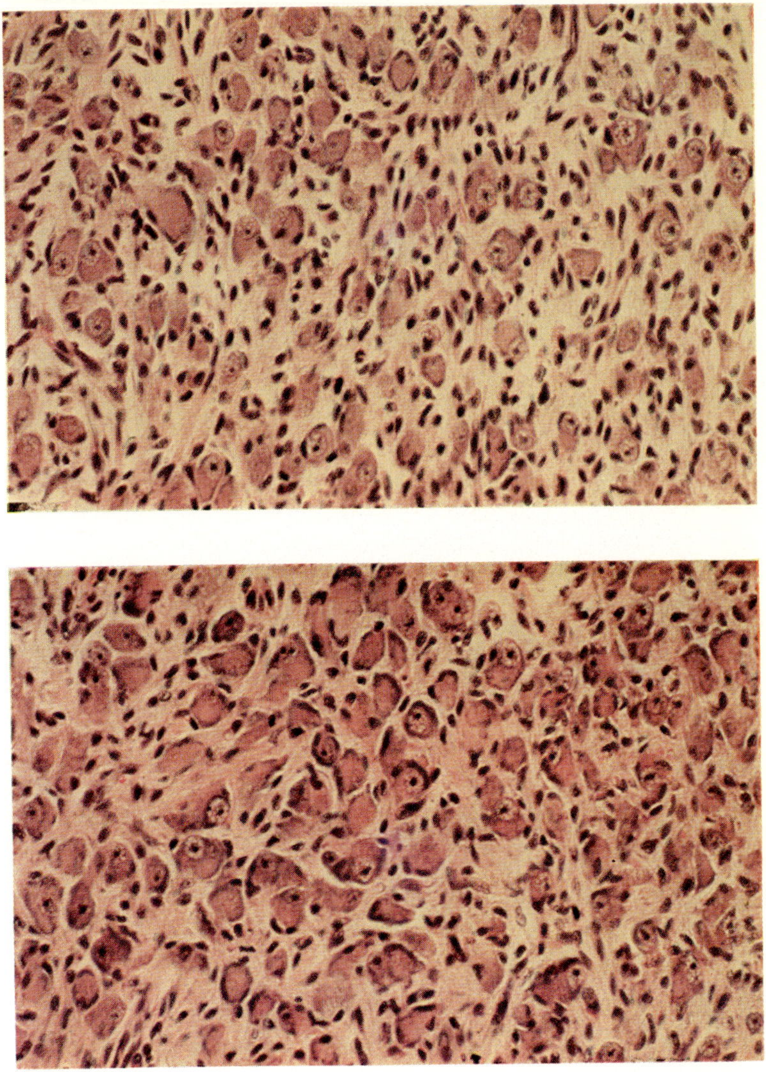

(a)

(b)

Fig. 5 Nine-day-old kittens: (*a*) control; (*b*) treated with mouse salivary gland NGF. Micrographs of sections through the superior cervical ganglion. Haematoxylin-eosin. (× 570)

PLATE V

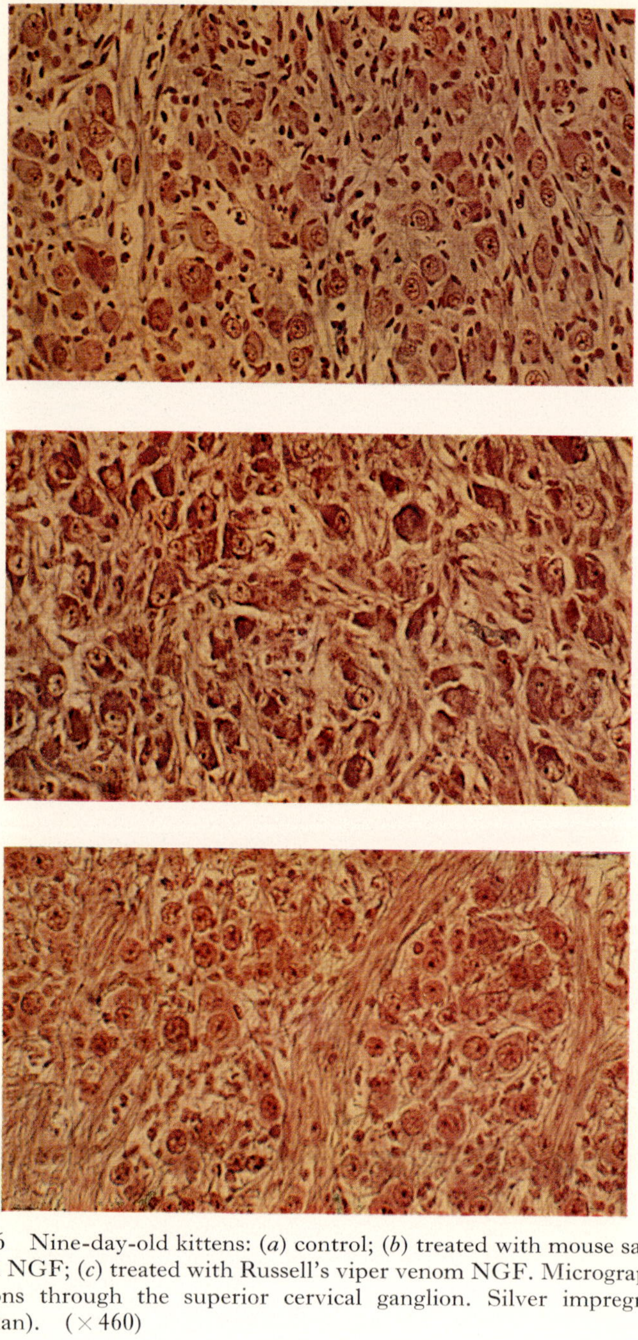

(a) (b) (c)

Fig. 6 Nine-day-old kittens: (*a*) control; (*b*) treated with mouse salivary gland NGF; (*c*) treated with Russell's viper venom NGF. Micrographs of sections through the superior cervical ganglion. Silver impregnation (Bodian). ($\times$460)

Plate VI

(*a*)

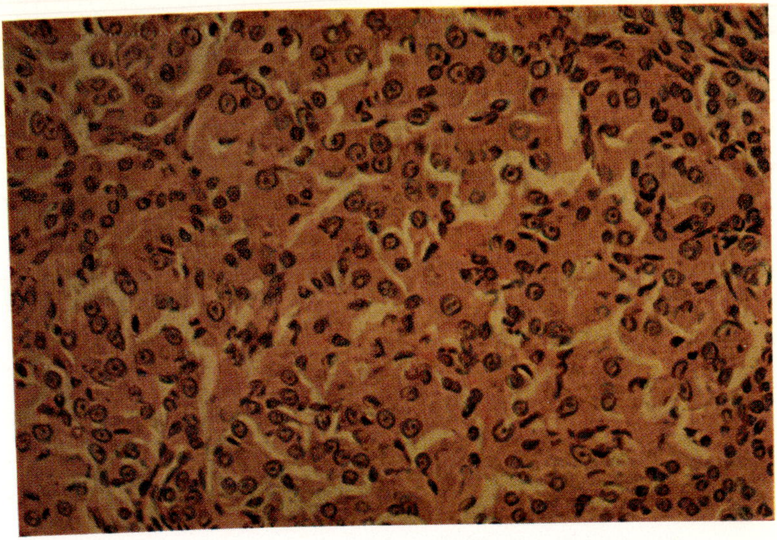

(*b*)

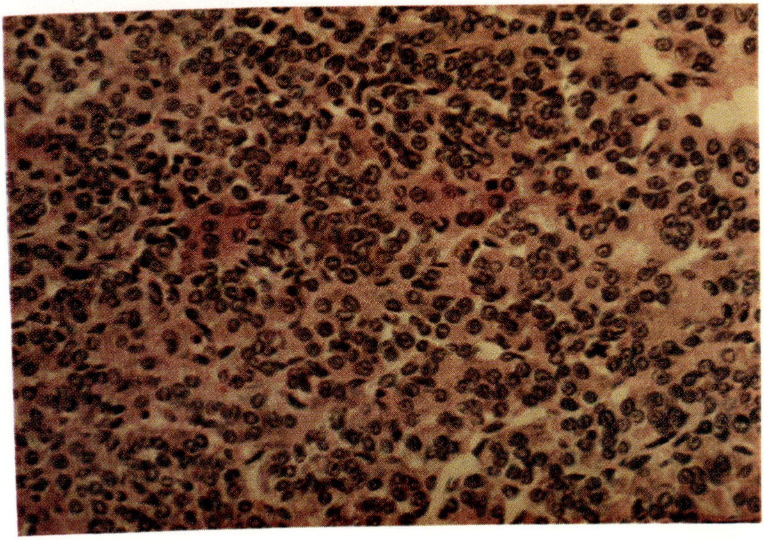

Fig. 7 Nine-day-old kittens: (*a*) control; (*b*) treated with mouse salivary gland NGF. Micrographs of sections through the adrenal medulla. Haematoxylin-eosin. (×450)

PLATE VII

Control NGF:RVV

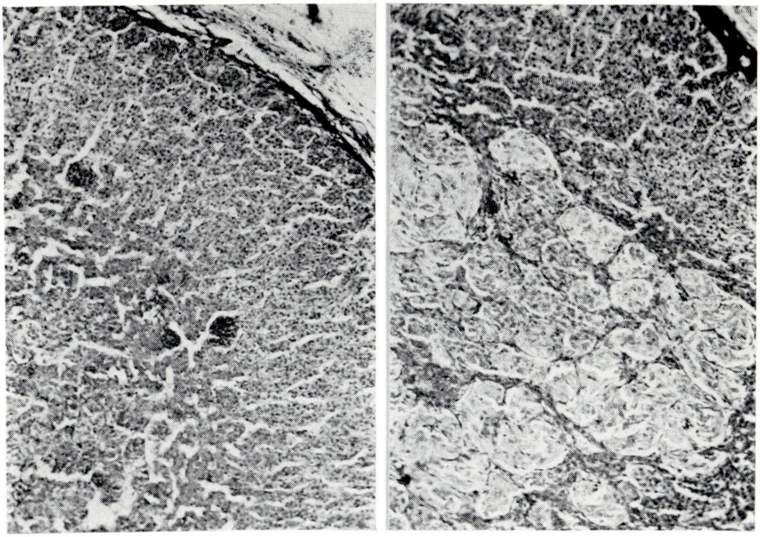

Fig. 8 Nine-day-old kittens: (*a*) control; (*b*) treated with Russell's viper venom (RVV) NGF. Micrographs of sections through the adrenal gland. PAS (periodic acid-Schiff reaction)-haematoxylin. (×82)

Plate VIII

Control NGF:MSG

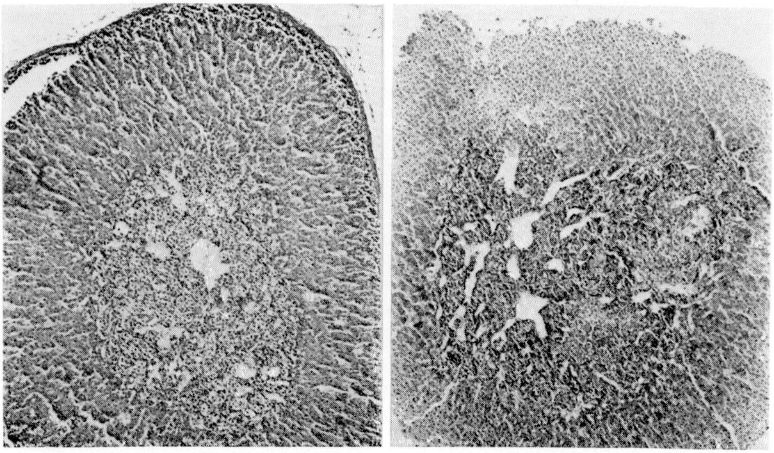

(a) (b)

Control NGF:MSG NGF:RVV

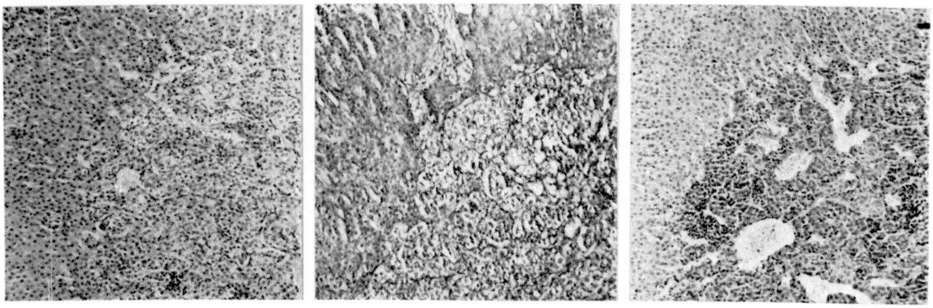

(a) (b) (c)

Fig. 9 Micrographs of sections through the adrenal glands of rats, treated for 14 days with: (a) saline; (b) NGF isolated from either mouse salivary glands (MSG) or (c) Russell's viper venom (RVV). PAS (periodic acid-Schiff reaction)-haematoxylin. ((a), (b) top: $\times 51$; (a)–(c) bottom: $\times 62$)

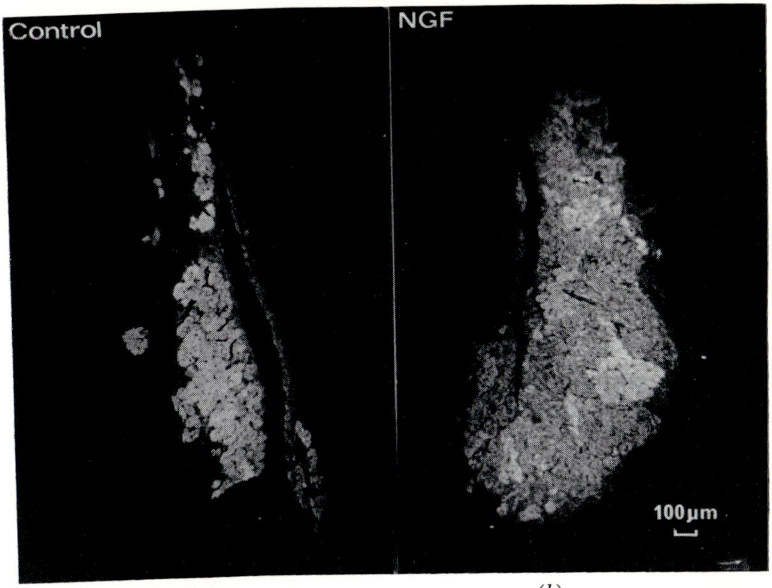

(*a*) (*b*)

Fig. 12 Nine-day-old kittens: (*a*) control; (*b*) treated with mouse salivary gland NGF. Fluorescence micrographs of formalin-fixed sections of the adrenal medulla.

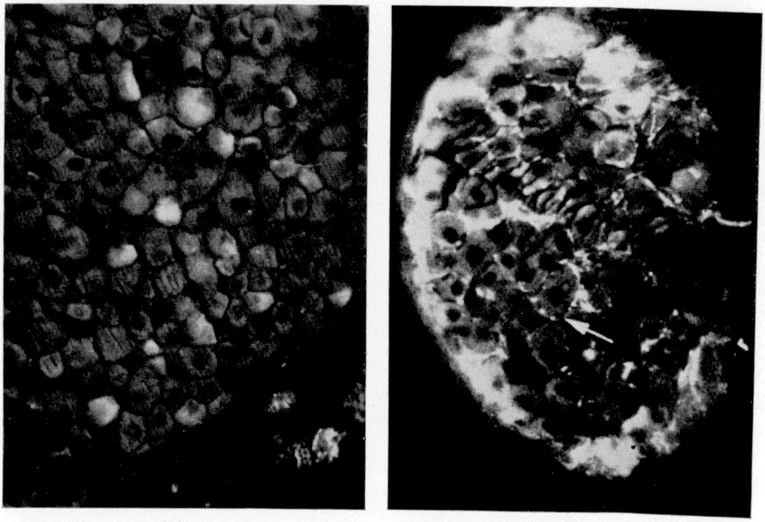

(*a*) (*b*)

Fig. 13 16-day-old mice; nodose ganglia: (*a*) control; (*b*) treated with mouse salivary gland NGF. Histochemical fluorescence technique. (×140) (From L. Olson, 1967.)

of between 5- and 10-fold. For this reason, the *in vitro* potencies included in Table 1 may not accurately represent the activity of NGF when injected into the intact animal.

Morphological changes

Sympathetic ganglia

The following methods were used in order to determine the tissue mass of the ganglia: (a) *Area measurements*: after the sectioning of the whole ganglion, each section was photographed and its contour drawn on transparent paper. All paper drawings from each ganglion were then weighed together. This weight is proportional to the volume of the ganglion. (b) *Wet weight*: within 30 min of dissection the ganglia were weighed on a torsion balance. They were then spread on pieces of non-fibrous paper and transferred to a fixative (Heidenhain's Susa or 10 per cent phosphate-buffered formaldehyde) for histological examination. The ganglia were left in the fixative for 3 to 24 hours; during this period they were photographed. The photographs provided a permanent record of the gross changes visible to the naked eye. (c) *Protein content*: the protein content of the ganglia was determined according to the method described by Lowry, Rosebrough, Farr & Randall (1951).

Both mouse salivary gland NGF and Russell's viper venom NGF produced a hypertrophy of all sympathetic ganglia in the *kitten* but the volume increase was not the same for the prevertebral and paravertebral ganglia. Fig. 1 shows the type of sympathetic ganglia studied and the relative increase in the size of each ganglion averaged for all animals treated with mouse salivary gland NGF. It is clear that the coeliac and the mesenteric ganglia show a significantly more pronounced hypertrophy than the stellate and the superior cervical. Mounts of these ganglia also illustrate these differences (Fig. 2). The percentage increases in mean weight for the superior cervical, stellate, coeliac and inferior mesenteric ganglia were respectively 63, 67, 127 and 81 per cent.

Similar results were obtained in *rats*. Treatment with either mouse salivary gland or Russell's viper venom NGF produced a hypertrophy of all sympathetic ganglia. Again the volume increase differed according to the type of ganglion; the prevertebral ganglia showing a significantly more pronounced hypertrophy than the paravertebral. This difference can be seen in Fig. 3, which shows whole mounts of the superior cervical, stellate and coeliac ganglia from one control rat and one rat treated with mouse salivary gland NGF for 14 days.

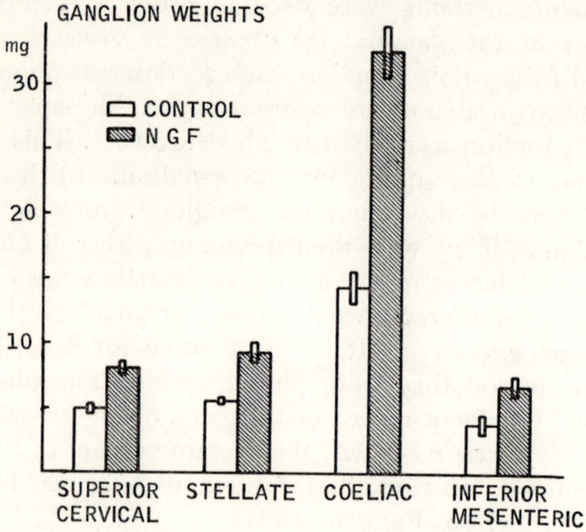

Fig. 1 Nine-day-old kittens: wet weights of sympathetic ganglia. Mean values and S.E.M. from 12 controls; and nine treated with mouse salivary gland NGF.

Microscopical examination of the sympathetic ganglia removed from NGF-treated kittens showed that the overall increase in size was the result primarily of cellular hypertrophy, although an increase in cell numbers was also present. In both the para- and prevertebral ganglia of the NGF-treated animals the cellular hypertrophy was accompanied by more advanced stages of differentiation. In the control nine-day-old kitten the sympathetic ganglia presented a histological picture of immaturity. Some neurones were large, with prominent nuclei and nucleoli and variable amounts of Nissl substance within the cytoplasm. Among these large cells, however, there were immature neurones which had smaller nuclei and reduced amounts of cytoplasm. Moreover, groups of small cells with basophilic nuclei and surrounded by very little cytoplasm appeared scattered among the more differentiated neurones. The administration of NGF produced marked changes. Microscopic examination of the same type of ganglia showed a majority of large mature neurones, uniform in size and clearly multipolar, with little evidence of immature or undifferentiated cells. The hypertrophic neurones also differed from the controls in the more intense basophilia and in the size of the nuclei, which were much larger than in the controls (Figs. 4 and 5). There was an increase in the amount of Nissl substance and in the size and number of nucleoli. The dendritic network surrounding the ganglia cells was highly developed; this could easily be seen in silver-stained sections which showed a markedly increased number of nerve processes. In the ganglia removed from animals treated with snake venom NGF there was a greater amount of neurofibrillar material. In addition, whereas in the ganglia removed from kittens treated with mouse salivary gland NGF, the silver-stained fibres appeared somewhat disordered with a random orientation of the fibres, in ganglia removed from animals treated with snake venom NGF the silver-stained fibres were not only more numerous but appeared to form bundles of fibres in almost parallel arrangement (Fig. 6). This finding, we think, is of some significance because an excessive amount of neurofibrillar material was found even when the total hypertrophy of the ganglia produced by the Russell's viper venom NGF was smaller than that produced by mouse salivary gland NGF.

Similar changes were observed in ganglia removed from NGF-treated rats. Moreover, in the superior cervical ganglion of the rat the hyperplasia was characterized by an overflow of sympathetic nerve cells into the preganglionic nerve trunk.

The increase in the amount of Nissl substance and in the size and number of nucleoli reflects a general increase in metabolic activity. This correlates well with the results of Dr Lucienne Papadaki (this volume, p. 89) who studied the fine structure of sympathetic ganglia dissected from the same animals. In the ganglia removed from NGF-treated rats and kittens, there was an increase in rough endoplasmic reticulum, an increase in polysomes, and an increasing involvement of the Golgi complex in dense-cored granule formation. There was also an increase in the number of nerve processes associated with each satellite cell and a greater number of neurotubules and neurofilaments within the processes.

These findings agree well with those of Levi-Montalcini & Booker (1960) who have described their results primarily in terms of morphological changes occurring in NGF-treated mice. There are, however, two main differences. First, the newborn mouse appears to be more sensitive to NGF than the kitten and the rat, the size of its superior cervical ganglion being increased on average four to six times or more after NGF treatment. Secondly, throughout our studies and in both kittens and rats the volume increase in the sympathetic ganglia was not of the same order; the prevertebral ganglia (coeliac and mesenteric) showing a significantly more pronounced hypertrophy than the paravertebral (stellate and superior cervical).

Adrenal medulla

In all animals, both rats and kittens, the size of the adrenal medulla relative to that of the cortex increased after treatment with NGF. This was found with both NGF preparations.

Area measurements of the cortex and the medulla were made in the adrenals removed from four control rats and five treated with mouse salivary gland NGF. In each case the whole adrenal was sectioned and each section was photographed, enlarged and the contour of the cortex and the medulla drawn on transparent paper. All drawings of the cortex were separated from those of the medulla and were then weighed independently. The weight of the total number of sections is proportional to the volume of the cortex or medulla. The results indicate that in the NGF-treated rats the medulla was 32.5 per cent of the total adrenal, while in the control rats it was only 25.5 per cent of the total. Microscopical examination of the adrenal showed that the hypertrophy of the adrenal medulla was the result of an increase in the number of medullary cells or an increase in their size or both. It is not possible to formulate a general pattern as it was found that in the same species and with the same NGF either one or the other process might prevail. However, in all cases the medullary cells of the NGF-treated animals seem to invade parts of the cortex, as if the area occupied by the medulla was not large enough to accommodate all the new or hypertrophied cells. The micrographs in Figs. 7, 8 and 9 illustrate these changes.

Catecholamine content

Experiments were also performed in order to correlate the morphological findings with catecholamine levels in peripheral organs. The catecholamine content of the salivary glands, heart, spleen, intestine, kidney, colon and adrenals was assayed fluorimetrically after extraction and ion-exchange purification (Bertler, Carlsson & Rosengren, 1958; Shore & Olin, 1958). After NGF treatment there was a significant increase in the catecholamine levels in all tissues examined. In addition, differential assays of adrenaline and noradrenaline showed that in the adrenals of the NGF-treated rats the increase in noradrenaline was significantly greater than that of adrenaline. In contrast, in NGF-treated kittens the percentage increase of adrenaline in the adrenal medulla was greater than that of noradrenaline. Fig. 10 summarizes the results obtained in kittens treated with mouse

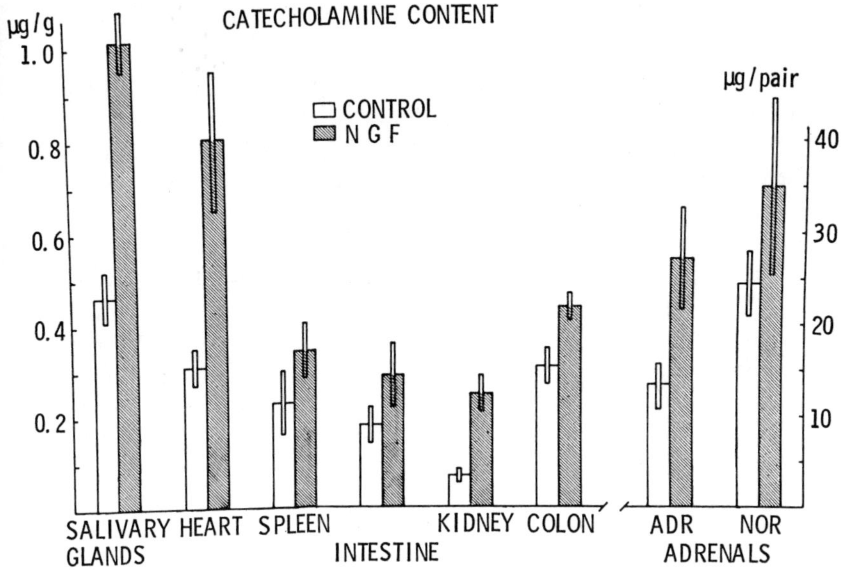

Fig. 10 Nine-day-old kittens. Catecholamine content of peripheral tissues. Mean values and S.E.M.

salivary gland NGF and Fig. 11, those in rats treated with the same type of NGF.

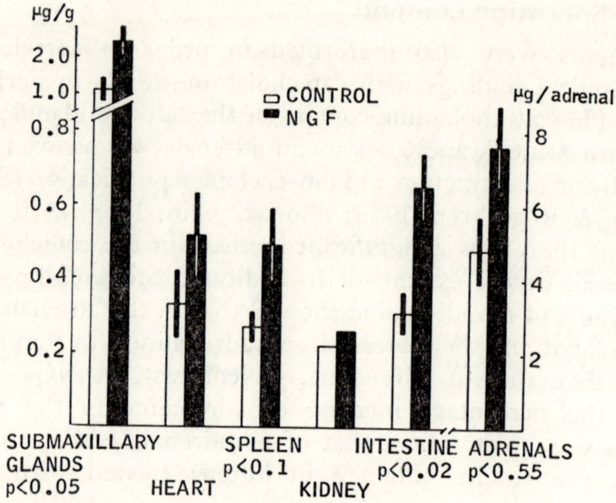

Fig. 11 14-day-old rats. Catecholamine content of peripheral tissues. Mean values and S.E.M.

The histochemical technique, developed by Falck, Hillarp and their collaborators (Falck, 1962; Falck, Hillarp, Thieme & Torp, 1962; Corrodi & Hillarp, 1963, 1964), based on the formaldehyde-induced fluorescence of catecholamines, was also used for the study of the effect of NGF on the adrenal medulla. The results showed an increase in the size of the adrenal medulla in both species and, in addition, a more intense fluorescence. Fig. 12 shows sections of adrenal medulla from one control kitten and one kitten treated with mouse salivary gland NGF. Additional information on the distribution and localization of catecholamines by means of the fluorescence histochemical technique is presented by Drs Nicolescu and Kakari (this volume, p. 108).

Hyperplasia in the absence of mitotic figures

From their studies in mice, Levi-Montalcini & Booker (1960) concluded that the increase in the number of sympathetic nerve cells in the NGF-treated animals was due to an increase in mitotic activity. They reached this conclusion because mitotic activity in mice is still high at birth and comes to an end at nine days. In our experimental animals it was difficult, at first sight, to explain the increase in the number of ganglion cells, since after many attempts, no evidence of mitotic figures was found. In the same ganglia, however, a large number of small-sized cells with basophilic nuclei surrounded by very little cytoplasm were seen. These small cells have previously been described as 'pluripotential' or 'primitive sympathetic cells' (Coupland, 1965; Levi-Montalcini & Booker, 1960); they are considered to be the precursors both of sympathetic neurones and of chromaffin cells.

In the ganglia removed from the NGF-treated kittens and rats, there was a decrease of about 26 per cent in the number of these small basophilic cells and an increase in the number of sympathetic cells ranging from 6 to 34 per cent. Although there was no dramatic change in the number of sympathetic nerve cells in some sections, when the large increase in the volume of the ganglia is taken into consideration, there must inevitably have been a significant increase in the sympathetic cell population of the whole ganglion. Cell counts were made: (*a*) with a grid mounted in the ocular of the microscope; (*b*) by projecting colour transparencies and by counting the cells of a predetermined area; and (*c*) from randomly selected fields of micrographs.

With light microscopy one can see very little morphological variation among the small cell population. They all have intensely basophilic nuclei and scarcely visible cytoplasm. However, from electron microscope examination of the normal ganglia, Dr Papadaki concluded that the small cell population may contain at least three types of cell (this volume, p. 97). One type of immature cell could be identified as a neuroblast with the chromatin mostly dispersed throughout the nucleoplasm. A second type of immature cell, surrounded by a basal lamina, had many pinocytotic vesicles present at the periphery of the plasma membrane and in continuity with it. The nucleus had an irregular profile with aggregations of nuclear chromatin occurring along the nuclear membrane and scattered in the nucleoplasm. It was concluded that this sort of cell could mature into a connective tissue cell of the fibroblast or endothelial cell type. The third cell type was somewhat similar with a partially formed basal lamina, but with no obvious pinocytotic activity and larger mitochondria. It is quite possible that this cell will become a satellite cell. At the electron microscope level, Dr Papadaki was unable to find immature cells of any of these three types in ganglia removed from NGF-treated animals.

I would therefore suggest that the increase in the number of ganglion cells is due to the rapid differentiation, and thus the rapid growth to maturity, of the primitive sympathetic cells under the influence of NGF. Such an interpretation is supported by the experimental findings of Olson (1967). Using the histochemical fluorescence technique, Olson examined various tissues from mice treated with NGF and was able to detect growth stimulation in all parts of the sympathetic adrenergic neurones. He also found, however, varicose adrenergic nerve terminals in areas normally devoid of adrenergic innervation. For example, fine fluorescent varicose nerve processes were seen in the nodose ganglia, known to consist of sensory nerve cells (Fig. 13). Another such example was provided by the small parasympathetic ganglia located in the hilar area of the submaxillary and sublingual glands. In the control mice these ganglia contained no structures with fluorescence for catecholamines. On the other hand, in NGF-treated animals, varicose fluorescent nerve terminals could, in most instances, be seen in these ganglia, sometimes forming synaptic structures around the nerve cell bodies. Olson obtained similar results with other structures, such as the larger ducts of the salivary glands or the normally non-innervated extraorbital lacrymal gland.

It is reasonable, therefore, to assume that multipotential cells exist in developing tissues in other parts of the body, and that they may be diverted into a variety of mature cells according to the type of stimulus they receive.

The increase in the number of medullary cells presents no problem, since mitotic figures and primitive sympathetic cells are both present in the adrenal medulla of most species after birth.

Conclusions

(1) Daily subcutaneous injections of either mouse salivary gland NGF, or Russell's viper venom NGF, in newborn kittens and

rats, resulted, after 8 to 14 days, in an increase in the size of the sympathetic ganglia and of the adrenal medulla.

(2) The volume increase of the sympathetic ganglia was not of the same order, the coeliac and the mesenteric ganglia showing a significantly more pronounced hypertrophy than did the stellate and the superior cervical.

(3) Microscopical examination of the ganglia showed that the overall increase in size was the result primarily of cellular hypertrophy, although an increase in cell numbers was also present. The increase in the number of sympathetic nerve cells did not stem from an increase in mitotic activity, because no mitotic figures could be found *in our animals*. However, in the sympathetic ganglia of the NGF-treated kittens, there was a decrease of about 26 per cent in the number of the small basophilic cells which have previously been described in the literature as multipotential, pluripotential or primitive sympathetic cells.

(4) The suggestion is therefore made that the increase in number of ganglion cells in the NGF-treated kitten and rat is due to the rapid differentiation, and thus the rapid growth to maturity, of these multipotential cells. Moreover, under the influence of NGF, the multipotential cells existing in developing tissues normally devoid of adrenergic innervation, may be diverted into mature sympathetic or chromaffin cells.

(5) Microscopical examination of the adrenal gland showed that the hypertrophy of the adrenal medulla was the result of an increase either in the number of medullary cells, or in their size, or in both. The increase in the number of medullary cells presents no problem as both mitotic figures and primitive sympathetic cells are present in the adrenal medulla of most species after birth.

(6) After NGF treatment there was a significant increase in the catecholamine levels of all tissues examined; moreover, studies by fluorescence microscopy showed an increase in the size of the medulla in both kittens and rats and, in addition, a more intense fluorescence.

Acknowledgements

My thanks are due to Dr L. Bitensky for many helpful discussions; and to Mr R. Owen and Mr P. Clayton for their most valuable technical assistance. The work was generously supported by grants from the Muscular Dystrophy Group of Great Britain, the Medical Research Council, and the Palisades Foundation, Inc. of the U.S.A.

Fig. 13 is reproduced from: Olson, L.: Outgrowth of Sympathetic Adrenergic Neurons in Mice Treated with a Nerve Growth Factor (NGF), *Z. Zellforsch.* **81**, 155–73 (1967) Berlin-Heidelberg-New York: Springer.

References

Bertler, A., Carlsson, A. & Rosengren, E. (1958). *Acta physiol. scand.* **44**, 273.

Cohen, S. (1959). *J. biol. Chem.* **234**, 1129.

Cohen, S. (1960). *Proc. natn. Acad. Sci. U.S.A.* **46**, 302.

Corrodi, H. & Hillarp, N.-Å. (1963). *Helv. chim. Acta* **46**, 2425.

Corrodi, H. & Hillarp, N.-Å. (1964). *Helv. chim. Acta* **47**, 911.

Coupland, R. E. (1965). *The Natural History of the Chromaffin Cell.* London: Longmans.

Edwards, D. C., Fenton, E. L., Kakari, S., Large, B. J., Papadaki, L. & Zaimis, E. (1966). *J. Physiol., Lond.* **186**, 10P.

Falck, B. (1962). *Acta physiol. scand.* **56**, Suppl. 197, 1.

Falck, B., Hillarp, N.-Å., Thieme, G. & Torp, A. (1962). *J. Histochem. Cytochem.* **10**, 348.

Fenton, E. L. (1970). *Expl. Cell Res.* **59**, 383.

Large, B. J. (1969). Ph.D. Thesis. University of London.

Lowry, O. H., Rosebrough, N. J., Farr, A. L. P. & Randall, R. J. (1951). *J. biol. Chem.* **193**, 265.

Levi-Montalcini, R. & Booker, B. (1960). *Proc. natn. Acad. Sci. U.S.A.* **46**, 373.

Levi-Montalcini, R. & Cohen, S. (1960). *Ann. N.Y. Acad. Sci.* **85**, 324.

Levi-Montalcini, R., Meyer, H. & Hamburger, V. (1954). *Cancer Res.* **14**, 49.

Olson, L. (1967). *Z. Zellforsch. mikrosk. Anat.* **81**, 155.

Papadaki, L. (1969). Ph.D. Thesis. University of London.

Shore, P. A. & Olin, J. S. (1958). *J. Pharmac. exp. Ther.* **122**, 295.

Zaimis, E. (1971). *J. Physiol., Lond.* **216**, 65P.

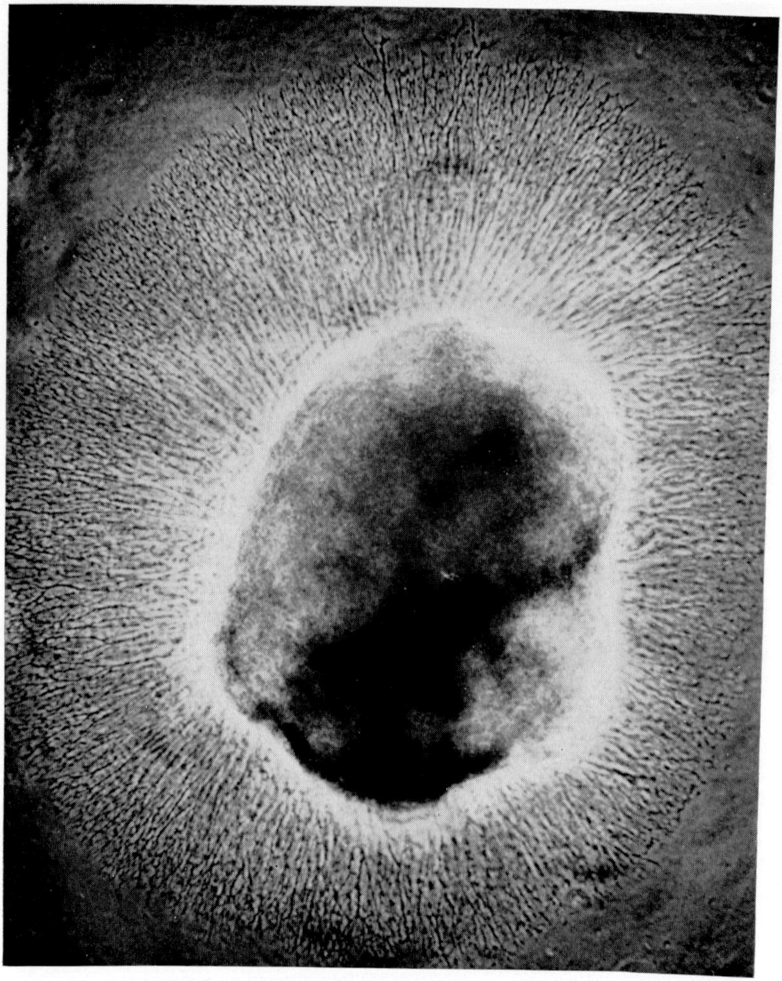

Fig. 1 Phase-contrast photograph of the halo of fibres growing from a sympathetic ganglion after incubation for 24 hours in the presence of NGF (1 μg/ml). (Partlow & Larrabee, 1971.)

In this and all other experiments in this paper, lumbar sympathetic ganglia were excised from chicken embryos (white Leghorn) and incubated at 37°C in modified McCoy's 5a culture medium, which was equilibrated with 5 per cent CO_2, 95 per cent O_2. In Figs. 1–10 inclusive, the excised ganglia were embedded in fibrin clots. The ganglia were typically from vertebral levels 25–30 or 26–30, identified by reference to the distinctive 25th vertebra. (Portmann, 1950.)

Metabolism During Development in Sympathetic Ganglia of Chickens: Effects of Age, Nerve Growth Factor and Metabolic Inhibitors

MARTIN G. LARRABEE

Thomas C. Jenkins Department of Biophysics, Johns Hopkins University, Baltimore, Md, USA

Our laboratory was introduced to the nerve growth factor (NGF) by Dr Giovanni Toschi, who arrived from Rome one day in 1965 bearing a generous gift of this fascinating material from Dr Rita Levi-Montalcini. Dr Toschi stayed with us to do many preliminary experiments with our methods and to introduce us to procedures in use in Rome. The results I shall describe come mainly from the doctoral dissertation of my student Dr Lester M. Partlow (1969; Partlow & Larrabee, 1969; 1971), and from experiments performed under his direction by a former undergraduate student, Mr William Ted Brown, who greatly assisted us in the development of methods.

All our experiments with NGF were performed on lumbar sympathetic ganglia excised from chicken embryos, the ganglia being embedded in fibrin clots. The embedding of the ganglia in clots permitted outgrowth of fibres to be observed in the same preparations in which metabolism was measured: this turned out to be essential to the conclusions that we reached. A newly devised quantitative and objective measure of the fibre outgrowth proved helpful. The measuring procedure can be explained by reference to Fig. 1, which shows a typical halo of fibres growing from an excised sympathetic ganglion in the presence of NGF. To express the extent of outgrowth we first determined the area occupied by the ganglion and the area included within the outer boundary of the halo. We then calculated radii for these two areas, under the pretext that they were circular, and used the difference between the radii to express the mean halo width. Elsewhere we have shown that this measure of fibre growth increased linearly with time for at least two days under our culture conditions, except for an initial lag (Larrabee, 1970; Partlow & Larrabee, 1971). Fig. 2 illustrates an application in a bioassay of NGF.

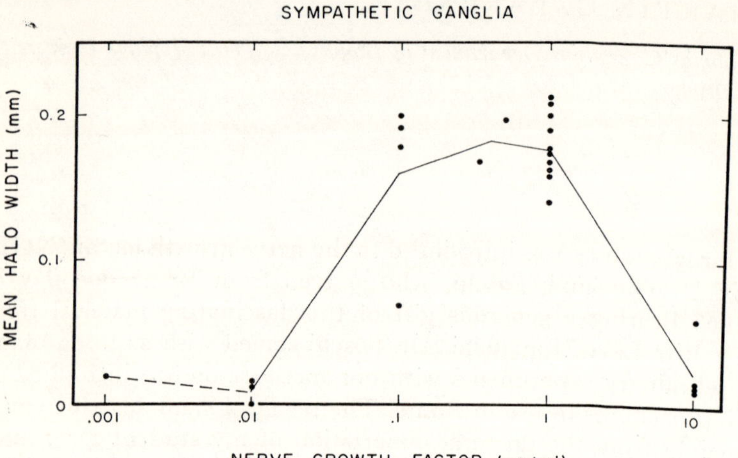

Fig. 2 Outgrowth of fibres from excised sympathetic ganglia, as a function of the concentration of NGF added to the culture medium. The ganglia were from 13- or 14-day chicken embryos. Incubation time, 24 hours (Brown, Partlow & Larrabee, unpublished results). The reduction of fibre outgrowth at high concentrations has been attributed to formation of a capsule by the growing fibres in the case of sensory ganglia (Levi-Montalcini & Angeletti, 1968*a*, *b*).

Metabolic effects of NGF

Several metabolic processes proceed at faster rates in excised ganglia in the presence of NGF than in its absence. This has been observed for the incorporation of labelled precursors into RNA, protein and lipids and for the release of labelled CO_2 from [^{14}C] glucose (Cohen, 1959; Angeletti, Liuzzi & Levi-Montalcini, 1964; Angeletti, Liuzzi, Levi-Montalcini & Gandini-Attardi,

1964; Angeletti, Gandini-Attardi, Toschi, Salvi & Levi-Montalcini, 1965; Angeletti, Levi-Montalcini & Calissano, 1968).

In our experiments the most conspicuous metabolic effects of NGF are best described as a sustaining of the initial rates with which the excised tissue starts off, rather than as a stimulation above the initial rate. Thus, these effects may be more closely related to the preservation of the morphology of the tissue (Levi-Montalcini & Angeletti, 1963) than to stimulation of fibre growth.

Fig. 3 shows the preservation of carbohydrate metabolism in sympathetic ganglia supplied with [1-^{14}C] glucose. The rate of output of labelled CO_2 is plotted against time after excision. The output from control ganglia without added NGF (dashed lines) at first rose progressively as the metabolic intermediates became equilibrated with the labelled carbon. Following this rise there

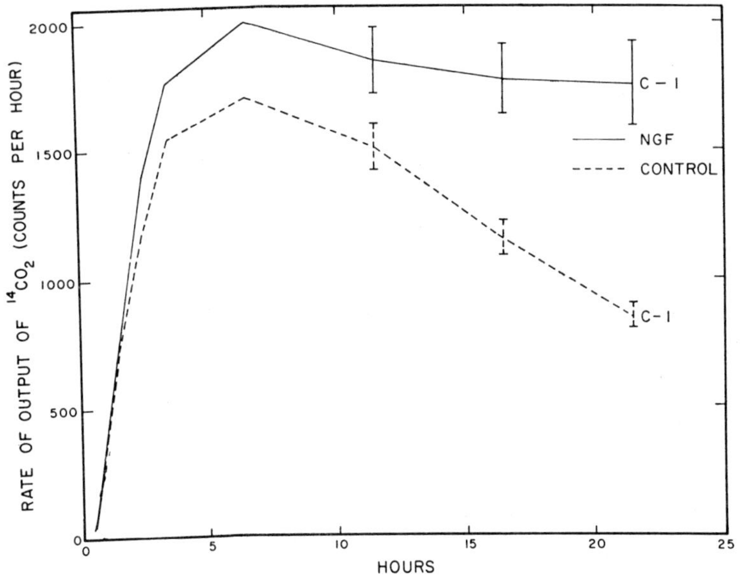

Fig. 3 Release of labelled CO_2 from sympathetic ganglia supplied with [1-^{14}C] glucose, in the presence or absence of the nerve growth factor (1 μg/ml). The ganglia were from 13- or 14-day embryos. Release of labelled CO_2 was measured continuously with the 'microbeaker respirometer' procedure of Horowicz & Larrabee (1962), modified in such a way that preparations in plastic culture dishes were gently rocked to keep the medium moving (Brown & Larrabee, quoted by Larrabee, 1969).

was a decline in rate as the control preparations progressively deteriorated during continued incubation. This deterioration was essentially eliminated in other ganglia that had been supplied with added NGF (solid lines). If we imagine that the later portions of the control and experimental curves in Fig. 3 are extrapolated back to zero time, it appears that there would have been little or no difference between the initial rates in the two preparations, if the beginnings had not been obscured by the experimental transition.

The maintenance of the rate of production of CO_2 from labelled glucose was more quickly obvious when the addition of NGF was delayed until the decline had already started (Fig. 4). In these cases there was clearly no stimulation above the pre-existing rate, but only a reduction in the subsequent decline.

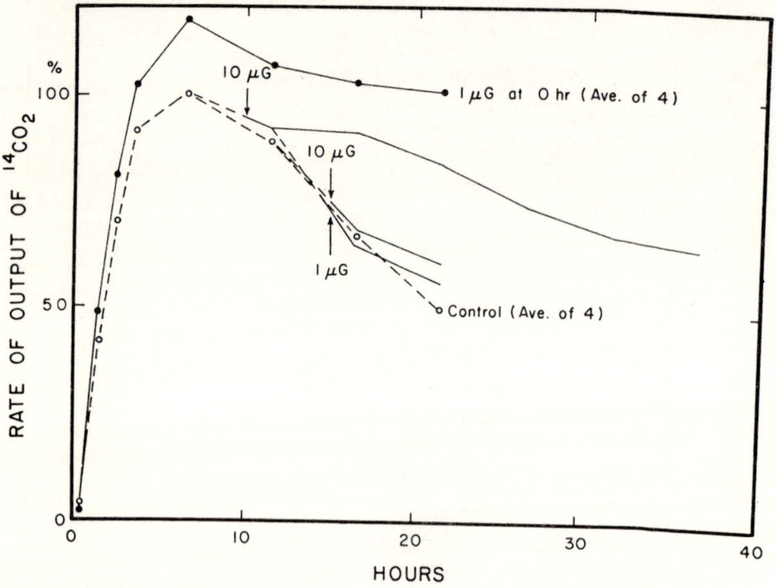

Fig. 4 Effects of delayed additions of the NGF on the release of labelled CO_2 from sympathetic ganglia supplied with [1-^{14}C] glucose. Other procedures as in Fig. 3. Points are averages for four preparations. Lines not drawn through points are for single preparations. Solid lines represent the presence of the growth factor, and dashed lines its absence. The indicated amounts of the factor were added to 1 ml of medium (Brown & Larrabee, unpublished results).

Other examples of the preservation of metabolic rates were found in the incorporation of labelled precursors into RNA and protein (Fig. 5). In these cases a reduction in rate of incorporation occurred quite abruptly in control ganglia after a few hours. This decline in rate was prevented or considerably delayed by addition of the growth factor.

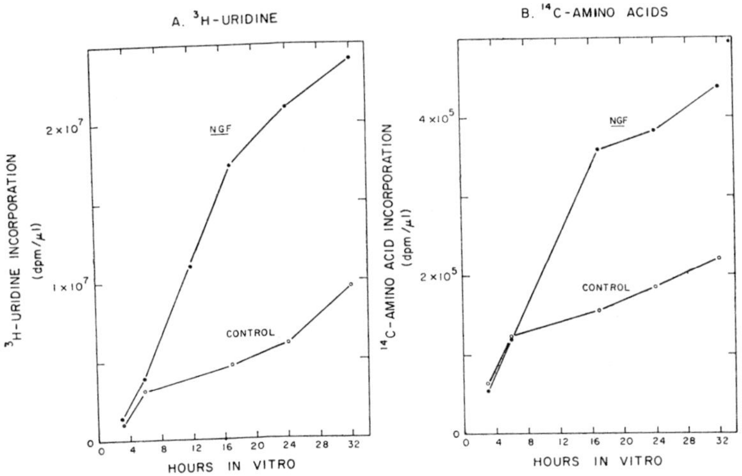

Fig. 5 Effects of NGF (1 μg/ml) on incorporation of labelled precursors into RNA (*a*) and into protein (*b*) in sympathetic ganglia from 13-day-old chicken embryos. Ordinates represent incorporation per unit volume of tissue (Partlow & Larrabee, 1971).

A reasonable explanation of the foregoing observations is that the freshly excised tissue contains some NGF derived from the embryo. Deterioration may then be supposed to set in when this endogenous material becomes degraded or washed out, unless it is replaced by exogenous growth factor supplied by the experimenter. From this point of view, NGF is a stimulator of metabolism, which declines in its absence. On the other hand there is no direct evidence that a ganglion, when freshly excised, actually contains enough growth factor to stimulate its own metabolism or that the amount of such endogenous growth factor declines during incubation. An alternative explanation is that metabolic decline may be due to depletion of other materials, whose loss is prevented or compensated by experimental addition of NGF. In this sense the growth factor is a preserver of the excised tissue, rather than a stimulator of its metabolism.

Separation of effects of NGF on fibre growth from those on RNA metabolism

We come now to the question of the mechanism by which NGF produces the well-known stimulation of fibre outgrowth. Probably the best theory we have had is that the factor influences the transcription of one or more messenger RNA's from DNA and that these messengers are translated into proteins which affect fibre growth. This concept derives from experiments on the effects of actinomycin D and puromycin on the incorporation of labelled precursors by ganglia in the presence of NGF (Angeletti *et al.*, 1965). Those metabolic measurements were made on sympathetic and sensory ganglia that were free-floating, so that

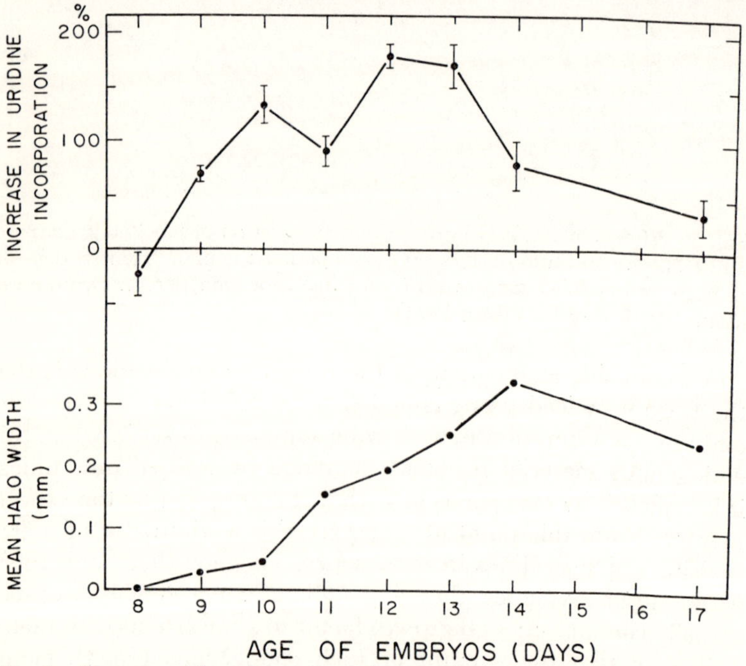

Fig. 6 Changes with embryonic age in the effects of NGF (1 μg/ml) on the incorporation of labelled uridine (*above*) and in the fibre growth elicited by the growth factor (*below*). Incubation time, 22 hours. Points and symbols in upper graph indicate means ± S.E.M. ($N = 4$) (Partlow & Larrabee, 1971).

fibre growth could not be observed simultaneously. We have made similar experiments on sympathetic ganglia, but with concurrent growth measurements.

Fig. 6 shows the effects of NGF on sympathetic ganglia from embryos of different ages. The upper curve shows the increase in labelling of RNA; the lower shows the outgrowth of nerve fibres in the presence of the growth factor. These two variables followed rather different time courses during development. For example, the increase in labelling was about as great in ganglia from 10-day-old embryos, where very little fibre outgrowth was caused, as it was at 12–13 days, where there was maximal outgrowth. This raised the question of how closely these two effects of the growth factor are really related.

We tried, therefore, the application of actinomycin D in a concentration of 1 μg/ml, which profoundly inhibits RNA synthesis in sympathetic neurones, as it does in other kinds of cells (Partlow, 1969; Partlow & Larrabee, 1971). To our surprise this did not prevent fibre outgrowth in the presence of NGF and did not even reduce the outgrowth significantly until more than 15 hours after the addition of the inhibitor (Fig. 7). However,

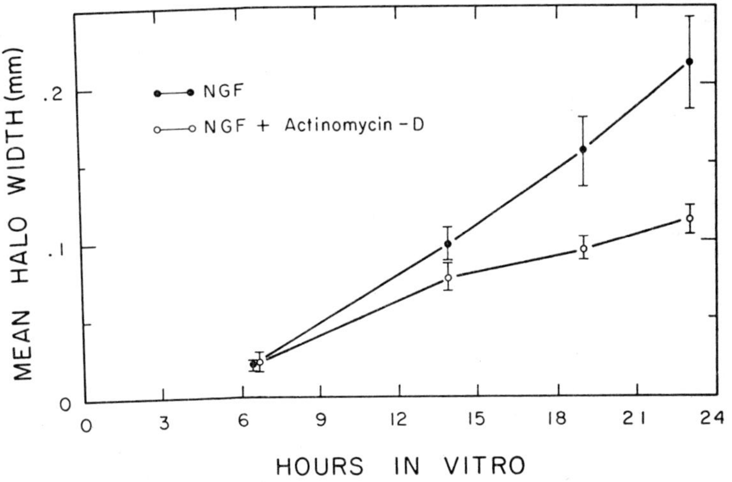

Fig. 7 Fibre growth from sympathetic ganglia in the presence of NGF (1 μg/ml) and in the presence or absence of actinomycin D (1 μg/ml). The ganglia were from 13-day chicken embryos. Each point and bar represents the mean ± S.E.M. (N = 4) (Partlow & Larrabee, 1971).

we did not feel that this experiment alone could be construed as unequivocal evidence that RNA metabolism was not essential for the stimulation of fibre outgrowth, because actinomycin D had been added simultaneously with the growth factor. It seemed possible that the growth factor might have altered RNA metabolism before it could be turned off by the inhibitor.

In our subsequent experiments actinomycin D was applied one hour before NGF was added. Labelled uridine was added together with the growth factor, so that RNA synthesis could be observed simultaneously with fibre growth. In these cases the incubation was terminated after 15 hours. The results are plotted against the concentration of the inhibitor in Fig. 8A. Fibres grew in abundance, although somewhat reduced in length (dashed lines), even when RNA synthesis was reduced to insignificant levels (solid lines). The RNA labelling is reproduced on a larger scale in Fig. 8B. The two higher concentrations

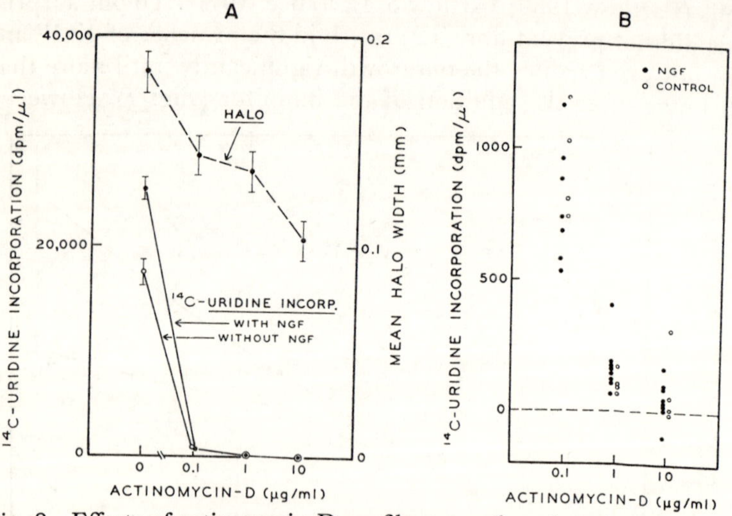

Fig. 8 Effects of actinomycin D on fibre growth and on incorporation of [^{14}C] uridine. Ganglia from 14-day chicken embryos were preincubated for one hour with the inhibitor before addition of the nerve-growth factor (1 μg/ml) and labelled uridine. Incubation was then continued for an additional 15 hours. (A) Each point and bar represents the mean ± S.E.M., for eight ganglia with the growth factor or for four controls without the factor. (B) Details of the data on labelling, plotted with an expanded scale of ordinates (Partlow & Larrabee, 1971).

of the inhibitor reduced the labelling below 1 per cent of the control. In this small residual synthesis there was no evidence of a difference between preparations with added NGF (filled points) and those without (unfilled points).

Although actinomycin D did not completely prevent the outgrowth of fibres, the growth was to some extent restricted after a number of hours. We guessed that this might be due to the well-known mechanisms by means of which the turning off of the RNA synthesis eventually decreases protein synthesis, as a result of the continual degradation of RNA. When the effects of

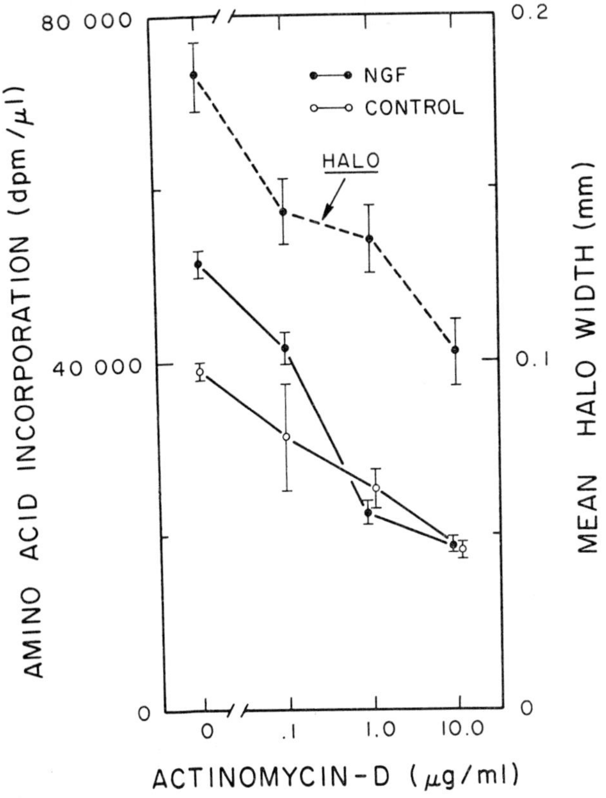

Fig. 9 Effects of actinomycin D on fibre growth (dashed line) and on incorporation of [^{14}C] leucine and [^{14}C] threonine (solid lines) by sympathetic ganglia. Procedures as in Fig. 8. Each point and bar represents the mean ± S.E.M. (N = 4) (Partlow & Larrabee, 1971).

actinomycin D were measured on the labelling of protein rather than on labelling of RNA, there was indeed a correlation between the degree of inhibition of growth and the inhibition of protein labelling (Fig. 9). Further evidence that the loss of fibre growth was due to loss of protein synthesis was obtained by comparing the effects of actinomycin D with those of another inhibitor, cycloheximide. The latter interferes with protein synthesis in an entirely different way, at the level of translation of RNA into protein (Sisler & Siegel, 1967). When incorporation of labelled amino acids into protein was reduced by a given amount by means of cycloheximide, the effects on fibre outgrowth were quantitatively indistinguishable from those accompanying the same reduction in labelling by actinomycin D (Fig. 10).

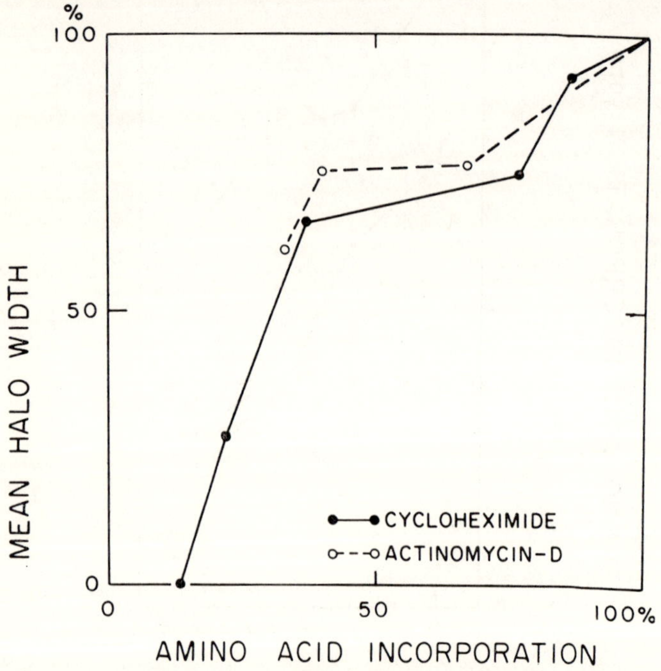

Fig. 10 Comparison of the inhibition of fibre growth by actinomycin D and by cycloheximide, as functions of the inhibition of labelling of protein. Growth and incorporation are both expressed as percentages of the values without an inhibitor. NGF was present in all cases. Procedures as in Figs. 8 and 9 (Partlow & Larrabee, 1971).

Thus the effect of either inhibitor on fibre growth can be ascribed to a generalized depression of protein metabolism.

The foregoing results are strong evidence that a change in RNA synthesis is not needed for the stimulation of fibre outgrowth by NGF. There is always, of course, the possibility that a few molecules of special messenger RNA might be produced in the presence of the inhibitor and not be detected. It is wishful thinking, however, to invoke undetected molecules. Instead there is a need for explanations of the growth effect which do not postulate an essential role of changes in RNA metabolism.

Carbohydrate metabolism in embryonic sympathetic ganglia

We have recently begun to study the developmental metabolism of sympathetic and dorsal root ganglia of the chicken embryo. This work has been undertaken partly in the hope of finding something in their history that might elucidate the action of NGF by explaining why its effectiveness changes so remarkably with embryonic age. Be this as it may, we are studying neuronal development in seemingly favourable preparations. The ganglia are simpler than brain tissue, which has usually been used for such studies, and they can be excised with relatively little damage, for well-controlled measurements *in vitro*. The sympathetic ganglia are readily available as early as one day after they are formed, and related developmental studies on enzymes are being carried out in other laboratories (Marchesio & Consolo, 1968; Giacobini, Marchesio, Giacobini & Koslow, 1970).

Probably the simplest measure of the development of a ganglion is its growth. Fig. 11A shows the dry weight of the lumbar paravertebral sympathetic chain of the chicken embryo as a function of age. The paravertebral chains are formed on the sixth day (Kuntz, 1910; Romanoff, 1960), after which there is relatively little growth for a few days. Then the size of the ganglia increases rapidly from 10 to 15 days, followed by a slower growth from 15 days to hatching, which occurs on the twenty-first day. Our histological preparations have shown that the sizes of the neuronal perikarya increase considerably during the growth period. It remains to be determined whether there is also some contribution to the size of the ganglia by cell migration or cell division during this period.

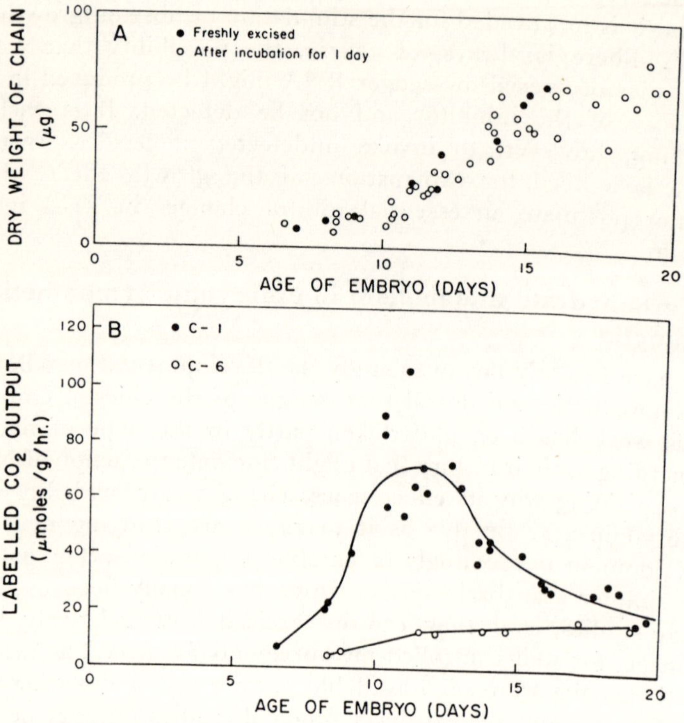

Fig. 11 Changes with age of embryo in (A) the weight of a chain of lumbar sympathetic ganglia (vertebral levels 25–30 or 26–30) and (B) the output of labelled CO_2 from [1-^{14}C] glucose or [6-^{14}C] glucose by these ganglia. (From Larrabee, 1970 with corrected scales of ordinates.)

Striking changes in carbohydrate metabolism were found during the period of rapid growth. One of these was revealed by the release of labelled CO_2 from specifically labelled glucose. In Fig. 11B the filled points demonstrate a great surge of carbon-1 into CO_2, with a maximum at 10–13 days. There was no accompanying surge of carbon-6 into CO_2 (unfilled points). This difference between the outputs of carbon-1 and carbon-6 into CO_2 implies activity of pentose pathways. This is presumably needed for pentose synthesis during growth, and perhaps also for the generation of reduced NADP for lipid synthesis, as other workers have suggested in the case of developing tissues.

A slightly earlier feature of ganglion metabolism was a high rate of glycolysis, revealed by the production of labelled lactate from glucose (Fig. 12). This faded as growth started and as the pentose pathway speeded up.

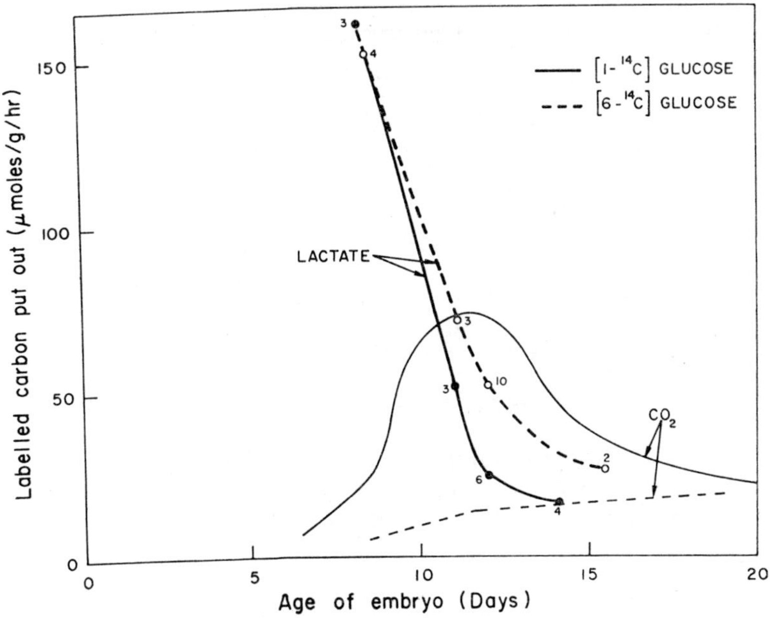

Fig. 12 Changes with age of embryo in the output of labelled lactate and labelled CO_2 from specifically labelled glucose. The curves for CO_2 production are copied from Fig. 11. Numerals beside points on the lactate curves indicate the numbers of observations which were averaged.

The existence of high rates of glycolysis, and that of pentose path activity, in developing nervous tissues, have previously been reported, but their time courses, and particularly their sequential relation to one another, do not seem to have been described (Liuzzi & Angeletti, 1964; Papaconstantinou, 1967; Davison & Dobbing, 1968).

Comparison of fibre growth 'in vitro' with ganglion growth 'in vivo'

It is well known that the extent to which fibres grow out of an excised sensory or sympathetic ganglion in the presence of the NGF depends upon the age of embryo from which the ganglion is obtained (Winick & Greenberg, 1965*a*; Levi-Montalcini &

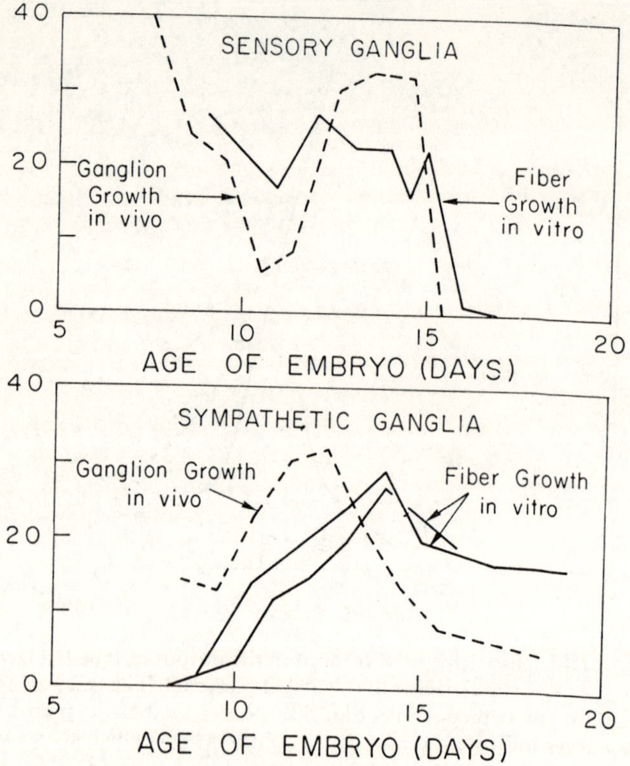

Fig. 13 Comparison of the rates of growth of sensory and sympathetic ganglia in the embryo with the growth of fibres from excised ganglia in the presence of the NGF (0.5 μg/ml). Ganglion growth *in vivo* (dashed lines) is expressed as the percentage increase in dry weight per day. The data for sensory ganglia were obtained by Wang & Larrabee (unpublished). Fibre growth *in vitro* (solid lines) is expressed as the mean width of the halo of fibres growing from excised ganglia, which were embedded in fibrin clots, during a period of 24 hours (Brown *et al.*, unpublished results). The width of the halo is given in μm divided by ten.

Angeletti, 1968*a*). In a systematic study of these changes with age we have confirmed the earlier reports that lumbar sensory ganglia from chicken embryos are responsive to the growth factor at an earlier age than are the lumbar sympathetic ganglia. In addition, a striking contrast was found between the ways in which the two kinds of ganglia lost responsiveness to NGF. The ability to grow fibres faded slowly in sympathetic ganglia after a maximum at 14 days, with some outgrowth still elicitable after hatching. The fibre growth from the sensory ganglia terminated with startling decisiveness at about the sixteenth day of embryonic life (Fig. 13).

The variations in fibre outgrowth with embryonic age are possibly related to the changes in the growth rates of the bodies of the ganglia in their natural situation in the embryo. In our studies, for example, fibre growth could be elicited only from ganglia that were increasing in size before they were excised. Moreover, the sudden loss of the response by sensory ganglia to the growth factor occurred at the same age as that at which these ganglia suddenly stopped growing in the embryo; at least the agreement was as precise as might be expected from two independent series of experiments. In sympathetic ganglia, on the other hand, both kinds of growth progressively tapered off (Fig. 13).

Speculations on the role of NGF in normal development

Before concluding I should like to offer a few speculations, not to be interpreted as in any sense compelling, but rather to turn attention in a direction that seems to deserve more thought and experimentation.

Clearly, NGF is not the only determinant of growth of sensory and sympathetic ganglia. This is shown by the difference in the ages of the embryo over which these two kinds of ganglia accomplish their fastest growth. Accordingly the time course of growth for both cannot be ascribed to systemic variations in the concentration of a single growth factor.

One might speculate that NGF influences the *rate* of growth during the period in which the cells of a ganglion are sensitive to it, but that the *amount* of growth is limited by other agents or by attributes of the tissue that terminate growth when a suitable size has been reached.

Another possibility refers to an idea presented earlier (p. 75) in connection with the *in vitro* metabolic experiments: namely that NGF may have essentially a preservative role. In this context it is relevant that in the normal development of the nervous system, many cells are destined to die before the adult state is reached (see Jacobson, 1970). Thus destructive forces are normally at work and may need regulation in order that a suitable balance in the numbers of the various cell types in the adult organism may be achieved. It does not seem impossible that NGF may serve as a normal antagonist of the destructive forces at critical stages of development. In other words, perhaps it is a prime deterrent of embryonic degeneration.

It is obvious that the function of the NGF in the normal development of the nervous system is still obscure. Much information must be gleaned before its role can be deduced. The following are a few very elementary questions that still await an answer: (*a*) How does the concentration of the growth factor vary with embryonic age in sympathetic and sensory ganglia and elsewhere in the embryo? There is evidence that NGF appears suddenly in the chicken embryo during the fourth to fifth day and remains relatively constant in concentration during days 6–8 (Winick & Greenberg, 1965*b*). What is its subsequent time course? What about particular tissues and other species? (*b*) How does the concentration of NGF that is normally present compare with those developed by the dosages typically used to cause overgrowth of the sympathetic nervous system? Is it possible that the dosages administered are excessive, and that they produce effects which, although spectacular and interesting, are misleading in terms of the normal role of the factor? (*c*) Would effects of the growth factor be discovered on other kinds of cells if all ages were thoroughly investigated, perhaps with particular attention paid to the ages at which cell sizes are normally increasing? Some effects have already been reported: for example, those on vestibular cells in tissue culture (Hillman & Sheikh, 1968).

The pioneers in this field have shown us exciting phenomena and given us powerful tools, which may have barely scratched the surface of problems that they may serve to attack. The possibilities are a challenge for new ideas, new imagination, and new ingenuity.

Acknowledgements

Investigations reported in this paper were supported by research grant no. NS–00702 from the National Institute of Neurological Diseases and Stroke and by training grant no. 5TI-GM-716 and predoctoral fellowship no. 5-F1-GM-31883 from the National Institute of General Medical Sciences.

References

Angeletti, P. U., Gandini-Attardi, D., Toschi, G., Salvi, M. L. & Levi-Montalcini, R. (1965). *Biochim. biophys. Acta* **95**, 111.

Angeletti, P. U., Levi-Montalcini, R. & Calissano, P. (1968). *Adv. Enzymol.* **31**, 51.

Angeletti, P. U., Liuzzi, A. & Levi-Montalcini, R. (1964). *Biochim. biophys. Acta* **84**, 778.

Angeletti, P. U., Liuzzi, A., Levi-Montalcini, R. & Gandini-Attardi, D. (1964). *Biochim. biophys. Acta* **90**, 445.

Cohen, S. (1959). *J. biol. Chem.* **234**, 1129.

Davison, A. N. & Dobbing, J. (1968). *Applied Neurochemistry*. Philadelphia: Davis.

Giacobini, G., Marchesio, P. C., Giacobini, E. & Koslow, S. H. (1970). *J. Neurochem.* **17**, 1177.

Hillman, H. & Sheikh, K. (1968). *J. Physiol., Lond.* **194**, 69P.

Horowicz, P. & Larrabee, M. G. (1962). *J. Neurochem.* **9**, 1.

Jacobson, M. (1970). *Developmental Neurobiology*. New York: Holt, Rinehart & Winston.

Kuntz, A. (1910). *J. Comp. Neurol.* **20**, 283.

Larrabee, M. G. (1969). In *Progress in Brain Research*, vol. **31**, p. 95. Ed. by Akert, K. & Waser, P. G. Amsterdam: Elsevier Publishing Co.

Larrabee, M. G. (1970). *Fedn Proc Fedn. Am. Socs exp. Biol.* **29**, 1919.

Levi-Montalcini, R. & Angeletti, P. U. (1963). *Devl Biol.* **7**, 653.

Levi-Montalcini, R. & Angeletti, P. U. (1968*a*). *Physiol. Rev.* **48**, 534.

Levi-Montalcini, R. & Angeletti, P. U. (1968*b*). In *Ciba Found. Symposium. Growth of the Nervous System*, p. 126. Ed. by Wolstenholme, G. E. W. & O'Connor, M. London: Churchill.

Liuzzi, A. & Angeletti, P. U. (1964). *Experientia.* **20**, 512.

Marchesio, P. C. & Consolo, S. (1968). *J. Neurochem.* **15**, 759.

Papaconstantinou, J. (1967). In *The Biochemistry of Animal Development*, vol. II, p. 57. New York: Academic Press.

Partlow, L. M. (1969). Doctoral Dissertation. Johns Hopkins University, Baltimore, Maryland, U.S.A.
Partlow, L. M. & Larrabee, M. G. (1969). *Fedn. Proc. Fedn. Am. Socs. exp. Biol.* **28**, 886.
Partlow, L. M. & Larrabee, M. G. (1971). *J. Neurochem.* In press.
Portmann, A. S. (1950). In *Traité de Zoologie*, tome XV, p. 78. Ed. by Grasse. P.-P. Paris: Masson.
Romanoff, A. L. (1960). *The Avian Embryo*. New York: Macmillan.
Sisler, H. D. & Siegel, M. R. (1967). In *Antibiotics*, vol. 1, p. 283. Ed. by Gottlieb, G. D. & Shaw, P. D. New York: Springer-Verlag.
Winick, M. & Greenberg, R. E. (1965*a*). *Nature, Lond.* **205**, 180.
Winick, M. & Greenberg, R. E. (1965*b*). *Pediatrics, Springfield* **35**, 221.

Fine Structural Changes in Sympathetic Ganglia of Animals Treated with Nerve Growth Factor

LUCIENNE PAPADAKI*

Department of Pharmacology, Royal Free Hospital School of Medicine, University of London, UK

The nerve growth factor (NGF) is known to stimulate a wide variety of metabolic processes within sympathetic ganglion cells: there is an increase in the synthesis of RNA, proteins and lipids and an increase in the oxidation of glucose (Angeletti, Liuzzi & Levi-Montalcini, 1964; Angeletti, Liuzzi, Levi-Montalcini & Gandini-Attardi, 1964; Angeletti, Gandini-Attardi, Toschi, Salvi & Levi-Montalcini, 1965). This stimulation of metabolic processes is accompanied by ultrastructural changes, a few of which have already been discussed by Drs Levi-Montalcini and Angeletti (this volume, pp. 46–58).

The fine structure of the *superior cervical ganglion* of both 14-day-old rats and 9-day-old kittens will be considered in this paper. Both species were treated daily, from immediately after birth, with NGF isolated either from Russell's viper venom or from mouse salivary glands (kindly provided by Professor C. A. Vernon, University College London and Dr D. C. Edwards, Wellcome Research Laboratories, respectively). The ganglia were dissected from the animals used by Professor Zaimis for her experiments (this volume, pp. 59–70). The excised ganglia were fixed in half strength Karnovsky fixative (1965), a formaldehyde-glutaraldehyde mixture (pH 7.4), and then post-fixed in osmium tetroxide (Millonig, 1961). After dehydration in ethanol,

* Present address: The School of Pathology, The Middlesex Hospital Medical School, University of London.

the ganglia were embedded in Epon 812 (Taab Laboratories, Reading, England). After thin sectioning, the material was contrast-stained with uranyl acetate and lead citrate (Reynolds, 1963) and was then examined by means of a Siemens Elmiskop I electron microscope.

On the whole, both species responded similarly to the nerve growth factors from both sources, so that reference either to the animal species, or to the source of NGF, will be made only where there was any particular difference.

Sympathetic ganglion cells

The general cytoplasmic features of the sympathetic neurone of a 9-day-old *kitten* can be seen in Figs. 1 and 2. Components of the Golgi complex were present, together with scattered mitochondria; there were small Nissl granules, made up of a few elements of rough endoplasmic reticulum and associated with these were rosetted ribosomes, known also as polysomes. Numerous microfilaments and microtubules occurred in the remaining cytoplasm.

In the NGF-treated kittens, the sympathetic neurones had the appearance of being highly stimulated cells (Fig. 3). The Golgi apparatus was greatly expanded and its stacked lamellae, with associated vesicles, could be seen in all parts of the neuronal perikaryon. Rough endoplasmic reticulum, the cisternal profiles of which were longer than were those in the control, filled most of the available cytoplasm. There was also a great increase in the number of polysomes. Dense-cored granules, rarely found in the control, were commonplace and could be seen, particularly in association with the Golgi apparatus. A few dense bodies were also apparent. These were probably lysosomes; they had a similar appearance to those seen in adult sympathetic ganglion cells. There was no apparent change in the number and size of the mitochondria, although in some cells there might have been an increase in the matrical density. The increase in total amount and lamellar length of the rough endoplasmic reticulum became more obvious at higher magnification (Fig. 4). The cisternae were plump and had a tendency to branch. There was a large number of polysomes which filled the spaces around and between the reticular profiles.

In sensory nerve cells of the chick embryo one of the most prominent effects of NGF, after twelve hours' incubation *in vitro*, was the abundance of aggregates of microfilaments in the perikaryon (Levi-Montalcini, Caramia, Luse & Angeletti, 1968). In our NGF-treated animals, however, there was an apparent lack of microfilaments and microtubules within the sympathetic cell cytoplasm. It is difficult to say whether this was really so, due to their migration to the many newly formed nerve processes, or whether their presence was masked by the increased density of ribosomes. Yamada & Wessells (1971) found no increase in microtubule protein synthesis in chick embryo dorsal root ganglia after sixteen hours' culture with NGF. Thus, the stimulated nerve process outgrowth was not preceded by an accumulation of microtubule protein, and Yamada & Wessells suggest that NGF may stimulate the 'growth cones' at the axon tips. It has been postulated that the fibrillar material carries the essential enzymes used at the nerve ending for synaptic transmission and formation of vesicles (De Robertis, 1964). The stronger probability is, therefore, that the process of axonal and denritic growth involves the formation *and* migration of neurofilaments and neurotubules, and that this process is stimulated by NGF.

In the control 14-day-old *rat* (Fig. 5) the cytoplasm of the sympathetic neurones appeared more active than did that of the 8-day-old kitten. The Golgi apparatus was prominent and there was a greater amount of rough endoplasmic reticulum, variable in lamellar length, together with an abundance of free ribosomes and polysomes. The scattered mitochondria were mainly small and rounded.

After treatment with NGF, the perikaryon of the sympathetic neurones of the rat had the well-developed and prominent Golgi apparatus characteristic of the mature neurone. The total amount of Nissl substance was considerably greater. In this species, however, NGF appeared to induce, in different cells, two different forms of Nissl granule. In one of these, there seemed to be a predominance of rough endoplasmic reticulum in which the long cisternal profiles could be seen in parallel array (Fig. 6). In the other, free polysome formation appeared to predominate (Fig. 7). This contrast is suggestive of different types of protein being synthesized within the various granules, and also of a relationship between the state of maturity of each cell and the manner in which it responds to the NGF. The immature neurone has many free ribosomes and polysomes, which occur in clusters and are related to the biosynthesis of material for the use of the cell itself, required in cytoplasmic expansion and in the formation of nerve processes. A large proportion of the protein synthesized apparently forms the subunits which make up the neurofilaments and neurotubules present in the axons and dendrites (Droz & Leblond, 1962). In later stages of maturation, the vacuolar system becomes highly developed and the rough endoplasmic reticulum is prominent, with a concurrent reduction in the number of ribosomal clusters (Kornguth, Walberg Anderson, Scott & Kubinski, 1967). Much of the newly synthesized protein is then transferred to the Golgi complex and becomes associated with lysosomes, neurosecretory vesicles, and other vesicular particles.

In the area of the Golgi complex there was a considerable number of dense-cored granules after NGF treatment (Fig. 8). This was especially noticeable when the animals had been treated with the mouse salivary gland NGF. These granules varied considerably in size—a finding supported by Hökfelt (1969) and Matus (1970). Dense-cored vesicles were seen in close proximity to almost every Golgi complex. They might be merely within the Golgi region; or in close association with the Golgi cisternae; or sometimes dense material was enclosed within the Golgi cisternae. The presence of a great number of dense-cored granules may help to explain the increased amount of specific catecholamine fluorescence found in sympathetic ganglia after NGF treatment (Olson, 1967). The perinuclear region, probably the Golgi apparatus, is considered to be the site of active synthesis and elaboration of the vesicular biogenic amines (Fuxe, Hökfelt, Nilsson & Reinius, 1966). Whether or not the cytoplasmic dense-cored granules found in the present material are catecholamine-containing vesicles is still a matter for conjecture. Both small and large dense vesicles have the capacity to take up and store exogenous amines, although their localization in the large dense-cored vesicles may not reflect storage of endogenous amines as the prime physiological function of these vesicles (Richards & Tranzer, 1970). There is some experimental evidence

CAPTIONS FOR FIG. 1–18 (PLATES XII–XVIII)

Fig. 1 Control kitten; sympathetic neurone. A general view of the cytoplasm is shown with two components of the Golgi apparatus (G) and scattered mitochondria (m). Free ribosomes and polysomes (p) are associated with a few short profiles of rough endoplasmic reticulum (rer). The intervening cytoplasm contains numerous microfilaments and microtubules (f). (× 16 400)

Fig. 2 Control kitten; sympathetic neurone. In the vicinity of the Golgi complex (G) a small Nissl granule (N) is apparent, made up of short strands of rough endoplasmic reticulum and polysomes. The mitochondria (m) are prominent as well as microfilaments and microtubules (f). (× 23 600)

Fig. 3 Treated kitten; mouse salivary gland NGF; sympathetic neurone. Elements of the Golgi complex (G) now extend around the periphery of the entire field. The central area is filled with rough endoplasmic reticulum (rer), the cisternal profiles of which are longer than in the control. The number of polysomes and free ribosomes (p) is also greatly increased. Some dense-cored vesicles (arrows) are apparent, particularly in association with the Golgi complex. Two dense bodies, lysosomes (l), can also be seen. (× 18 200)

Fig. 4 Treated kitten; mouse salivary gland NGF; sympathetic neurone. The cytoplasm in the immediate vicinity of the Golgi apparatus (G) is filled with polysomes (p), free ribosomes and rough endoplasmic reticulum (rer), whose lamellar length is longer than in the control and with a tendency toward branching (arrows). Mitochondria (m). (× 22 800)

Fig. 5 Control rat; sympathetic neurone. The cytoplasm appears more active than that of the 9-day-old kitten. A Golgi complex (G) can be seen in the centre of the field and throughout are scattered mitochondria (m) with a moderate amount of rough endoplasmic reticulum (rer) and associated polysomes (p). (× 23 800)

Fig. 6 Treated rat; snake venom NGF; sympathetic neurone. A Nissl granule is shown in which the long cisternal profiles of the rough endoplasmic reticulum extend diagonally across the field. The space between the cisternae is filled with polysomes (p) and free ribosomes. (× 12 700)

Fig. 7 Treated rat; mouse salivary gland NGF; sympathetic neurone. This large Nissl granule is made up primarily of polysomes, in contrast to that seen in Fig. 6. The elements of rough endoplasmic reticulum (rer) are short and scattered. A few long microtubules (t) can be seen. (× 10 900)

Fig. 8 Treated rat; mouse salivary gland NGF; sympathetic neurone. Many dense-cored granules (markers) are seen in close association with the Golgi complex (G). Notice the dense material still enclosed within the Golgi cisternae (arrow) and the variation in size of the granules. (× 38 200)

Fig. 9 Control kitten; nerve cell processes. Five processes can be seen in cross-section, each surrounded by its own satellite cell. One is probably a dendritic process (d) since there are ribosomes scattered within the cytoplasm. Notice also the large amount of extracellular space and the paucity of neurofilaments and neurotubules within the processes. (× 6350)

Fig. 10 Treated kitten; mouse salivary gland NGF; nerve cell processes. Many axons are occupying a single satellite cell; about half have become separated from each other by arms of satellite cell cytoplasm (arrow), but some still lie next to each other (double arrow). A general increase in density of the axoplasm is apparent, due mainly to the increased numbers of neurofilaments and neurotubules. Mitochondria (m). (× 8200)

Fig. 11 Control rat; synapse. Two developing synapses can be seen with some thickening of the pre- and post-synaptic membranes. There are very few synaptic vesicles (v) either in the presynaptic bag area or in relation to the areas of membrane specialization. (× 41 000)

Fig. 12 Treated rat; mouse salivary gland NGF; synapse. The presynaptic bag area is filled with synaptic vesicles (v) and there is a dense packing of these vesicles along the presynaptic membrane (arrow). There is also a greater density of the fibrillar material along the postsynaptic membrane. (× 27 250)

Fig. 13 Treated kitten; snake venom NGF; synapse. There is a similar picture to that in the NGF-treated rat. Notice that in the synaptic bag area to the left, even at some distance from the synapse, there is a mass of packed vesicles (v). A few dense-cored vesicles (arrow) are also apparent. (× 25 400)

Fig. 14 Treated rat; mouse salivary gland NGF; intermediate cells. Portions of several cells can be seen with interdigitating plasma membranes (arrow). The nucleus (nuc) has peripheral aggregations of chromatin. Many dense-cored granules (g) are present in the peripheral cytoplasm and the mitochondria (m) are relatively large. There are also synaptic junctions (s) between nerve processes and the chromaffin cells. (× 15 900)

Fig. 15 Treated kitten; snake venom NGF; sympathetic neurones. One neurone is intact while the other exhibits distended cisternae of the rough endoplasmic reticulum (rer) with only a few ribosomes remaining attached to the membranes. Many mitochondria (m) are also swollen, showing loss of matrix and cristal structure. (× 14 350)

Fig. 16 Control rat; small cell. This cell is identified as a neuroblast. There is a large nucleus with little surrounding cytoplasm; the chromatin is dispersed throughout the nucleoplasm and the nucleolus (nucl) is of the reticular form. In the lower part of the field where the plasma membrane is clear, part of a satellite cell can be seen beginning to circumscribe the young neurone (arrow). (× 12 100)

Fig. 17 Control kitten; small cell. An immature cell which is surrounded by a basal lamina (bl). Many pinocytotic vesicles are present (arrows). The nuclear membrane is irregular with aggregations of chromatin along the inner surface. This is probably a connective tissue cell. (× 12 300)

Fig. 18 Control kitten; small cell. This is probably a developing satellite cell with a partially formed basal lamina (bl). The mitochondria (m) are large and a small process (arrow) of cytoplasm is beginning to sprout. (× 17 100)

Plate XII

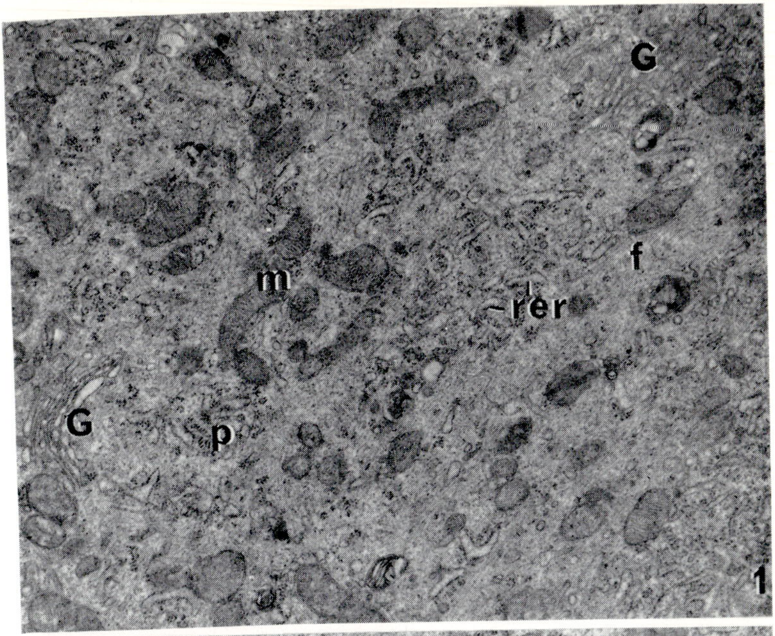

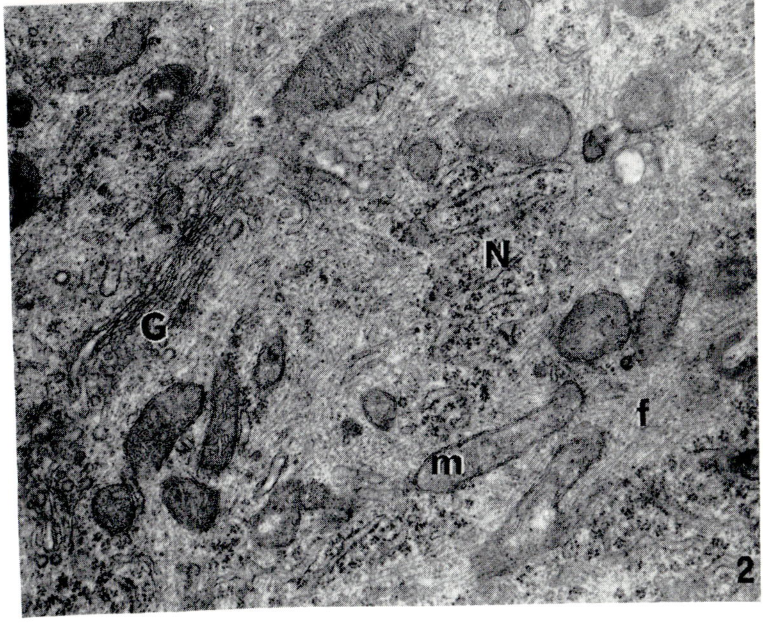

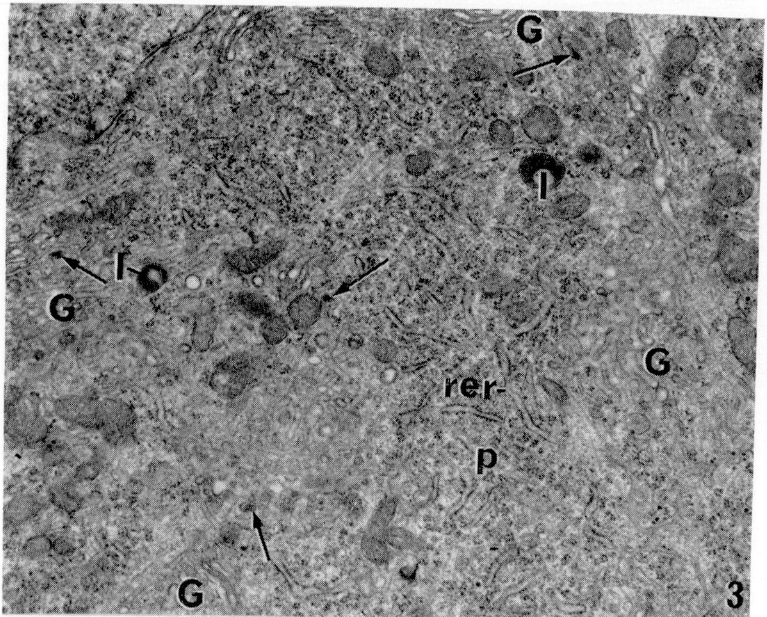
G
l
l
G
G
rer-
p
G
3

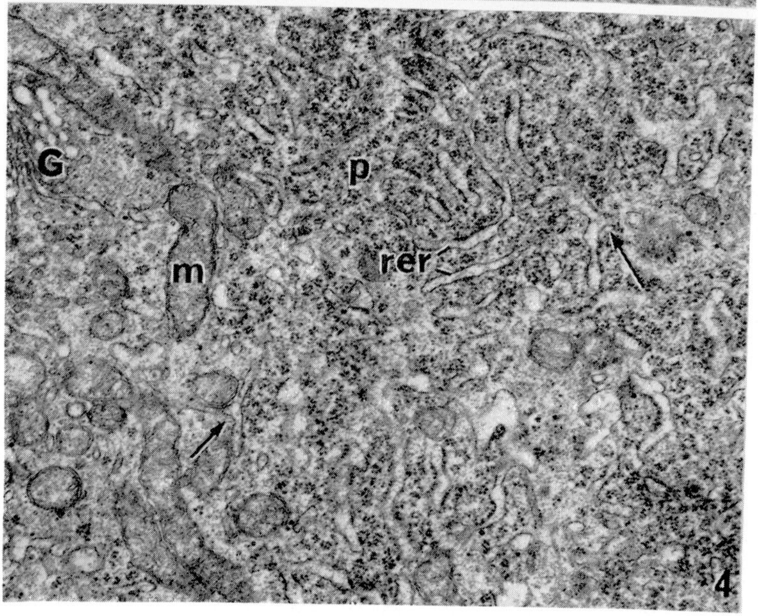
G
p
m
rer
4

PLATE XIV

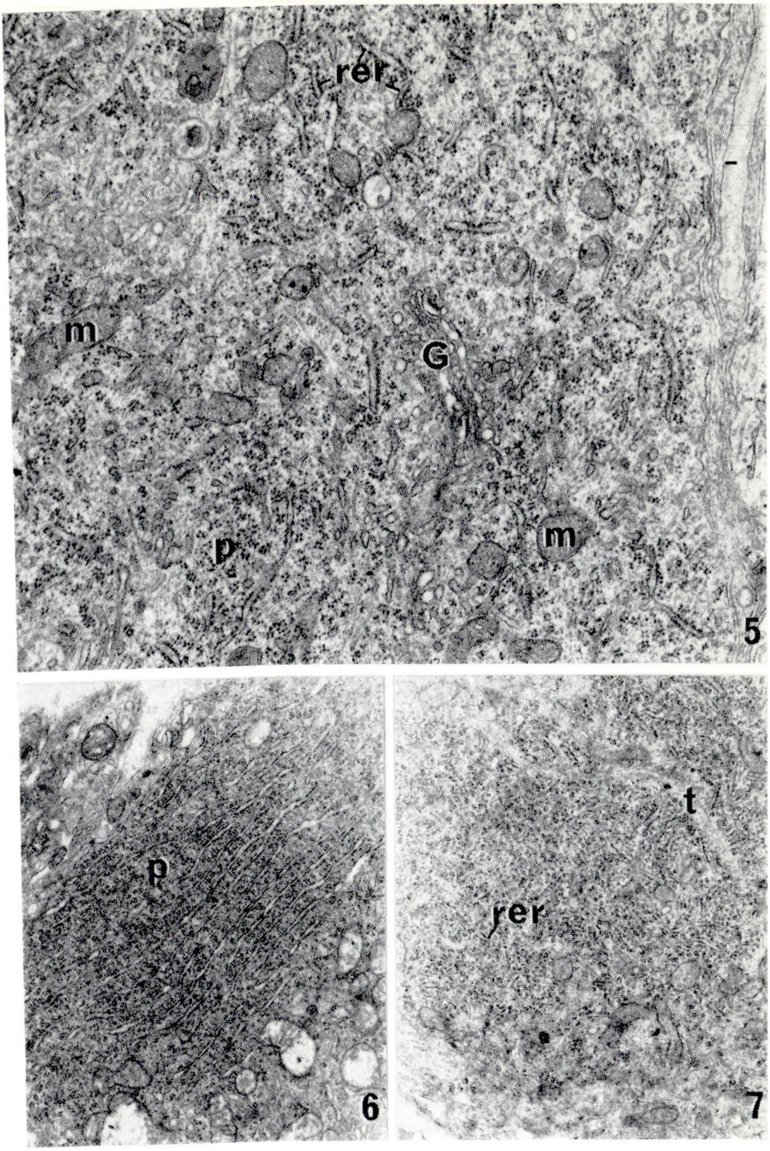

Plate XV

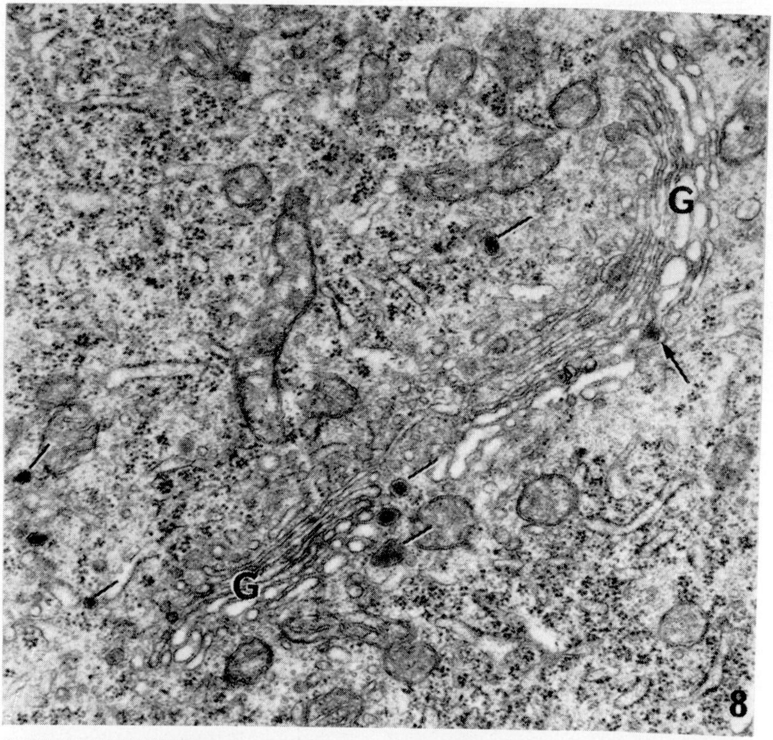

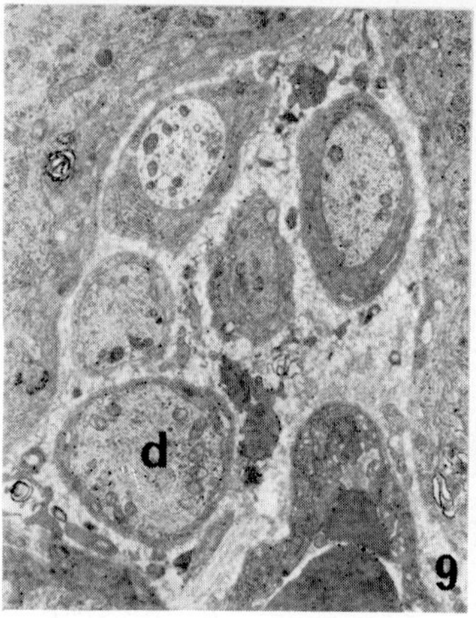

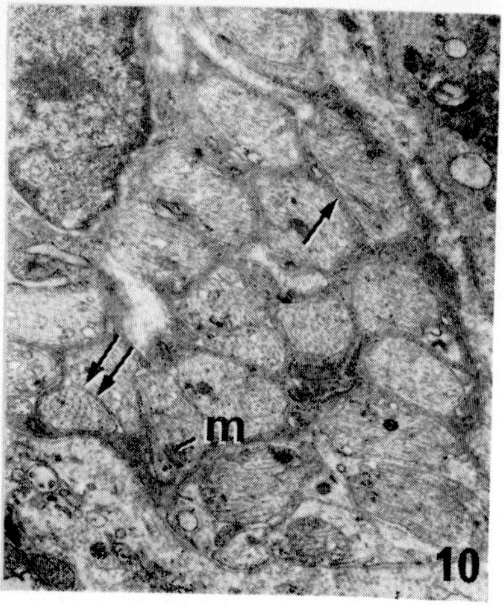

Plate XVI

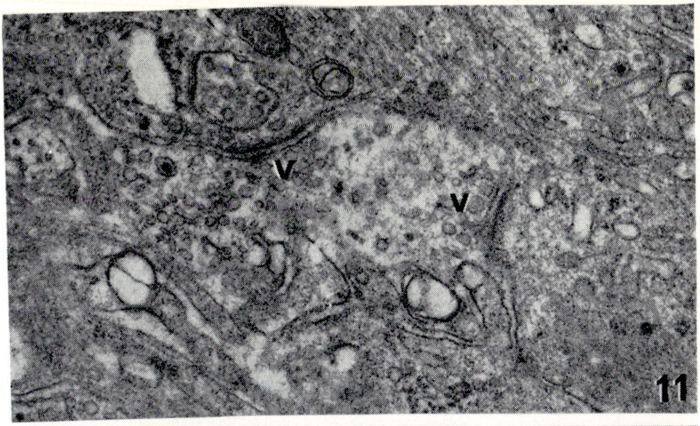

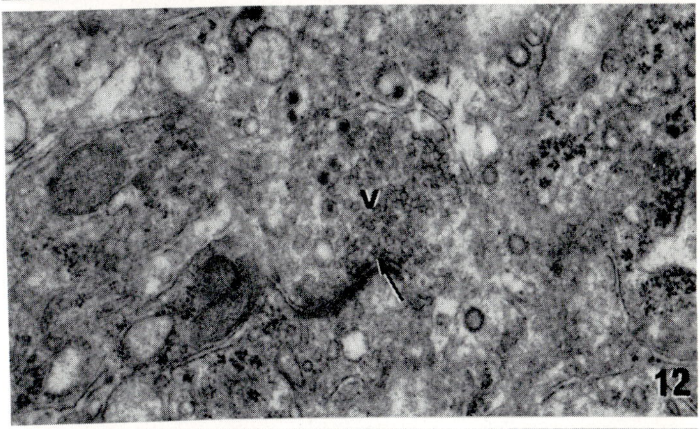

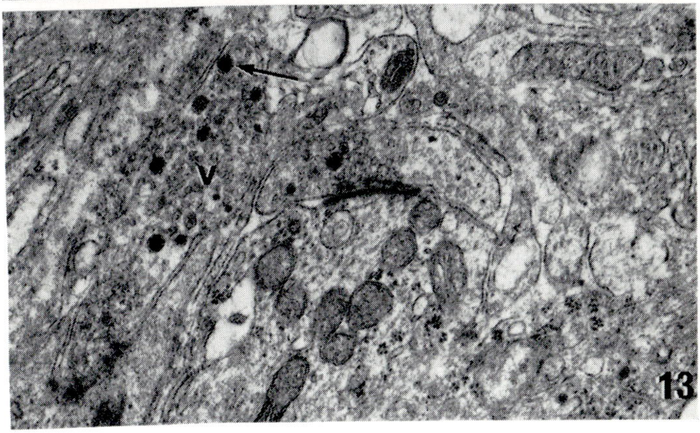

Plate XVII

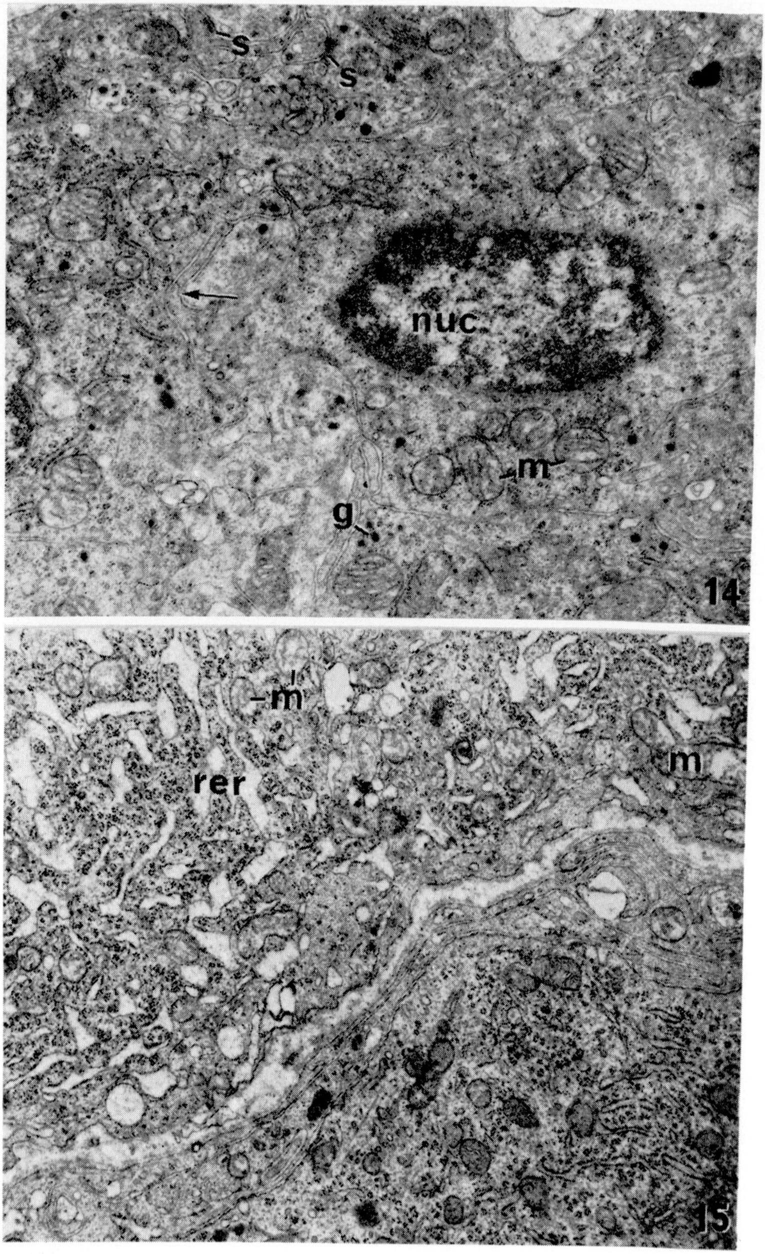

Plate XVIII

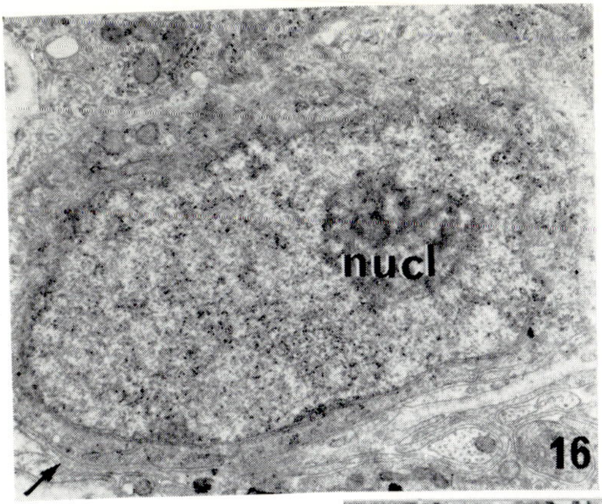

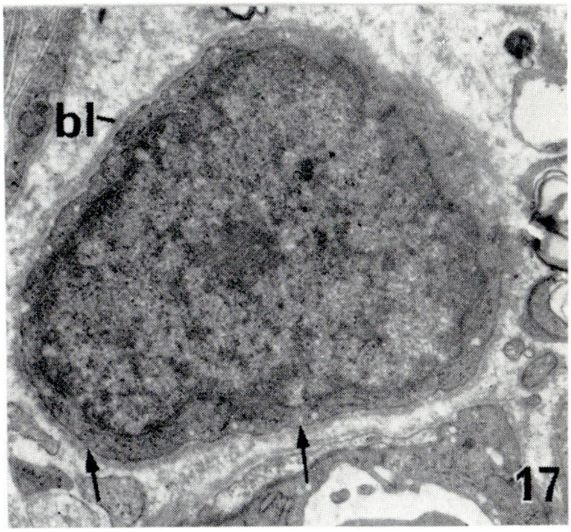

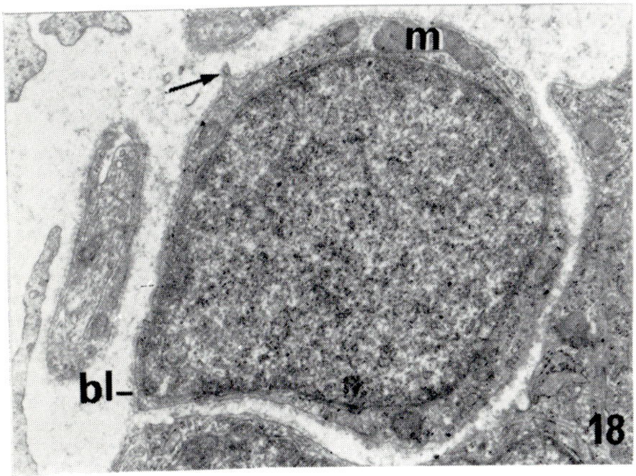

to suggest that an RNA may be an important component of the large dense-cored particle and may participate in differentiation (Kornguth *et al.*, 1967). Bloom & Aghajanian (1968*a*, *b*) found that the dense core of the large vesicles consists of a protein matrix, which may be some form of particle-bound enzyme concerned with monoamine metabolism. Biochemically, the major proportion of the noradrenaline in the superior cervical ganglion is apparently localized in the soluble and not in the microsomal fraction (Fischer & Snyder, 1965). More recently, Descarries & Droz (1970) have shown that exogenous noradrenaline is distributed throughout the perikaryon of labelled nerve cell bodies and that it could not be related to any particular cytoplasmic organelle. Finally, they suggest that a cytoplasmic macromolecular complex could be the binding site for noradrenaline; and that this complex, rather than the preformed synaptic vesicles, migrates into the axon.

It is appropriate at this juncture to comment on some of the unusual morphological effects of NGF observed by other workers. After incubation of chick embryo dorsal root ganglion cells with NGF, Crain, Benitez & Vatter (1964) reported the appearance of 'crystalline arrays' in the neuronal perikaryon, and thought that these arrays were early evidence of the formation of nerve processes. These structures have now, however, been demonstrated to be ribosomal crystals and may be found only in hyperchromatic degenerating neuroblasts (Weis, 1971). The existence was also reported of 'peculiar extra-nuclear membranes' which projected into the cytoplasm as long whip-like extensions, after one hour's exposure to NGF *in vitro* (Blood, 1971). This may well be the result of a stimulated production of the endoplasmic reticular membrane system.

Nerve processes

There appeared to be more nerve cell processes in the 14-day-old rat than in the 8-day-old kitten. In the superior cervical ganglion of both species, the cytoplasm within many of these processes had a very light appearance, since it contained so few neurofilaments and neurotubules. In control animals, especially the kitten, single axons were often surrounded by their own satellite cells (Fig. 9). All the satellite cells were separated from the relatively large extracellular space by a fairly complete basal lamina. This great quantity of extracellular space, which would be expected to decrease with age and development, was only scantily infiltrated by a connective tissue matrix: a situation typical of developing nervous tissue (Pick, Gerdin & Delemos, 1964; Johnson & Armstrong-James, 1970).

After NGF treatment, the general picture was one of greater maturity. The amount of extracellular space was much reduced and there was an obvious increase in the number of nerve cell processes, which formed an extensively branching network. The cytoplasm of most of the nerve cell processes was characterized by a tight aggregation of neurofilaments and neurotubules, arranged parallel to the long axis of the process. This resulted in an overall increase in the density of the axoplasm. Small mitochondria, and both clear and dense-cored granules, could also be seen. Many of the dendritic processes also contained profiles of smooth endoplasmic reticulum, as well as glycogen and an occasional multivesicular body. In the kitten, many axons occupied a single satellite cell (Fig. 10). In any one bundle, many of the nerve cell processes had become separated from each other by arms of satellite cell cytoplasm, but there were some which still lay next to each other. Collagen fibres were now the prominent extracellular structures, along with the frequent appearance of fibroblasts of varying shape and cytoplasmic organization.

Synapses

In relation to function, it is important to consider the synaptic regions within the ganglion. In the superior cervical ganglion, most synapses are axodendritic in nature (Elfvin, 1963). Synaptic regions that could be so defined in the developing nervous tissue (Armstrong-James & Johnson, 1970), were rare in the 9-day-old kitten. The superior cervical ganglion of the 14-day-old rat contained more easily demonstrable synapses than that of the 9-day-old kitten (Fig. 11). There was some thickening of the pre- and postsynaptic membranes, with some dense fibrillar material extending into the cytoplasm of the postsynaptic process; but this subsynaptic web was not as dense as in the adult (De Robertis, Pellegrino de Iraldi, Rodriguez de Lores

Arnaiz & Salganicoff, 1961). The pre- and postsynaptic membranes had surfaces slightly curved toward the postsynaptic membrane. There were very few synaptic vesicles in relation to the areas of membrane specialization, and few vesicles in the area of the presynaptic bag itself. Because of the large extracellular space, the relative volume occupied by nerve cell processes was small and there was less opportunity for contact between processes. In some areas, however, there was a suggestion of a developing synapse. An electron-lucent swelling on a dense fibre could sometimes be seen where there was some thickening of the adjacent membranes.

In the NGF-treated animal there was an obvious increase in the number of synapses. Both the pre- and postsynaptic membranes were increased in thickness and electron density, and the dense fibrillar material of the subsynaptic web was more extensive in the cytoplasm of the postsynaptic process. The whole presynaptic area was filled with synaptic vesicles, which were densely packed, even at some distance from the synaptic area (Figs. 12 and 13). Synaptic vesicles could also be seen lined up along the presynaptic membrane. The same variety of vesicular shapes and sizes occurred in both the treated and control animals; some were cylindrical or disc-shaped, the others were spherical (300 to 500 Å) and some were of the large dense-cored variety (800 to 1000 Å). The large dense-cored vesicles always seemed to occur in the company of clear synaptic vesicles, usually in small numbers and located away from the synaptic junction. Many workers have found a variety of vesicles in the presynaptic area which may result from aldehyde fixation (Elfvin, 1963 Gray, 1969; Bodian, 1970; Dennison, 1971).

It has been postulated that the capacity of neuronal membranes to form specialized cell junctions is maximal at a certain stage of differentiation (Mugnaini, 1970). It therefore seems likely that the effect of NGF in stimulating a greater degree of maturity in the developing sympathetic ganglion could in itself contribute to the increase in the number of synapses observed. Furthermore, the effect of NGF in increasing the number of nerve cell processes will obviously add to the possibilities for contact between them; and this must also be associated with an increase in the number of synapses. It has been shown recently that a phase of rapid nervous development occurs between seven and fourteen days of age in the rat (Armstrong-James & Johnson, 1970). During a similar period, there is a vast increase in the number of synapses in the mouse superior cervical ganglion (Black, Bloom, Hendry & Iversen, 1971). Thus, in the sympathetic ganglion, the preganglionic innervation of the adrenergic neurones probably influences the maturation of these neurones in the same way as afferent axons in the forebrain influence the differentiation of the dendrites destined to receive them (Morest, 1970). Would it not, therefore, be reasonable to find the same reciprocal relationship in reverse when the animals had been treated with NGF? This is certainly true when newborn animals have been treated with the NGF-*antiserum* (Berk, Filipe & Zaimis, 1965; Zaimis, 1967; Papadaki, 1969). Together with the almost complete destruction of the superior cervical ganglion and its postganglionic nerve trunk, there is a 40 per cent reduction in the diameter of the preganglionic cervical sympathetic trunk.

Whether or not more synapses are formed under the influence of NGF than would ultimately have been formed when maturity had been reached, is impossible to say; but such a situation was not obviously apparent in either the cat or rat.

Chromaffin or intermediate cells

An interesting finding in the NGF-treated *rats* was the appearance of groups of small intermediate neurones (Fig. 14). These cells were small, about one-third the size of sympathetic neurones, were closely packed together to form compact groups with interdigitating plasma membranes, and were usually positioned near fenestrated capillaries. The nucleus, unlike that of the sympathetic neurones, was more centrally positioned and had peripheral aggregations of dense chromatin. In the cytoplasm, the mitochondria were larger than those in the primary neurones, and the endoplasmic reticulum was comparatively poorly developed; but free ribosomes and polysomes were numerous. Dense-cored granules of variable size were usually located in the peripheral cytoplasm. Nerve processes, some containing synaptic vesicles, could be observed making contact with the cell body or another process. Satellite cells did not completely surround each individual cell; usually each group was surrounded by a common sheath of satellite cells. Morphologically, these cells show many features which place them in a category between the chromaffin cells of the adrenal medulla and the primary sympathetic neurones. These groups of cells have been described in the superior cervical ganglion of the adult rat in several electron microscopical studies (Siegrist, Dolivo, Dunant, Foroglou-Kerameus, De Ribaupierre & Rouiller, 1968; Matthews & Raisman, 1969; Williams & Palay, 1969); and it is suggested that these cells are involved in an intraganglionic regulatory system. At what age these groups of cells appear is not known, so it may be significant that with the 14-day-old rat they were only apparent in the NGF-treated animals.

These small intermediate neurones are probably the same as the highly fluorescent groups of cells seen in sympathetic ganglia after formaldehyde treatment; and they probably contain a primary catecholamine (Eränkö & Härkönen, 1965; Norberg, Ritzén & Ungerstedt, 1966; Jacobowitz & Woodward, 1968). There appear to be fewer clusters of these fluorescent cells in the cat superior cervical ganglion than in that of the rat (Jacobowitz, 1970). It is probable that the small intermediate neurones seen at the ultrastructural level are similar to the highly fluorescent groups of cells. Thus, the appearance of these groups of cells in the 14-day-old NGF-treated rats may help to explain the increased amount of noradrenaline found in the sympathetic ganglia of NGF-treated mice (Crain & Wiegand, 1961).

Small cell population

I would like now to comment on the small cell population discussed by Professor Zaimis elsewhere in this volume (pp. 59–70). With the light microscope, one can see few differences among them. Under the electron microscope, however, differences in these cells become apparent which may characterize them as belonging to at least three types of cell. One type could be identified as a neuroblast (Fig. 16). In this cell, as in most immature cells, there is a large nucleus in relation to the amount of cytoplasm, although it is smaller than that found in the fully developed sympathetic neurone. The chromatin is mostly dispersed throughout the nucleoplasm. The nucleolus may be either of the reticular form or in the form of aggregates of fine and coarse granules—depending on whether the cell is in a state of quiescence or of activity for maturation. There is little surrounding cytoplasm, which forms a crescent-shaped thin envelope around the nucleus. In many instances the satellite cells were just beginning to send arms of cytoplasm between neighbouring neuroblasts. Very few of these young neuroblasts were fully circumscribed by their satellite cells. Similar observations have been made on developing sympathetic neurones in man (Pick *et al.*, 1964).

Fig. 17 shows another type of immature cell which is surrounded by a basal lamina. Many pinocytotic vesicles are present at the periphery of the plasma membrane and in continuity with it. In the scanty cytoplasm of these cells are a few short lamellae of rough and smooth endoplasmic reticulum, as well as a number of glycogen granules. The nucleus has an irregular profile with aggregations of nuclear chromatin occurring along the nuclear membrane and scattered in the nucleoplasm. These characteristics suggest that this sort of cell could mature into a connective tissue cell of the fibroblast or endothelial cell type. It may be more likely that these cells will be endothelial, since it has recently been found that cerebral cortical vessels develop as a network of mesodermal cells (Caley & Maxwell, 1970). Furthermore, there appear to be very few patent capillaries in the cerebral cortex during the first ten days of life in the rat and it is between ten and twenty days that the majority of blood vessels develop patent lumina.

The third cell type (Fig. 18) is somewhat similar with a partially formed basal lamina, but with no obvious pinocytotic activity and larger mitochondria. It is quite possible that this cell will become a satellite cell, since many of them appear to give off tiny processes which are not yet large enough to affect axonal invagination or to surround a sympathetic neurone. I should emphasize that no cells in such a state of immaturity were seen in the ganglia from the NGF-treated animals. It is quite possible that NGF stimulated development of the satellite cells as well as the sympathetic neurones, since there is such a close metabolic relationship between the two cells. Pevzner (1965) has suggested that the satellite cells actually support their neurones metabolically during prolonged activity. Further evidence for this close relationship has been provided by Schwyn (1967), who has shown that the satellite cells in the superior cervical ganglion of the cat respond to increased synaptic activity by proliferating. Furthermore, Dr E. M. Shooter (unpublished results) has found that the γ-subunits of the NGF molecule will stimulate both mitosis and growth of fibroblast cells in tissue culture.

Cellular damage

Finally, one aspect of the *snake venom* factor that should be mentioned is that in both species of animals there were sympathetic neurones in which cisternae of the rough endoplasmic reticulum were distended and sometimes vesiculated with an electron transparent interior (Fig. 15). When this occurred there was frequently a loss of ribosomes, to such an extent that few of the ribonucleoprotein particles were attached to the membranes of the endoplasmic reticulum. The mitochondria were often swollen and showed loss of matrix and internal cristal structure. Whether this is a direct toxic effect of the snake venom factor, or whether the factor has made particular neurones more susceptible to fixation artifacts, is impossible to say. One might perhaps favour the former explanation, since these observations are typical of cellular injury to sympathetic neurones and are the characteristic changes which follow axon sectioning (Dixon, 1970). This damage, however, was not confined to the neurones themselves, but was also apparent in some of the satellite cells.

Summary

I have presented some of the ways in which the fine structure of the superior cervical ganglion reflects the biochemical activity stimulated by NGF, particularly that of RNA and protein synthesis: there is an increase in rough endoplasmic reticulum, an increase in polysomes, and an increasing involvement of the Golgi complex in dense-cored granule formation. There is also an increase in the number of nerve processes associated with each satellite cell and a greater number of neurotubules and neurofilaments within the processes. Synaptic development is also stimulated. Finally, with regard to the small cell population, it seems likely, because of the close relationship that exists between the satellite cell and the neurone, that NGF has stimulated maturation of the supporting cells as a consequence of its effects on the sympathetic neurones. In the excised ganglion NGF may be a preserver rather than a stimulator of metabolism, as has been suggested by Dr Larrabee (this volume, pp. 71–88). In the intact animal, however, when NGF is administered during development, the nerve growth factor is conspicuously a metabolic stimulator, morphologically speaking. The overall result is, therefore, enhanced development of the sympathetic ganglion generally as well as specifically.

Acknowledgement

I am grateful to Mr J. T. Wilkes for his skilled technical assistance.

References

Angeletti, P. U., Liuzzi, A. & Levi-Montalcini, R. (1964). *Biochim. biophys. Acta* **84**, 778.

Angeletti, P. U., Liuzzi, A., Levi-Montalcini, R. & Gandini-Attardi, D. (1964). *Biochim. biophys. Acta* **90**, 445.

Angeletti, P. U., Gandini-Attardi, D., Toschi, G., Salvi, M. L. & Levi-Montalcini, R. (1965). *Biochim. biophys. Acta* **95**, 111.

Berk, L., Filipe, I. & Zaimis, E. (1965). *J. Physiol., Lond.* **177**, 1P.

Armstrong-James, M. & Johnson, R. (1970). *Z. Zellforsch. mikrosk. Anat.* **110**, 559.

Black, I. B., Bloom, F. E., Hendry, I. A. & Iversen, L. L. (1971). *J. Physiol., Lond.* **215**, 24P.

Blood, L. A. (1971). *J. Anat.* **108**, 204.

Bloom, F. E. & Aghajanian, G. K. (1968*a*). *Experientia* **24**, 1225.

Bloom, F. E. & Aghajanian, G. K. (1968*b*). *J. Pharmac. exp. Ther.* **159**, 261.

Bodian, D. (1970). *J. Cell Biol.* **44**, 115.

Caley, D. W. & Maxwell, D. S. (1970). *J. comp. Neurol.* **138**, 31.

Crain, S. M. & Wiegand, R. G. (1961). *Proc. Soc. exp. Biol. Med.* **107**, 663.

Crain, S. M., Benitez, H. & Vatter, A. E. (1964). *Ann. N.Y. Acad. Sci.* **118**, 206.

De Robertis, E. (1964). *Histophysiology of Synapses and Neurosecretion*, p. 99. Oxford: Pergamon Press.

De Robertis, E., Pellegrino de Iraldi, A., Rodriguez de Lores Arnaiz, G. & Salganicoff, L. (1961). *Anat. Rec.* **139**, 220.

Dennison, M. E. (1971). *J. Cell Sci.* **8**, 525.

Descarries, L. & Droz, B. (1970). *J. Cell Biol.* **44**, 385.
Dixon, J. S. (1970). *Acta anat.* **76**, 473.
Droz, B. & Leblond, C. P. (1962). *Science* **137**, 1047.
Elfvin, L.-G. (1963). *J. Ultrastruct. Res.* **8**, 441.
Eränkö, O. & Härkönen, M. (1965). *Acta physiol. scand.* **63**, 511.
Fischer, J. E. & Snyder, S. (1965). *J. Pharmac. exp. Ther.* **150**, 190.
Fuxe, K., Hökfelt, T., Nilsson, O. & Reinius, S. (1966). *Anat. Rec.* **155**, 33.
Gray, E. G. (1969). *Prog. Brain Res.* **31**, 141.
Hökfelt, T. (1969). *Acta physiol. scand.* **76**, 427.
Jacobowitz, D. (1970). *Fedn Proc. Fedn. Am. Socs exp. Biol.* **29**, 1929.
Jacobowitz, D. & Woodward, J. K. (1968). *J. Pharmac. exp. Ther.* **162**, 213.
Johnson, R. & Armstrong-James, M. (1970). *Z. Zellforsch. mikrosk. Anat.* **110**, 540.
Karnovsky, M. J. (1965) *J. Cell Biol.* **27**, 137A.
Kornguth, S. E., Walberg Anderson, J., Scott, G. & Kubinski, H. (1967). *Expl Cell Res.* **45**, 656.
Levi-Montalcini, R., Caramia, F., Luse, S. A. & Angeletti, P. U. (1968). *Brain Res.* **8**, 347.
Matthews, M. R. & Raisman, G. (1969). *J. Anat.* **105**, 255.
Matus, A. I. (1970). *Brain Res.* **17**, 195.
Millonig, G. (1961). *J. appl. Physics* **32**, 1637.
Morest, D. K. (1970). *Z. Anat. EntwGesch.* **130**, 265.
Mugnaini, E. (1970). *Brain Res.* **17**, 169.
Norberg, K.-A., Ritzén, M. & Ungerstedt, U. (1966). *Acta physiol. scand.* **67**, 260.
Olson, L. (1967). *Z. Zellforsch. mikrosk. Anat.* **81**, 155.
Papadaki, L. (1969). Ph.D. Thesis. University of London.
Pevzner, L. Z. (1965). *J. Neurochem.* **12**, 993.
Pick, J., Gerdin, C. & Delemos, C. (1964). *Z. Zellforsch. mikrosk. Anat.* **62**, 402.
Reynolds, E. S. (1963). *J. Cell Biol.* **17**, 208.
Richards, J. G. & Tranzer, J.-P. (1970). *Brain Res.* **17**, 463.
Schwyn, R. C. (1967). *Am. J. Anat.* **121**, 727.
Siegrist, G., Dolivo, M., Dunant, Y., Foroglou-Kerameus, C., De Ribaupierre, Fr. & Rouiller, Ch. (1968). *J. Ultrastruct. Res.* **25**, 381.
Weis, P. (1971). *J. comp. Neurol.* **141**, 117.
Williams, T. H. & Palay, S. L. (1969). *Brain Res.* **15**, 17.
Yamada, K. M. & Wessells, N. K. (1971). *Expl Cell Res.* **66**, 346.
Zaimis, E. (1967). In *Scientific Basis of Medicine Annual Reviews*, p. 59. London: Athlone Press.

Apparent Orientating Effects Produced by Nerve Growth Factor

KATHARINE A. CHARLWOOD, D. MARGARET LAMONT and BARBARA E. C. BANKS*

Departments of Chemistry and Physiology, University College, London, UK*

It has been observed that when the sensory ganglia of chick embryos are cultured on rat tail collagen, in a liquid medium, with tissues containing nerve growth factor (NGF), such as explants of mouse sarcoma 180 or mouse adrenal gland (Bueker, 1948; Lamont, 1968), the outgrowth of nerve fibres from each ganglion is greater from the side facing the source of NGF than from the opposite side. The effect is not observed when the ganglia are cultured in the presence of explants of mouse adrenal cortex or chick embryo heart muscle—that is, tissues which are believed not to contain NGF.

This result could be explained by the concentration of NGF being greater on the side of the ganglion closer to the source. However, when two ganglia are cultured in the presence of a single source, as is illustrated in the diagram, the outgrowth of fibres from the side of the more distant ganglion facing towards the source is greater than the outgrowth from the side of the nearer ganglion facing away from the source.

It would appear that the fibre growth follows not the concentration of NGF but the concentration gradient. The effect may therefore be an example of chemotaxis; and it is suggested that NGF, as well as playing some role in the *growth* of nerve fibres, may also have some part in determining the course that nerve fibres take during development and regeneration. This effect has been further investigated by culturing sensory ganglia in the presence of a glass capillary tube containing an aqueous solution of purified NGF. Typical fibre outgrowths are shown in Figs. 2–5.

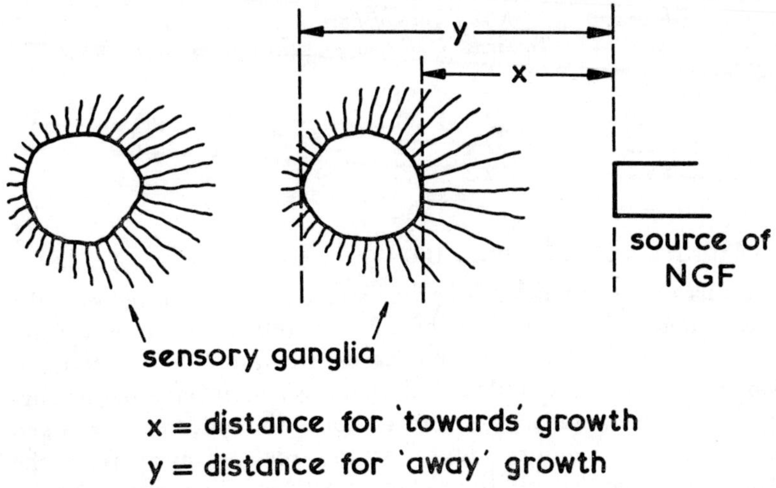

Fig. 1 Outgrowth of nerve fibres from sensory ganglia in the presence of a source of NGF.

Culture with adrenal medulla explants

Sensory ganglia of eight-day chick embryos were cultured, on collagen, in liquid medium [Medium 199 (1 part), rabbit serum (1 part) and 0.9 per cent sodium chloride buffered with 0.02 M-phosphate buffer pH 7.4 (1 part)] in the presence of an explant (1 mm^3) of the adrenal medulla of a male mouse. The distances of the near and far sides of the ganglia from the source (x and y in Fig. 1) were measured using a travelling microscope. Fibre outgrowth towards and away from the source was scored, after 24 hours, on an arbitrary scale from 0 to 10. Usually, two ganglia were cultured with a single source, giving four measurements of growth and distance for each culture. The results of about 50 cultures and some two hundred measurements are given in Table 1. The difference in fibre outgrowth towards and away from the source for equal distances is statistically significant for distances up to 1.5 mm. The effect is not significant beyond this limit.

Table 1 Fibre outgrowth produced by sensory ganglia cultured in the presence of mouse adrenal medulla

Distance	*Mean score of fibre outgrowth* ± S.E.M.	
mm	*Towards NGF source*	*Away from NGF source*
0–0.5	3.4 ± 0.1	—
0.5–1.0	3.2 ± 0.1	2.2 ± 0.3
1.0–1.5	2.8 ± 0.2	2.0 ± 0.1
>1.5	2.2 ± 0.3	1.8 ± 0.1

Culture with sarcoma 180

Cultures were set up as described above but the adrenal medulla was replaced by an explant of sarcoma 180 taken directly from the mouse: the liquid medium used [Medium 199 (3 parts) and chicken serum (1 part)] was chosen because it gave better survival of the sarcoma. After 30–44 hours the cultures were fixed and stained, the fibre outgrowth towards and away from the tumour was scored and the distances between the tumour and the ganglia were measured. Fifty-four ganglia were used for the final analysis and the results are given in Table 2.

Table 2 Fibre outgrowth from sensory ganglia cultured in the presence of sarcoma 180

Distance	*Mean score of fibre outgrowth* ± S.E.M.	
mm	*Towards NGF source*	*Away from NGF source*
0–0.9	5.5 ± 0.3	2.6 ± 0.2
1.0–1.9	4.6 ± 0.2	2.3 ± 0.1
2.0–2.9	4.1 ± 0.2	1.7 ± 0.2
>3.0	1.0 ± 0.1	1.2 ± 0.1

The effect of the sarcoma extended further than that of the adrenal medulla, the difference in outgrowth of fibres towards and away from the tumour being statistically significant up to 2 mm from the explant.

Capillary tube source of NGF

Sensory ganglia of eight-day chick embryos were cultured, on collagen, in liquid medium [Medium 199 (1 part), rabbit serum

Plate XIX

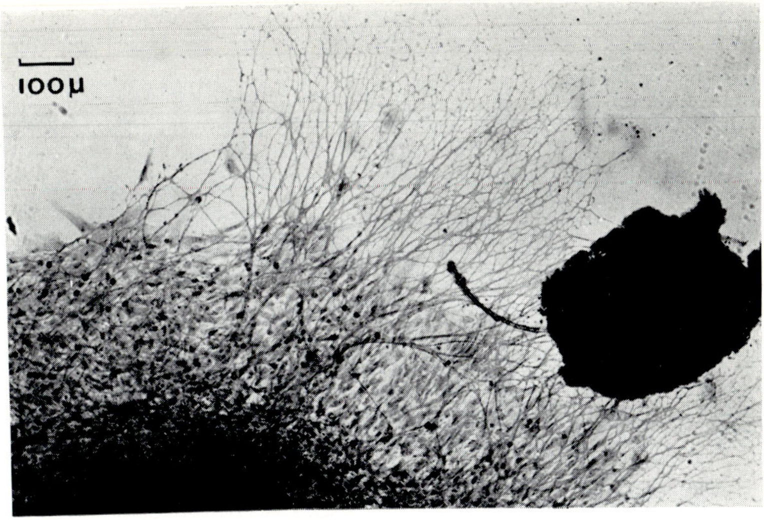

Fig. 2 Outgrowth of nerve fibres from a sensory ganglion towards a mouse adrenal medulla explant (right).

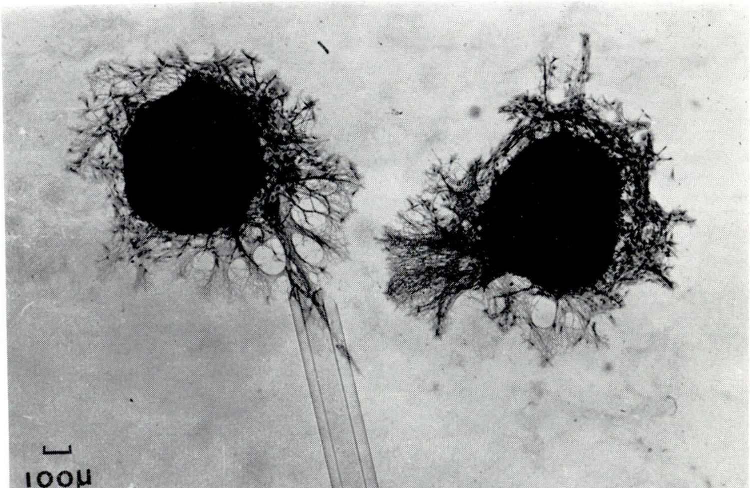

Fig. 3 Outgrowth of nerve fibres from sensory ganglia cultured in the presence of a capillary tube containing NGF at a concentration of 30 μg/ml.

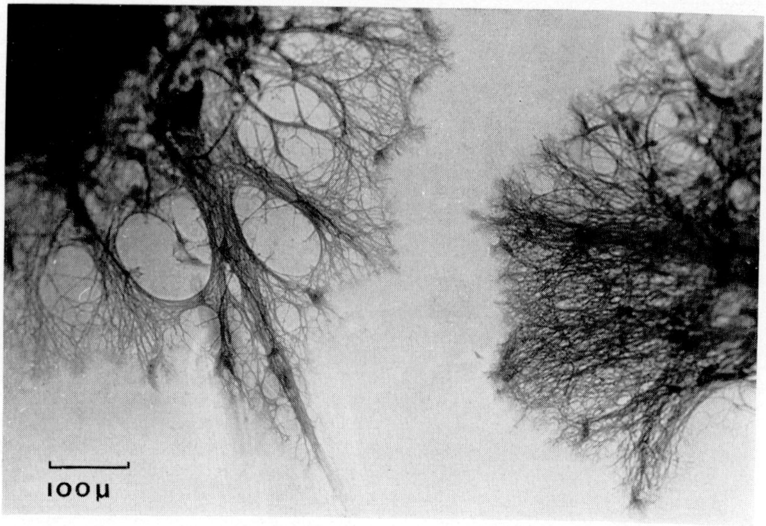

Fig. 4 Outgrowth of nerve fibres from sensory ganglia towards a capillary tube containing NGF at a concentration of 30 μg/ml.

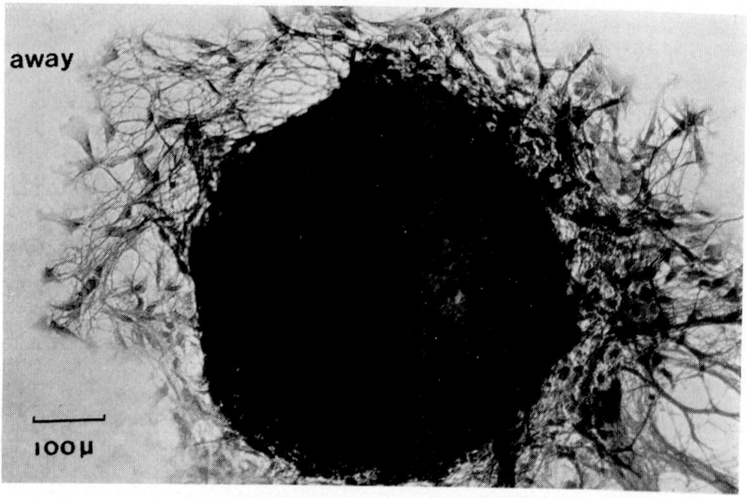

Fig. 5 Outgrowth of nerve fibres from the side of a sensory ganglion facing away from a capillary tube containing NGF at a concentration of 30 μg/ml.

(1 part) and 0.9 per cent sodium chloride buffered with 0.02 M-phosphate buffer pH 7.4 (1 part)] in which a glass capillary tube of known diameter was fixed horizontally. The capillary was filled with an aqueous solution of purified NGF (usually 30 μg/ml). After 24 hours in culture, fibre outgrowth from the sides of each ganglion facing towards and away from the capillary tip was scored on an arbitrary scale from 0 to 10. The corresponding distances from each side of the ganglion to the end of the capillary were measured using a travelling microscope. The cumulative results of some 350 measurements for capillary tubes of varying diameter are given in Table 3. Differences between

Table 3 Response of sensory ganglia to a capillary tube containing NGF at 30 μg/ml

Distance mm		*Mean score ± S.E.M. of fibre outgrowth for various capillary diameters*				
		0–10[1]	11–15	16–20	21–25	>25
0–1	Towards	3.3 ± 0.3	3.7 ± 0.5	3.7 ± 0.4	4.4 ± 0.5	4.6 ± 0.6
	Away	1.4 ± 0.3	1.3 ± 0.2	1.4 ± 0.3	1.7 ± 0.5	1.5 ± 0.3
1–2	Towards	3.3 ± 0.4	3.1 ± 0.3	3.5 ± 0.3	3.9 ± 0.5	4.3 ± 0.5
	Away	1.6 ± 0.2	1.8 ± 0.2	1.8 ± 0.3	1.0 ± 0.6	1.7 ± 0.4
>2	Towards	1.3 ± 0.2	1.3 ± 0.2	1.7 ± 0.3	1.7 ± 0.4	3.0 ± 0.4
	Away	1.4 ± 0.2	1.5 ± 0.2	1.4 ± 0.2	1.2 ± 0.3	1.2 ± 0.3

[1] Capillary diameters in unit divisions (1 division = 6.25 μm).

'towards' and 'away' scores are highly significant for distances from ganglion edge to capillary tip of up to 2mm for all sizes of capillary. For distances greater than 2mm, the difference between growth towards and away from the source is only significant for the largest capillary diameters. For equal distances between ganglion edge and source, the differences in the scores for growth towards the source are significant only when the smallest and the largest diameter sources are compared; they are not significant when a comparison is made of the scores for consecutive capillary diameters.

The difference in fibre outgrowth towards and away from the capillary tube is not observed when the capillary is filled with saline solution, with a solution of heat-inactivated NGF, or with very dilute solutions of active NGF. If the liquid culture medium is supplemented with NGF, at a low concentration, so that total fibre outgrowth is increased above that observed in control cultures, the difference in growth towards and away from a capillary source of NGF (at 30 μg/ml) is maintained.

It might be argued that the fibres from the side of the ganglion facing the capillary tip might be drawn into the tube by convection currents resulting from physicochemical differences between the culture medium and the liquid inside the capillary. Alternatively, there might be an effective pumping or suction action due to the capillary. Fibres that had entered the tube for any of these reasons might then not be able to escape by random movement, so that the accumulation of fibres around the capillary tip might not be due to a specific orientating effect of NGF. However, in many cases the outgrowing fibres did not actually reach the capillary and, in these cases, these objections would not be valid.

The results cannot be taken as unambiguous evidence for chemotaxis. It is possible that the side of each ganglion facing away from the source of NGF is completely screened from the influence of the source by the bulk of the ganglion. Since the cultures were made in a liquid medium, it is unlikely that the fibres were following lines of tension between the ganglion and the source.

Attempts are now being made to determine the direction and rate of growth of fibres from ganglia by time-lapse cinephotomicroscopy. The effect of a localized source of NGF on the growth of fibres from single cells, obtained by dispersion of sensory ganglia, is also being studied. Preliminary results indicate that the response is complex because the cells, at this stage in their development, are bipolar. It appears that fibres from single cells do accumulate around the tip of a capillary source of NGF but that the cell bodies do not.

Acknowledgements

Generous financial support from the Whitehall Foundation, New York, is gratefully acknowledged. One of us (K.A.C.) also wishes to thank the Medical Research Council for a Research

Fellowship during the tenure of which most of this work was carried out.

References

Bueker, E. D. (1948). *Anat. Rec.* **102**, 369.
Lamont, D. M. (1968). Ph.D. Thesis, University of London.

Studies of Tissue Monoamines by Fluorescence Microscopy

ELENA NICOLESCU,* SOPHIA KAKARI† and ELEANOR ZAIMIS

Department of Pharmacology, Royal Free Hospital School of Medicine, University of London

Levi-Montalcini and her co-workers (for references see Levi-Montalcini, 1964) have demonstrated that sympathetic ganglia can hypertrophy, or conversely be destroyed, after treatment of the newborn mouse with a protein or its antiserum. This protein, known as nerve growth factor (NGF), is isolated at present from either mouse salivary glands or snake venom. The observations made by Levi-Montalcini and her co-workers have been confirmed in our department; and they have been extended to other species.

Methods and results

Daily subcutaneous injections of either mouse salivary gland NGF or Russell's viper venom NGF in newborn kittens and rats resulted after 8 to 14 days in an increase in the size of the sympathetic ganglia and of the adrenal medulla (Zaimis, this volume, p. 61). Microscopical examination of the ganglia showed that the overall increase in size was the result primarily of cellular hypertrophy, although an increase in cell numbers was also present. Microscopical examination of the adrenal gland showed that the hypertrophy of the adrenal medulla was the

* *Present address:* Department of Physiology, Faculty of Medicine, Bucharest, Rumania.

† *Present address:* Department of Experimental Neurosurgery, New York University School of Medicine, New York.

Plate XXI

KITTEN: Spleen

Control

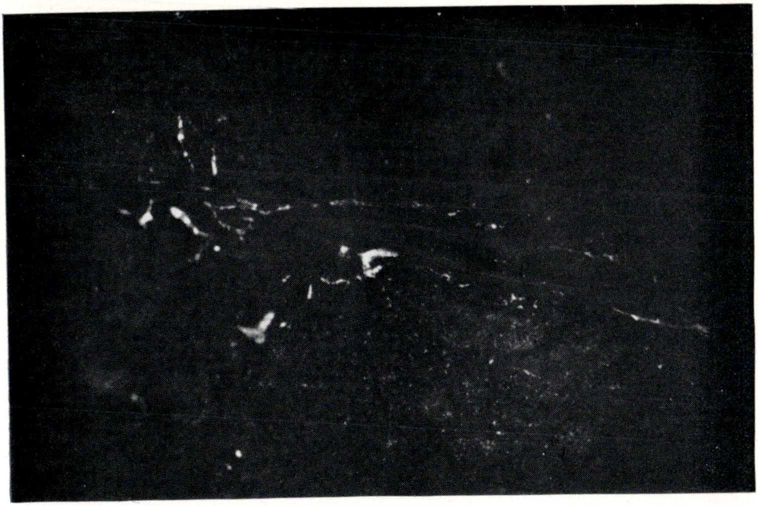

(*a*)

NGF

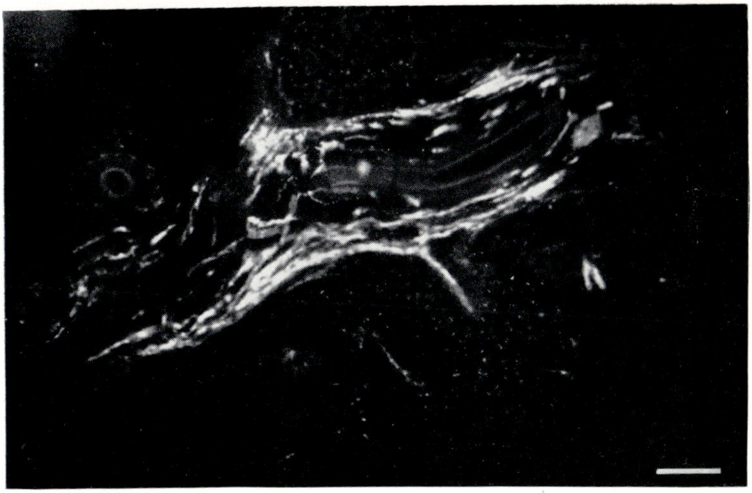

(*b*)

100 μm

Figs. 1, 2 and 3 Kittens; nine days old. Fluorescence micrographs representing three types of tissue (spleen, salivary gland and heart atrium) removed from (*a*) controls; and (*b*) animals treated with mouse salivary gland NGF.

Plate XXII

KITTEN: Salivary glands

Control

(a)

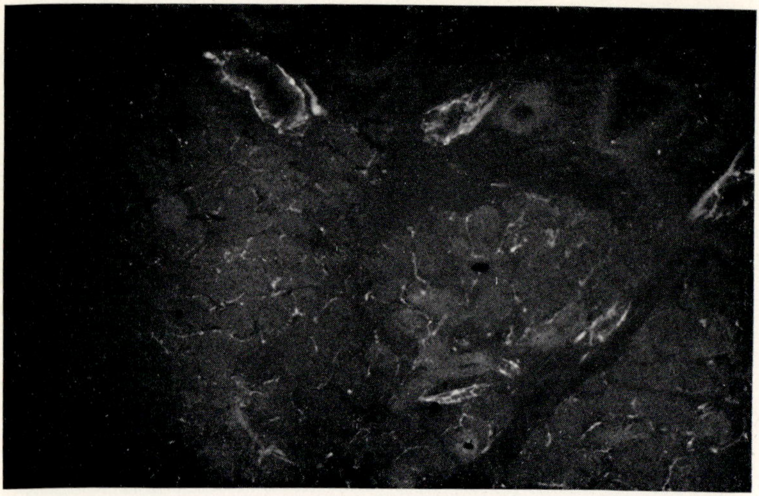

NGF

(b)

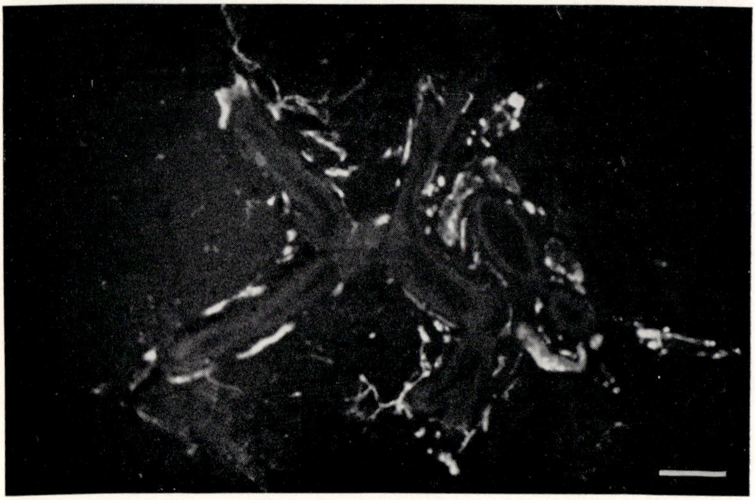

100 μm

Plate XXIII

KITTEN: Atria

Control

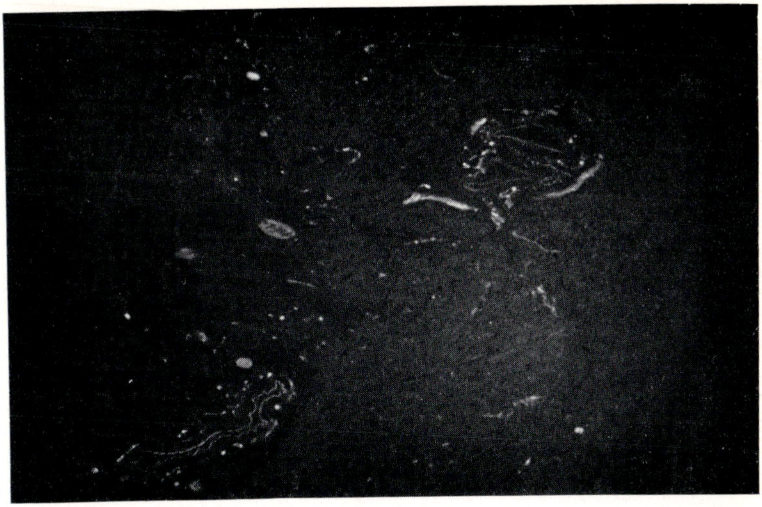

(*a*)

NGF

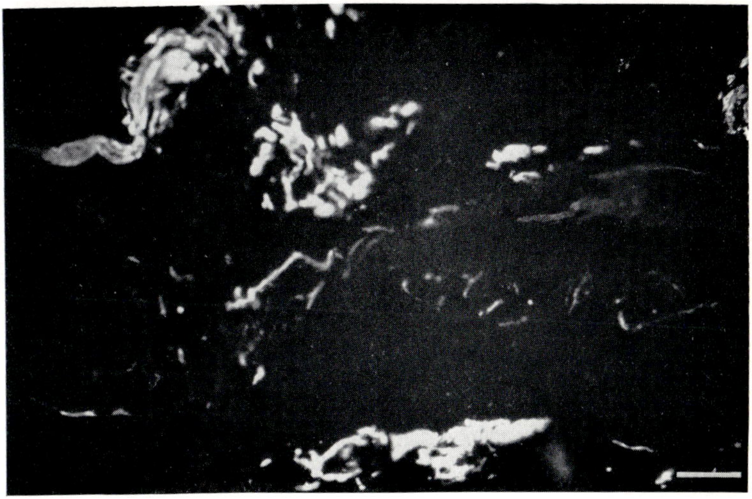

(*b*)

100 μm

PLATE XXIV

RAT: Vas Deferens

Control

(*a*)

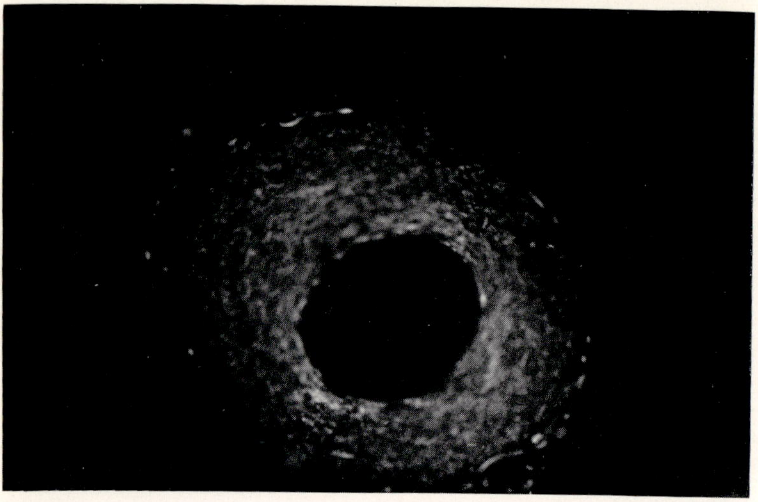

NGF

(*b*)

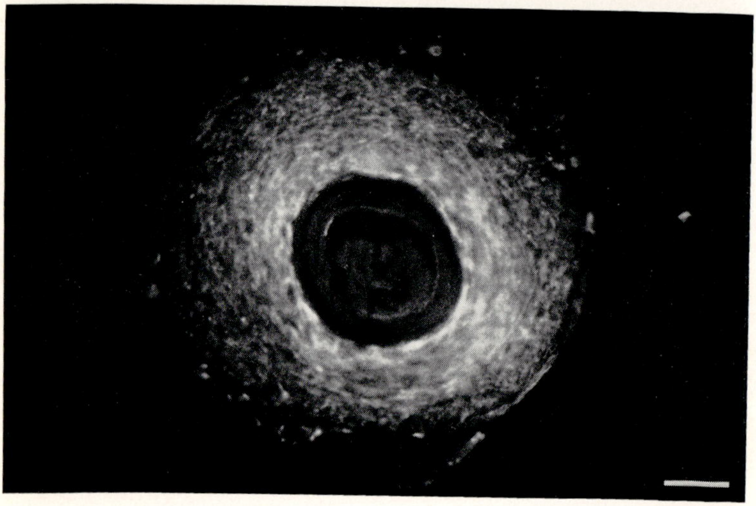

100 μm

Fig. 4 Rats; 15 days old. Fluorescence micrographs of sections of vas deferens removed from (*a*) control; and (*b*) a rat treated with mouse salivary gland NGF.

PLATE XXV

RAT: Adrenal

Control

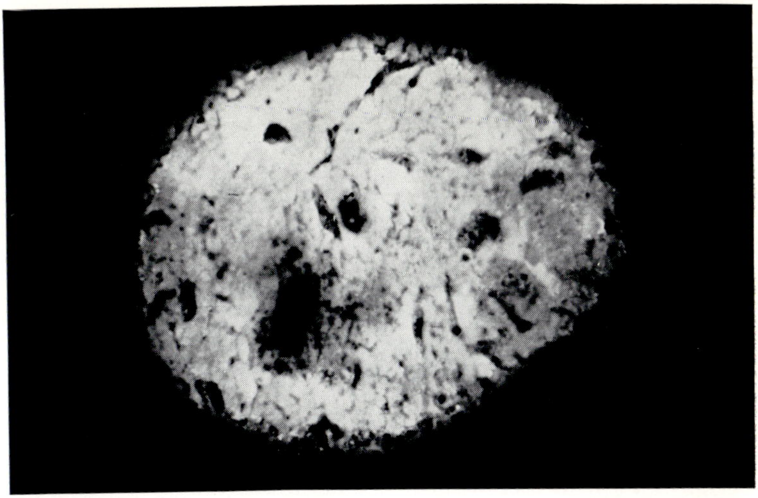

(*a*)

NGF

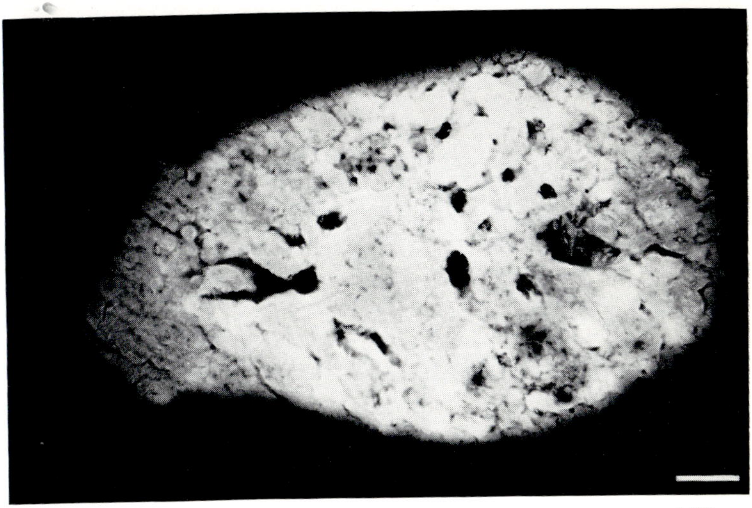

(*b*)

100 μm

Figs. 5, 6 and 7 Fluorescence micrographs of sections of adrenal medulla removed from rats treated for 11–14 days after birth with (*a*) saline (control); or (*b*) NGF. The treated rat in Fig. 5 received mouse salivary gland NGF, and those in Fig. 6 and 7 NGF prepared from Russell's viper venom.

Plate XXVI

RAT: Adrenal

Control

(*a*)

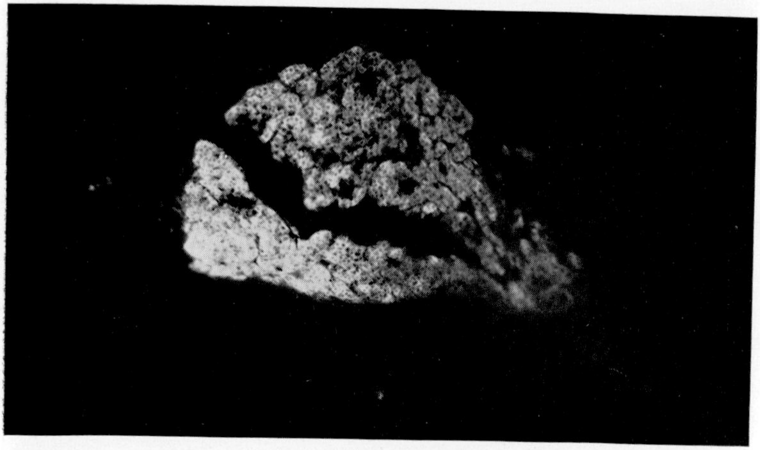

NGF

(*b*)

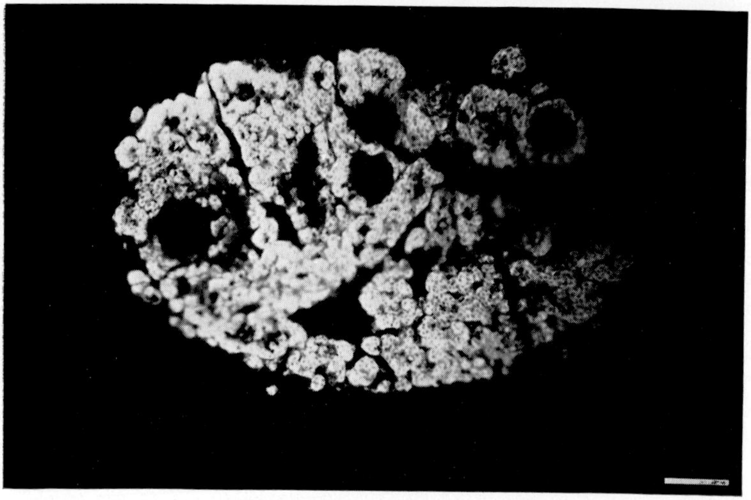

100 μm

Plate XXVII

RAT: Adrenal

Control

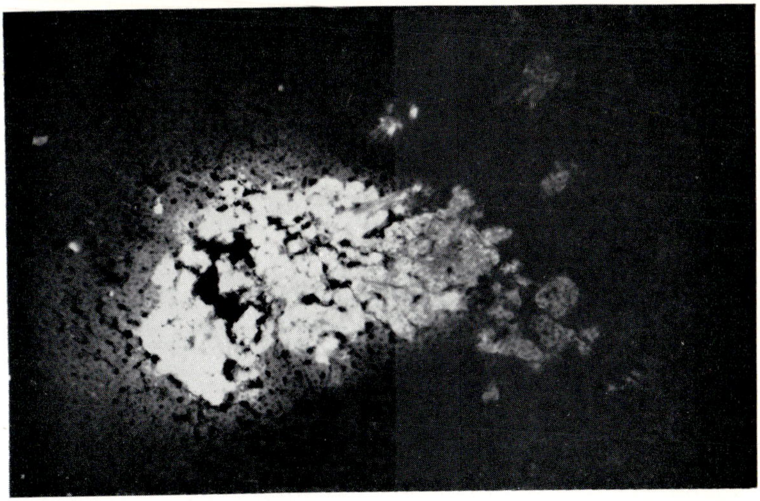

(*a*)

NGF

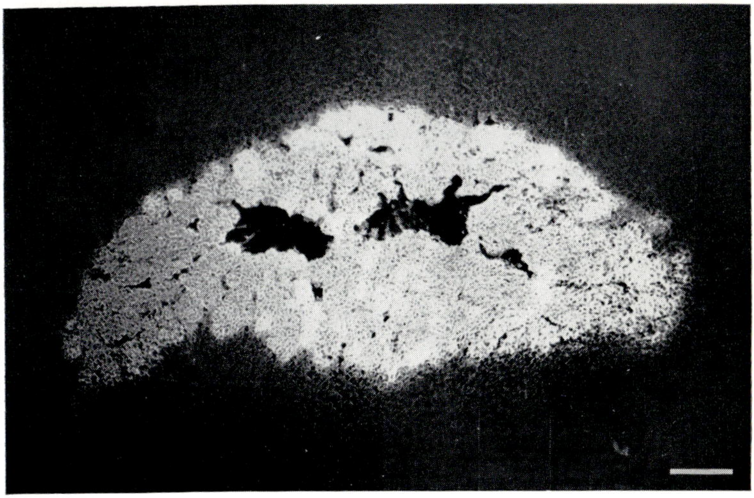

(*b*)

100 μm

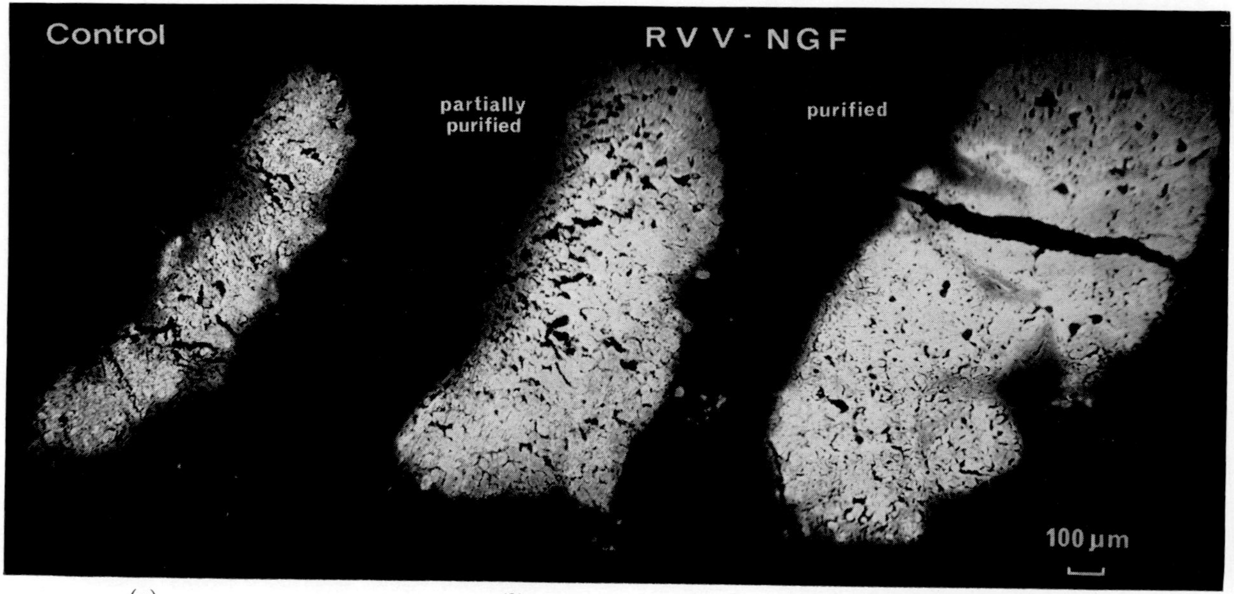

(*a*) (*b*) (*c*)

Fig. 8 Kittens; nine days old. Fluorescence micrographs of sections of adrenal medulla from animals treated with saline (*a*); or Russell's viper venom (RVV) NGF, partially purified (*b*), or purified (*c*).

MOUSE:
Adrenal

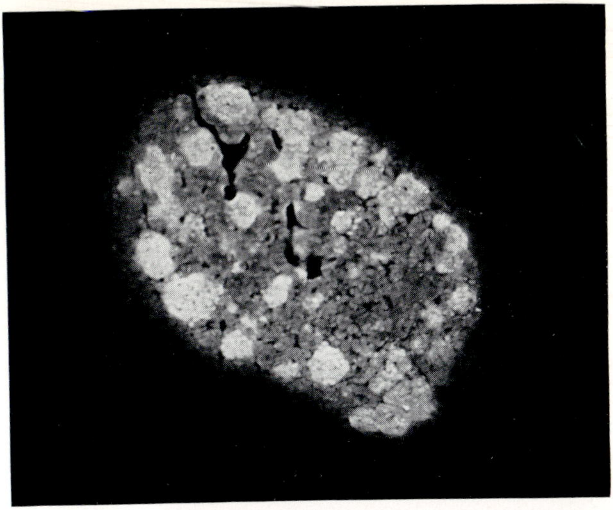

(*a*)
Control

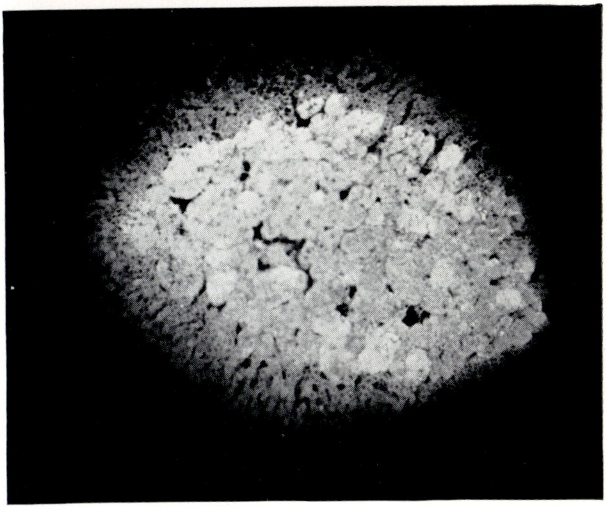

(*b*)
NGF

Fig. 9 Mice; 10 days old. Fluorescence micrographs of sections of adrenal medulla removed from animals treated for 10 days with (*a*) saline (control); and (*b*) mouse salivary gland NGF. In the sections from the control a strong fluorescence is present in the typical noradrenaline cell islets, while the adrenaline-containing cells are weakly fluorescent. ($\times$ 100)

Plate XXX

RAT: Atria

Control

(*a*)

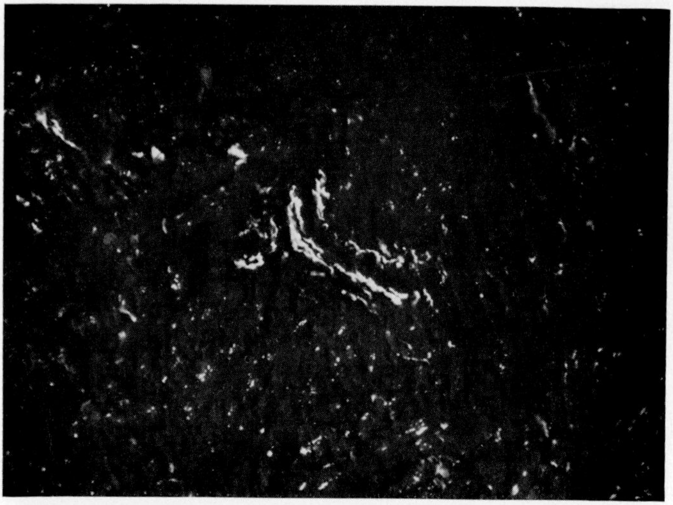

Immunosympathectomized

(*b*)

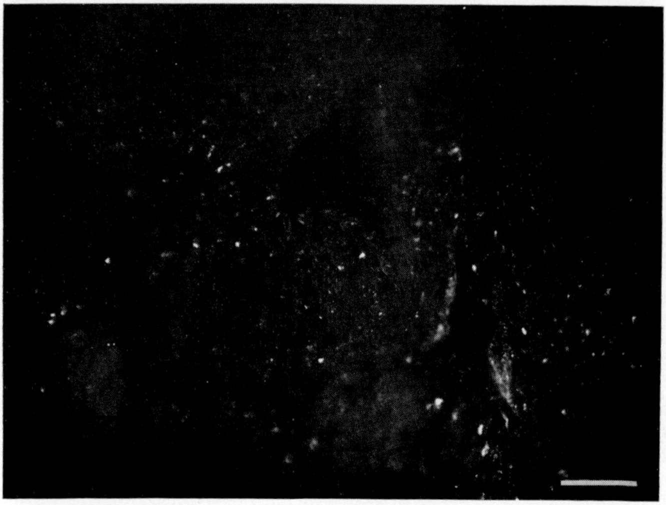

100 μm

Fig. 10 Rats; three months old. Fluorescence micrographs of atria removed from (*a*) control; and (*b*) animal treated for the first five days after birth with NGF-antiserum.

Plate XXXI

RAT: Spleen

Control

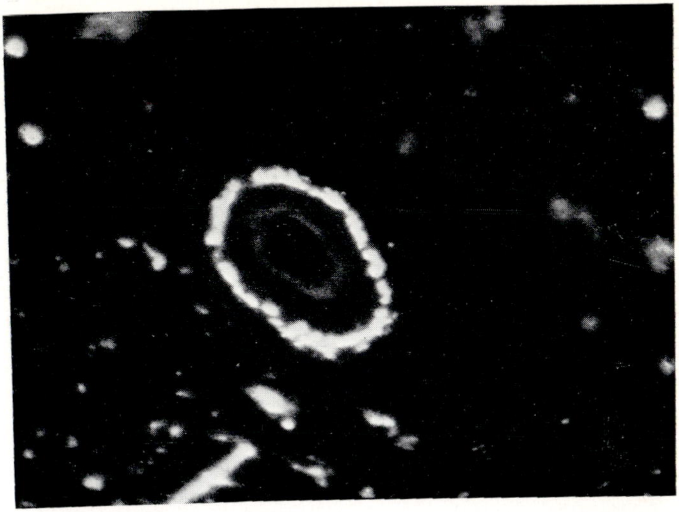

(*a*)

Immunosympathectomized

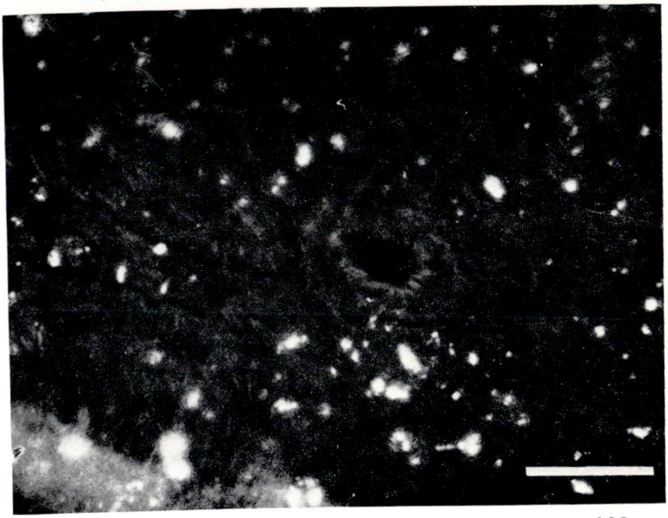

(*b*)

100 μm

Fig. 11 Rats; two months old. Fluorescence micrographs of spleen removed from (*a*) control; and (*b*) animal treated for the first five days after birth with NGF-antiserum.

Plate XXXII

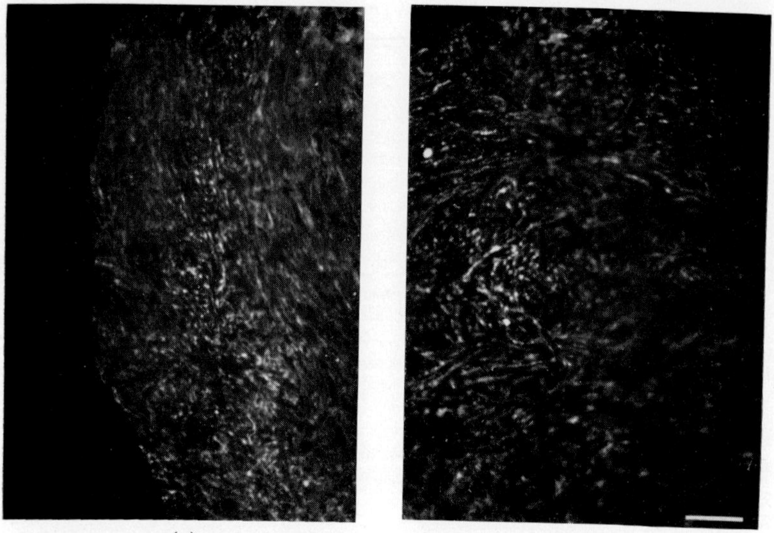

(*a*) (*b*) 100 μm

Fig. 12 Rats; two months old. Fluorescence microphotographs of vas deferens removed from (*a*) control; and (*b*) animal treated for the first five days after birth with NGF-antiserum.

result of an increase either in the number of medullary cells, or in their size, or in both. In contrast, treatment of newborn rats with NGF-antiserum resulted in almost complete destruction of the paravertebral ganglia, and severe atrophy of the coeliac ganglion, but had a very limited effect on the mesenteric ganglion (Zaimis, Berk & Callingham, 1965). In both NGF- and NGF-antiserum-treated animals there was a good correlation between the hypertrophy or atrophy of the sympathetic ganglia and the catecholamine content of the tissues innervated by these ganglia.

In the present study, an attempt was made by means of the fluorescence histochemical technique to obtain additional information on the distribution and localization of catecholamines in tissues removed from both NGF-treated kittens and rats and NGF-antiserum-treated rats. The animals used were the same, or belonged to the same groups, as those used by Zaimis (this volume, p. 60) and Papadaki (this volume, p. 89).

Eränkö (1951, 1952) observed in adrenals fixed with *formaldehyde solution* a green fluorescence in certain groups of cells in the medulla. Analysis with specific chemical methods showed subsequently that the medullary cells exhibiting this kind of fluorescence contained a high concentration of noradrenaline. Later on it was independently observed in several laboratories (Eränkö, 1961; Falck & Torp, 1961; Lagunoff, Phillips & Benditt, 1961) that aromatic monoamines became intensely fluorescent in freeze-dried tissues when they were exposed to *formaldehyde vapour*. Finally, Falck, Hillarp and their colleagues (Carlsson, Falck & Hillarp, 1962; Falck, 1962; Falck, Hillarp, Thieme & Torp, 1962) were the first to report the successful demonstration of catecholamines by formaldehyde vapour in nervous tissues.

During exposure to formaldehyde vapour the catecholamines condense with formaldehyde in a two-step reaction to intensely fluorescent 3,4-dihydroisoquinolines. The second step can be reversed by treatment with sodium borohydride (Corrodi, Hillarp & Jonsson, 1964); the fluorescence disappears but can be regenerated by renewed treatment with formaldehyde vapour.

Thus, with the help of this method, we were able to distinguish formaldehyde-induced fluorescence from non-specific fluorescence due to compounds other than aromatic monoamines. In addition, the catecholamine content of the tissues was estimated biochemically, in order to establish the nature of the fluorogenic substances.

Because the emission spectra of noradrenaline and adrenaline are essentially similar, other means must be used to discriminate between them. Adrenaline differs from noradrenaline in being, as a secondary amine, more slowly condensed with formaldehyde (Eränkö, 1964, 1967; Falck, 1962). Thus primary and secondary catecholamines can be distinguished from each other histochemically; for instance exposure of tissues to formaldehyde gas for one hour at 50°C is sufficient to show the presence of noradrenaline, whereas more than one hour at 80°C is needed for the demonstration of adrenaline. In order to demonstrate both adrenaline and noradrenaline, the dried tissues of our experimental animals were exposed to formaldehyde vapour at 80°C for 1 to 2 hours.

The formaldehyde-induced fluorescence can demonstrate not only catecholamines such as dopamine, noradrenaline and adrenaline, but also 5-hydroxytryptamine. Moreover, formaldehyde also renders fluorescent the precursors of these compounds. The formaldehyde-induced fluorescence reaction of noradrenaline-containing adrenergic nerve fibres is green, while that of 5-hydroxytryptamine is yellow. However, special care is necessary when colour differences are used as guides to the nature of the amines demonstrated with the formaldehyde-induced fluorescence method. Both the eye and the photographic colour emulsion tend to 'see' the green colour, due to noradrenaline, as progressively more yellow when the intensity of the fluorescence is increased.

NGF-treated rats and kittens

The distribution of catecholamines was studied in the heart, spleen, salivary glands, vas deferens and the adrenals. In the NGF-treated kittens and rats the specific fluorescence was generally increased, although variation in intensity was observed.

Fluorescence microphotographs of different types of tissue are illustrated in Figs. 1, 2 and 3. In the spleen, salivary glands, and the atrium of the newborn kitten, adrenergic fibres are normally thin and weakly fluorescent. In sections of tissues removed from NGF-treated kittens, accumulations of strongly fluorescent material can be seen. Similar changes were observed in the NGF-treated rats. These results are in good agreement with those of Olson (1967) in the mouse.

In the rat, the muscle layer of the vas deferens is richly innervated by adrenergic fibres (Fig. 4). After NGF treatment a marked overgrowth of these fibres was found.

Figures 5–8 show sections of adrenal medulla removed from either control or NGF-treated animals. In both species and with both NGF preparations there was an increase in the size of the adrenal medulla and, in addition, a more intense fluorescence. The catecholamine content of these tissues was assayed fluorimetrically after extraction and ion-exchange purification by our colleagues Lucienne Papadaki and B. Large. After NGF treatment there was a significant increase in the catecholamine content of all tissues examined. In addition, differential assays of adrenaline and noradrenaline showed that in the adrenals of the NGF-treated rats the increase in noradrenaline was significantly greater than that of adrenaline. In contrast, in NGF-treated kittens the percentage increase of adrenaline in the adrenal medulla was greater than that of noradrenaline.

In mice treated with NGF (kindly provided by Dr D. C. Edwards) there was a much stronger fluorescence in the adrenal medulla but the hypertrophy was less than that found in the adrenals of rats and kittens (Fig. 9).

NGF-antiserum-treated rats

Previous investigations (Zaimis *et al.*, 1965) have demonstrated that treatment of newborn rats with NGF-antiserum results in almost complete destruction of the paravertebral ganglia, and severe atrophy of the coeliac ganglion, and has little effect on the mesenteric ganglion. This lack of uniformity in the destruction of the various sympathetic ganglia was reflected in the catecholamine content of the tissues innervated by them. The noradrenaline content of the heart and spleen was almost zero, that of the small intestine was about 25 per cent of normal, while the noradrenaline content of the vas deferens was 65 per cent of that of the controls.

The present histochemical findings are in accordance with the morphological and biochemical results: in the rats treated with

NGF-antiserum the fluorescence normally existing in organs innervated by the paravertebral sympathetic ganglia or the coeliac ganglion was significantly decreased or completely absent. Fig. 10 shows sections of left atrium from a control rat and from a rat treated with NGF-antiserum. In the atrium of the immuno-sympathectomized rat there is very little fluorescence left. Fig. 11 shows a complete absence of fluorescence in the blood vessels of the spleen removed from a rat treated with NGF-antiserum. In contrast, fluorescent adrenergic terminals persisted in the vas deferens (Fig. 12). Similar results were obtained by Hamberger, Levi-Montalcini, Norberg & Sjöqvist (1965).

Summary

Using fluorescence microscopy the distribution of catecholamines was studied in the heart, spleen, salivary glands, vas deferens and adrenals of newborn kittens and rats treated with either NGF or its antiserum. The fluorescence attributed to the presence of catecholamines was increased in organs removed from the NGF-treated animals. In contrast, a great reduction or almost complete absence of this fluorescence was observed in the organs of animals treated with NGF-antiserum. In both groups of animals there was good correlation between the fluorescence histochemical findings and the catecholamine content of the tissues.

Acknowledgements

This investigation was supported in part by research grants (to E. Z.) from the Muscular Dystrophy Group of Great Britain, the Medical Research Council, and the Wellcome Foundation. Our thanks are due to Mr R. Owen and Mr P. Clayton for their valuable technical assistance.

References

Carlsson, A., Falck, B. & Hillarp, N.-Å. (1962). *Acta physiol. scand.* **56**, Suppl. 196.

Corrodi, H., Hillarp, N.-Å. & Jonsson, G. (1964). *J. Histochem. Cytochem.* **12**, 582.

Eränkö, O. (1951). *Acta physiol. scand.* **25**, Suppl. 89.
Eränkö, O. (1952). *Acta anat.* **16**, Suppl. 17.
Eränkö, O. (1961). Personal communication acknowledged in Falck & Torp (1961).
Eränkö, O. (1964). *J. Histochem. Cytochem.* **12**, 487.
Eränkö, O. (1967). *Ann. Rev. Pharmac.* **7**, 203.
Falck, B. (1962). *Acta physiol. scand.* **56**, Suppl. 197.
Falck, B., Hillarp, N.-Å., Thieme, G. & Torp, A. (1962). *J. Histochem. Cytochem.* **10**, 348.
Falck, B. & Torp, A. (1961). *Med. Expl, Basle* **5**, 429.
Hamberger, B., Levi-Montalcini, R., Norberg, K.-A. & Sjöqvist, F. (1965). *Int. J. Neuro-pharmacol.* **4**, 91.
Lagunoff, D., Phillips, M. & Benditt, E. V. (1961), *J. Histochem. Cytochem.* **9**, 534.
Levi-Montalcini, R. (1964). *Science* **143**, 105.
Olson, L. (1967). *Z. Zellforsch. mikrosk. Anat.* **81**, 155.
Zaimis, E., Berk. L. & Callingham, B. A. (1965). *Nature, Lond.* **206**, 1220.

Lipid Metabolism in Chick Embryo Sensory Ganglia Stimulated with Nerve Growth Factor

ANTONIA LIUZZI,* G. D'AGNOLO and F. H. FOPPEN

Laboratori di Biologia Cellulare, C.N.R., Rome; Laboratori di Chimica Biologica, Istituto Superiore di Sanità, Rome, Italy*

It has been shown that nerve growth factor (NGF) stimulates the incorporation of labelled precursors into cellular metabolites of sensory and sympathetic ganglia (Angeletti, Gandini-Attardi, Toschi, Salvi & Levi-Montalcini, 1965; Toschi, Dore, Angeletti, Levi-Montalcini & De Haën, 1966; Angeletti, Liuzzi & Levi-Montalcini, 1964). However, a thorough investigation of ganglionic metabolism in the presence of NGF has demonstrated that the only cellular constituents significantly affected are neutral lipids (Foppen, Liuzzi & D'Agnolo, 1969). In view of the striking enhancement of triglyceride synthesis, we have measured the activity of enzymes concerned with the synthesis of neutral lipids.

Two hundred chick embryo sensory ganglia were incubated for four hours at 37°C in a CO_2-conditioned incubator, each suspended in 1 ml of Eagle's basal medium with or without NGF (0.01 μg/ml). At the end of the incubation period the ganglia were harvested, washed in cold saline solution and homogenized in buffer. The following enzymes were measured in the whole homogenate: fatty acid synthetase by the method of Pugh, Saver, Waite, Toomey & Wakil (1966); acyl CoA:1,2-diglyceride-*O*-acyltransferase (EC 2.3.1.20) by the method of Young & Lynen (1969); 1,2-diacyl-sn-glycero-3-phosphate phosphohydrolase (EC

3.1.3.4) by the method of Wilgram & Kennedy (1961); acyl CoA:sn-glycero-3-phosphate-*O*-acyltransferase (EC 2.3.1.15) according to Kuhn & Lynen (1965).

1, 2-diacyl-sn-glycero-3-phosphate phosphohydrolase and fatty acid synthetase were stimulated by about 60 per cent. The activities of both transferases, on the other hand, more than doubled in the presence of NGF. Acyl Co A:1,2-diglyceride-*O*-acyltransferase activity increased from 0.6 nmol of substrate transformed/100 ganglia/hour for the controls to 1.6 nmol of substrate transformed/100 ganglia/hour for the NGF-treated ganglia; the activity of acyl CoA:sn-glycero-3-phosphate-*O*-acyltransferase was 47 nmol of substrate transformed/100 ganglia/hour for the controls and 115 nmol of substrate transformed/100 ganglia/hour for the ganglia treated with NGF.

These results support our earlier hypothesis on neutral lipid synthesis (Foppen *et al.*, 1969). The principal biochemical property of NGF is a direct or mediated action on one or both transferases involved in the synthesis of triglycerides.

References

Angeletti, P. U., Gandini-Attardi, D., Toschi, G., Salvi, M. L. & Levi-Montalcini, R. (1965). *Biochim. biophys. Acta* **95**, 111.

Angeletti, P. U., Liuzzi, A. & Levi-Montalcini, R. (1964). *Biochim. biophys. Acta* **84**, 778.

Foppen, F. H., Liuzzi, A. & D'Agnolo, G. (1969). *Biochim. biophys. Acta* **187**, 414.

Kuhn, N. J. & Lynen, F. (1965). *Biochem. J.* **94**, 240.

Pugh, E. L., Saver, F., Waite, M., Toomey, R. E. & Wakil, S. J. (1966). *J. biol. Chem.* **241**, 2635.

Toschi, G., Dore, E., Angeletti, P. U., Levi-Montalcini, R. & De Haën, C. (1966). *J. Neurochem.* **13**, 539.

Wilgram, G. F. & Kennedy, E. P. (1961). *J. biol. Chem.* **238**, 2615.

Young, D. L. & Lynen, F. (1969). *J. biol. Chem.* **244**, 377.

Lack of Effect of Nerve Growth Factor on Peripheral Sensory Nerve Regeneration

N. R. SAUNDERS

Department of Physiology, University College London, UK

In spite of the large amount of work which has been done on the nerve growth factor (NGF), it is not clear whether it affects the regeneration of any neurones. The only relevant published work is that of Scott & Liu (1963, 1964) and Scott, Gutmann & Horsky (1966); but, as will be considered in the discussion, these experiments do not appear to provide convincing evidence that NGF can affect the outgrowth of spinal neurones after damage. In the present study the problem has been investigated by estimating in rats and rabbits, injected with NGF or with saline, the distance grown by sensory fibres following crushing of peripheral nerves. The results were negative. Nevertheless, it seems worth while to report the details, in order to avoid future waste of valuable material in repetition of the same experiments, especially as relatively large amounts of NGF are required for this type of experiment.

Methods

Two experiments were carried out. In the first, twelve female white rats (240–270 g) were operated on in sterile conditions and under ether anaesthesia. Standard 'crushes' (Evans & Saunders, 1967) were made in the left sural and left lateral popliteal nerves. The crushes were marked with carbon black, and the mark was found to remain in position throughout the experiment. The rats were assigned randomly to two groups. One group (control) received a daily injection of 1.0 ml sterile 0.9 per cent saline solution, while the other group (experimental) received daily 400 units of NGF per g body weight. All injections were administered intraperitoneally. The NGF used was 7S mouse salivary gland NGF, kindly supplied by the Wellcome Research Laboratories. Seven days after operation the rats were re-anaesthetized, the crushed nerves were exposed, and the rats were placed in a standard position. Estimates were made of the farthest distance below the crush to which the regenerating sensory axons had grown. The method used depends upon the high sensitivity of regenerating sensory nerve endings to mechanical stimuli, which was first described by Tinel (1917) in man and was used (e.g. Konorski & Lubinska, 1946) to estimate the rate of regeneration of sensory fibres in experimental animals. After being immersed in light paraffin oil, the nerve was tapped distal to the crush with a glass stylus. The impulses thus set up were detected central to the crush, using platinum electrodes and a suitable high-gain amplifier system ('Isleworth' preamplifier and 'Tektronix' 502A oscilloscope). Signals were monitored through a loudspeaker, displayed on the oscilloscope screen, and recorded on a S.E. Laboratories 2005 U.V. recorder.

The maximum point distal to the crush at which impulses could be initiated was determined by tapping with the glass stylus back and forth along the nerve. This point was marked with carbon black and its distance distal to the crush was measured by placing a size 5/0 thread alongside the path of the nerve. Each estimation was repeated five times. Tests with Plasticine and wire models suggest that the standard error of the mean of repeated observation was <1 mm. The crushed nerves were then fixed in 10 per cent formol in 0.9 per cent saline solution and examined histologically.

The superior cervical ganglia were removed and each of the pair weighed. The rats were examined in pairs (control and experimental) without the experimenter being aware from which group each came.

In the second experiment NGF was injected intrathecally into rabbits and similar measurements were made of the distance of sensory fibre regeneration following crushing of peripheral nerves. The rabbits were anaesthetized with 5 per cent thiopentone, injected intravenously, under sterile conditions.

Cannulae were made from No 12 stainless steel syringe needles cut to 7–8 mm length and fixed into a nylon holder with an external thread. These were implanted chronically into one lateral ventricle of 26 young New Zealand white rabbits (8 weeks old, 1100–1400 g body weight) using the method of Oldendorf & Davson (1967). Each cannula was cemented in position with 'Surgical Simplex' (North Hill Plastics Ltd.). Between injections a cap with a central stylet was screwed over the nylon holder. For injection this was replaced by a syringe connecting piece. Standard crushes were made of the whole sciatic nerve (Evans & Saunders, 1967); NGF injected into a lateral ventricle would be expected to reach the lumbar dorsal root ganglia via the subarachnoid space and via the central spinal canal, which is patent in the rabbit (this was confirmed by injecting dye).

The rabbits were divided randomly into three groups. Each rabbit received daily one of the following injections into its ventricular cannula:

(1) 0.4 ml 0.9 per cent saline solution (control)
(2) 15 000 units NGF/kg body weight (high NGF)
(3) 1500 units NGF/kg body weight (low NGF)

After ten days the rabbits were re-anaesthetized and estimates were made of the farthest distance grown by the regenerating sensory nerves.

Results

The results from the experiments on rats are shown in Table 1. There was no significant difference in the maximum distance of

Table 1 Regeneration of peripheral sensory nerve fibres of four-month-old rats

	Sural nerve		*Lateral popliteal nerve*	
	Control	*NGF*	*Control*	*NGF*
Mean (mm)	12.8	13.4	11.5	10.6
S.E.M.	1.3	1.6	1.0	1.0
N	6	5	6	5

Mean values shown are mm distal to crush reached by fastest fibres, 7 days after crushing.

Control rats received 1.0 ml of 0.9 per cent saline solution intraperitoneally daily.

Experimental rats received 400 units/g body weight NGF intraperitoneally daily.

regeneration between the control animals and those treated with NGF. It is important to emphasize that the electro-physiological method used estimates the distance regenerated by the fastest growing fibres. Estimates of the distance regenerated, made on histological material from these experiments, gave similar values (Dr K. E. Webster, unpublished results). That biologically significant amounts of NGF were injected is shown by the observation that the superior cervical ganglia of the NGF-treated animals weighed significantly more than those of the control rats. In five pairs of rats the mean values, expressed as the weight of one ganglion, were 1.9 mg (S.E.M. = 0.2) for controls; and 2.7 mg (S.E.M. = 0.2; $P = <0.02$) for the NGF-treated rats.

Only a few of the experiments on rabbits were successful. Four of the eight controls and twelve of the eighteen NGF-treated animals died before the end of the ten-day experimental period. Most of the deaths took place within 48 hours of operation; and they occurred in rabbits which had been operated on during a time of exceptionally hot weather. Because of the small number of animals in each group, no useful conclusions can be drawn about the toxicity of intrathecally injected NGF. Four control rabbits, and three in each treated group, survived, and the mean maximum regeneration distances in the nerves examined at ten days are shown in Table 2. The values for all three

Table 2 Regeneration of peripheral sensory nerve fibres of two-month-old rabbits ten days after crushing

	Mean maximum regeneration distance (mm)		
	Sural nerve	*Medial popliteal*	*Lateral popliteal*
Control (N = 4)	19.8	23.0	23.2
	Mean for all nerves = 22.0; S.E.M. = 3.8; N = 9		
'Low' NGF (N = 3)	21.2	20.2	18.4
	Mean for all nerves = 19.8; S.E.M. = 3.2; N. = 8		
'High' NGF (N = 3)	23.5	23.2	23.2
	Mean for all nerves = 23.4; S.E.M. = 3.2; N = 8		

'Low' NGF rabbits: 1500 units NGF/kg body weight by intrathecal injection, daily.

'High' NGF rabbits: 15 000 units NGF/kg body weight by intrathecal injection, daily.

'Control': 0.4 ml of 0.9 per cent saline solution by intrathecal injection, daily.

nerves in each group have also been pooled: the differences between each group are not statistically significant.

Discussion

There was no evidence in these experiments of an effect of NGF on the maximum distance of sensory nerve regeneration following a crush injury, when the NGF was injected either intraperitoneally (in rats) or intrathecally (in rabbits). That the NGF was administered to the rats in adequate amounts was shown by the fact that the superior cervical ganglia of the treated animals were significantly larger than were those of the controls. However, the lack of effect of NGF in rats could have been due to its failure to reach the dorsal root ganglion cells: the relatively large NGF molecule would not be expected to cross the blood-brain barrier. This does not appear to occur, since intrathecal injection of NGF in rabbits was also without effect.

These negative results are not surprising, since there is evidence that the effect of NGF on sensory ganglia is confined to a restricted period of development (Levi-Montalcini & Angeletti, 1968). However, since clinical recovery from nerve injury is frequently poor it seems important that substances which affect neurone growth should be investigated for possible effects on nerve regeneration.

The claim of Scott & Liu (1963, 1964) that NGF has a positive effect in promoting regeneration of spinal neurones does not seem to have been borne out by their evidence. Scott & Liu investigated three kittens which were given different amounts of NGF following crush lesions of the dorsal funiculus. The lesions were made 'through the dura'. From the description of the postoperative state of the animals, it seems that the lesions may have been different in each case. Since there is evidence (e.g. Nathaniel & Pease, 1963) that the central processes of dorsal root ganglion cells *do* regenerate following injury, it is surprising that none of the four control kittens showed any signs of regeneration, whereas the three NGF-treated animals did. Scott & Liu describe in the histological preparations from two of the NGF-treated kittens, axons and growth cones which were several millimetres rostral to the site of injury 30–50 days after injury. They also give conduction velocities of up to 65 metres/second in these fibres.

These results do not seem to be mutually compatible for two reasons:

(1) The histological illustrations show fibres of diameter less than 2 μm. Even allowing for considerable shrinkage, this is surely far too small to account for the velocities recorded (cf. Erlanger & Gasser, 1937).

(2) Previous work has shown that regenerating axons only develop to the degree implied by such fast conduction velocities when they successfully innervate another cell (Gutmann & Sanders, 1943; Sanders & Young, 1946; Sanders & Whitteridge, 1946).

Measurements of conduction velocity, at different distances along the dorsal funiculus, would have given more convincing evidence of a continuing process of regeneration in the fibres from which records were taken. Sanders & Whitteridge have shown that the conduction velocity of a crushed nerve decreased markedly at the site of a crush, and that it decreases even more sharply towards the ends of the regenerating fibres. The conduction velocity of these regenerating fibres only approached normal after several months of regeneration with successful innervation of peripheral end organs.

The paper of Scott and his co-workers (1966) concerns the uptake of [^{3}H] leucine into rat dorsal root ganglion cells (estimated from radioautographic grain counts) following lesions either of peripheral nerves or of dorsal roots. These workers found no effect of NGF following crushing of sciatic and femoral nerves; and this is in agreement with our results. They did, however, find a small increase in grain count (14 per cent) in NGF-treated animals after dorsal root crush, compared with the uncrushed control side. The significance of this finding is not clear.

Thus far, there is no evidence that NGF can affect the regeneration of sensory neurones. However, the fibres investigated in the present experiments grow at the very rapid rate of 5 to 6 mm/day, after an initial delay of about five days in the crush. The possibility that NGF affects the regeneration rate of more slowly growing fibres has not been excluded: information on this may become available from further examination of the histological material.

A more profitable approach might take the form of an investigation of the effect of NGF on regeneration of axons in the foetus, since this would be at a time when the sensory ganglia are believed to respond to NGF.

Acknowledgements

I should like to thank the Wellcome Research Laboratories for a generous supply of NGF, and the Central Research Fund of the University of London for an equipment grant.

References

Erlanger, J. & Gasser, H. S. (1937). *Electrical Signs of Nervous Activity*, Philadelphia: University of Pennsylvania Press.
Evans, C. A. N. & Saunders, N. R. (1967). *J. Physiol., Lond.* **192**, 79.
Gutmann, E. & Sanders, F. K. (1943). *J. Physiol., Lond.* **101**, 489.
Konorski, J. & Lubinska, L. (1946). *Lancet* **i**, 609.
Levi-Montalcini, R. & Angeletti, P. U. (1968). *Physiol. Rev.* **48**, 534.
Nathaniel, E. J. H. & Pease, D. C. (1963). *J. Ultrastruct. Res.* **9**, 533.
Oldendorf, W. H. & Davson, H. (1967). *Archs Neurol. Psychiat.* **17**, 196.
Sanders, F. K. & Whitteridge, D. (1946). *J. Physiol., Lond.* **105**, 152.
Sanders, F. K. & Young, J. Z. (1946). *J. exp. Biol.* **22**, 203.
Scott, D. Jr., Gutmann, E. & Horsky, P. (1966). *Science* **152**, 787.
Scott, D. Jr. & Liu, C. N. (1963). *Expl Neurol.* **8**, 279.
Scott, D. Jr. & Liu, C. N. (1964). *Progr. Brain Res.* **13**, 127.
Tinel, J. (1917). *Nerve Wounds*, London: Ballière, Tindall & Cox.

SECTION II

NGF-Antiserum

Effects of Immunosympathectomy on Biogenic Amines and Cholinesterases

GERDA I. KLINGMAN
and JACK D. KLINGMAN

Departments of Biochemical Pharmacology, School of Pharmacy and Biochemistry, School of Medicine, State University of New York at Buffalo, USA

We were introduced to the nerve growth factor (NGF) and its antiserum during the McCollum-Pratt Symposium at Johns Hopkins University in 1958 by Drs Rita Levi-Montalcini and Stanley Cohen. Since then we have considered the discovery of NGF and its antiserum one of the most fascinating developments of the two and a half decades that began with the publications by Dr Elmer D. Bueker (1948*a*, *b*).

In this paper we present a few highlights from studies which span a six-year period, from 1963 to 1969. The bovine NGF antiserum from Abbott Laboratories, Inc. was used to immunosympathectomize rats, 300 units/g per day being administered subcutaneously for five to six days, the first dose being given a few hours after birth. Sprague-Dawley Charles River descendent rats, bred and raised in our laboratories, were used. The effectiveness of the antiserum treatment was checked by making cell counts of the superior cervical ganglia and occasionally of other sympathetic ganglia. This dose schedule resulted in reproducible immunosympathectomy with residual cell populations in superior cervical ganglia of 7–12 per cent. Swiss Webster and DBA–1 mice were also used in some experiments.

Concentration and content of catecholamines and enzymes associated with catecholamine metabolism in peripheral tissues and sympathetic ganglia

In the course of these studies it became apparent that the postganglionic sympathetic cells were not uniformly destroyed by NGF-antiserum, since some tissues had lower residual noradrenaline concentrations and contents than had others. In the submaxillary glands 1.5 per cent, heart and ventricles 4–6 per cent, right atrium 14.1 per cent and left atrium 15.7 per cent of noradrenaline remained, while 30–40 per cent remained in the upper small intestine (duodenum and jejunum), liver and lungs (Klingman, 1964; 1965*a*).

Other investigators (Zaimis, Berk & Callingham, 1965; Visscher, Lee & Azuma, 1965; Iversen, Glowinski & Axelrod, 1966) made similar observations in antiserum-treated rats and mice. These studies were done with NGF-antiserum from the following sources: Zaimis and co-workers received antiserum from Dr Levi-Montalcini and Abbott Laboratories, Iversen and co-workers used bovine antiserum from Abbott Laboratories and Visscher and co-workers prepared their own NGF and NGF-antiserum by procedures adapted from Cohen (1960) and Levi-Montalcini & Angeletti (1961).

There is a misconception regarding the effect of the antiserum on the sympathetic innervation of the uterus. Contrary to various statements, the majority of these neurones are destroyed in rats and mice, since the uterine noradrenaline content of immunosympathectomized rats decreased to 20 per cent in our study (Klingman, 1965*a*), and to 15 per cent in the study of Iversen and co-workers (1966). The latter decrease was not statistically significant, owing to the fact that the standard errors were a third and a quarter of the means. In mice the uterine noradrenaline concentration decreased by 90 per cent after postnatal treatment with NGF-antiserum (Klingman & Klingman, 1967*a*).

The uptake *in vivo* of [^{3}H]noradrenaline by the uterus of immunosympathectomized mice and rats (Zaimis *et al.*, 1965; Sjöqvist, Titus, Michaelson, Taylor & Richardson, 1965; Iversen *et al.*, 1966) was no different from that of control animals when the total radioactivity or the specifically labelled noradrenaline was measured. These observations have probably contributed to the misconception. In only a few peripheral organs, such as the heart and the spleen, does good agreement exist between the uptake of labelled noradrenaline and the extent of sympathetic denervation as assessed by the residual amounts of noradrenaline. No such agreement was obtained with other peripheral tissues, notably the lungs, portions of intestine, submaxillary glands and uterus. The results from the latter tissues are more variable when different studies are compared (Levi-Montalcini & Angeletti, 1962; Klingman, 1965*a*; Klingman & Klingman, 1965; Iversen, Glowinski & Axelrod, 1965; Sjöqvist *et al.*, 1965; Visscher *et al.*, 1965; Zaimis *et al.*, 1965; Iversen *et al.*, 1966; Klingman & Klingman, 1967*a*).

These earlier studies left uncertain the effects of the antiserum on the catecholamines of the adrenal medulla. Some investigators reported increases (Carpi & Oliverio, 1964; Visscher *et al.*, 1965; Berk, Filipe & Zaimis, 1965; Iversen, quoted by Berk *et al.*, 1965), while others found no changes (Klingman, 1965*a*, Hamberger, Levi-Montalcini, Norberg & Sjöqvist, 1965; Klingman, 1966*b*; Iversen *et al.*, 1966; Klingman & Klingman, 1967*b*). The results of a recent study by Mueller, Thoenen & Axelrod (1969) may have resolved this controversy (see p. 130).

In rats and mice the central catecholamines were not affected by NGF (Crain & Wiegand, 1961) or by its antiserum (Levi-Montalcini & Angeletti, 1962; Klingman, 1964; 1965*a*; Zaimis *et al.*, 1965; Visscher *et al.*, 1965; Iversen *et al.*, 1966; Klingman, 1966*b*; Klingman & Klingman, 1967*a*). However, no exhaustive studies of discrete areas of the central nervous system have been made.

The activities of the various enzymes of catecholamine metabolism have been investigated in organs and ganglia from immunosympathectomized animals. Early in our studies, it became apparent that the non-specificity of the available assay procedures for enzymes such as monoamine oxidase and L-amino acid decarboxylase (dopa decarboxylase), would make such studies quite unproductive in terms of yielding information on the metabolism of the catecholamines in most intact and sympathetically denervated tissues. These assay procedures do not allow us to discriminate between the enzymes specifically involved in the endogenous metabolism of these amines and those enzymes which metabolize the same substrate but are not specifically involved in the amine metabolism.

Partial agreement was noted between the results of several studies of tissue monoamine oxidase activity after immunosympathectomy (Levi-Montalcini & Angeletti, 1962; Klingman, 1965*b*; 1966*a*; Iversen *et al.*, 1966) and surgical sympathectomy (Armin, Grant, Thompson & Tickner, 1953; Burn & Robinson, 1953; Burn, Philpot & Trendelenburg, 1954; Håkanson & Owman, 1965; Potter, Cooper, Willman & Wolfe, 1965; Snyder, Fischer & Axelrod, 1965; Nagatsu, Rust & De Quattro, 1969). In our study the monoamine oxidase activity decreased markedly in sympathetic ganglia and moderately in the spleen, submaxillary glands, kidneys and liver (Klingman, 1965*b*; 1966*a*). In the study by Iversen and co-workers (1966), using a different assay procedure and substrate, only the activity in the submaxillary glands was reduced, while the activity of the heart, jejunum, liver and brain was no different from that of controls.

After immunosympathectomy L-amino acid decarboxylase activity was reduced in sympathetic ganglia, submaxillary glands, spleen, uterus and right and left atria (Klingman, 1964; 1965*a*). A correlation was noted between the superior cervical and stellate ganglia in terms of residual cell populations, noradrenaline levels and enzyme activity (Table 1). These values, as percentages of controls, were 11.8 per cent, 8 per cent and 4.6 per cent for the superior cervical ganglion and 19.1 per cent, 17.2 per cent and 9.9 per cent for the stellate ganglion. Other data also suggested a possible correlation between the innervation (number of nerve endings), noradrenaline levels and L-amino acid decarboxylase activity. Thus, in control rats, the right atrium contained significantly more noradrenaline and the enzyme activity was three times greater than that of the left atrium. After immunosympathectomy the noradrenaline level and the decarboxylase activity of the right and left atrium decreased in proportion to the control values. Iversen and co-workers (1966) reported a reduction in L-amino acid decarboxylase activity in the submaxillary glands, heart and jejunum.

Table 1 Cell population and noradrenaline and L-amino acid decarboxylase activity of superior cervical and stellate ganglia of control and immunosympathectomized rats

Ganglion	*Number of rats*	*Cell population total number and* S.E.M.	*Number of rats*	*Noradrenaline ng/ ganglion (right) and* S.E.M.	*Number of rats*	L-*amino acid decarboxylase activity: dopamine formed/ hr/ ganglion (left) and* S.E.M.
Control, superior cervical	4	39 206 ± 499	7	29.8 ± 4.2	8	0.175 ± 0.015
Immunosympathectomized superior cervical	4	4643 ± 341[1]	7	2.4 ± 0.4[1]	8	0.008 ± 0.006[1]
Control, stellate	3	60 575 ± 5190	8	40.7 ± 3.8	6	0.243 ± 0.029
Immunosympathectomized stellate	4	11 586 ± 245[1]	8	7.0 ± 1.7[1]	6	0.024 ± 0.004[1]
Superior cervical, percentage of control	—	11.8	—	8.0	—	4.6
Stellate, percentage of control	—	19.1	—	17.2	—	9.9

[1] $P < 0.001$. (Klingman, 1965*a*; Klingman & Klingman, 1965.)

The localization of catechol-*O*-methyltransferase in peripheral tissues is almost exclusively extraneuronal, even though activity has been found in sympathetic ganglia (Axelrod, Albers & Clements, 1959; Klingman, 1965*b*) and other neuronal tissues (Axelrod *et al.*, 1959). For this reason, significant reductions could not be expected in peripheral organs after sympathectomy. After treatment with NGF-antiserum the activity in sympathetic ganglia was reduced when the activity was expressed in terms of tissue wet weight. When the activity was expressed in terms of the protein concentration of the supernatant (used in the assay procedure), the decrease was statistically not significant (Klingman, 1965*b*). In the study of Iversen and co-workers (1966) no statistically significant changes occurred in catechol-*O*-methyltransferase activity of the heart, submaxillary glands, jejunum, liver and brain from immunosympathectomized rats.

Iversen and co-workers (1966) presented evidence of decreased dopamine-β-hydroxylase activity in salivary glands, heart and jejunum of immunosympathectomized mice.

L-Tyrosine hydroxylase is the rate-controlling enzyme in the biosynthesis of the catecholamines. After chemical sympathectomy (6-hydroxydopamine) the activity of this enzyme doubled; and phenylethanolamine-*N*-methyltransferase activity increased slightly in rat adrenal glands (Mueller *et al.*, 1969). The increased activities of these enzymes in the presence of unchanged adrenal catecholamine concentrations indicates an increased turnover of catecholamine. This recent study by Mueller and co-workers (1969) brings to mind three observations reported by Iversen and co-workers (1966) which at that time could not be explained. In immunosympathectomized mice a 50 per cent reduction in the accumulation of [^{3}H]-noradrenaline and a doubling in the turnover of adrenal catecholamines were noted, while the concentration and content of catecholamines in the adrenals were unchanged. One may therefore speculate that immunosympathectomy produces similar increases in enzyme activity to chemical sympathectomy. The enhanced activity of the rate-controlling enzyme observed after chemical sympathectomy is probably a compensatory mechanism which together with the supersensitivity of sympathetically denervated tissues, could explain why animals with extensive sympathectomies (immunological, chemical or surgical) but intact adrenal medullae, function relatively normally under most conditions.

The NGF-antiserum and ontogenesis of the peripheral sympathetic nervous system

The potentiality of the NGF-antiserum for studying ontogenesis of the sympathetic nervous system was demonstrated several years ago (Klingman, 1966*b*; Klingman & Klingman, 1967*a*) but only a few investigations have been made so far. For example, Wragg and co-workers (Wragg, Machado & Machado, 1968; Machado, Machado & Wragg, 1969; Machado, Wragg & Machado, 1969) used the antiserum postnatally to explore the circadian rhythm of 5-hydroxytryptamine in the pineal gland of neonatal rats.

Several basic questions were answered in the course of our studies, in which mouse foetuses were exposed by maternal injection during several gestational periods to different dose levels of the NGF-antiserum (Klingman, 1966*b*; Klingman & Klingman, 1967*a*).

(1) The antibody seems to cross the placental barrier readily, at least during the later stages of gestation.

(2) Since the antiserum is capable of producing immunosympathectomy *in utero*, it is a suitable tool with which to study the embryonic development of the sympathetic nervous system.

(3) The destruction of postganglionic neurones *in utero* is similar in distribution and extent to but perhaps less severe than postnatal immunosympathectomy. However, this may be a matter of dose rather than an actual difference in effectiveness (Table 2).

(4) Sympathetic postganglionic neurones differed in their prenatal susceptibility to the antibody. For instance, the innervation of the spleen and the heart could be partially destroyed during the early stages of gestation (7–12 days), whereas the neurones that innervate the submaxillary glands and the uterus were not affected. The repair or regeneration of these developing neurones cannot be ruled out. Evidence accumulated during the past decade supports the view that the postganglionic neurones are more susceptible to the effect of NGF and its antibody at certain stages of neuronal development. However, our knowledge

Table 2 Noradrenaline (ng/g of wet weight and S.E.M.) in peripheral tissues of mice after prenatal and/or postnatal exposure to NGF-antiserum

	Prenatal (*900 units*) *Control*	*Prenatal* (*900 units*) *Antiserum*	*Postnatal* (*450 units*) *Control*	*Postnatal* (*450 units*) *Antiserum*	*Prenatal* (*900 units*) *and postnatal* (*450 units*) *Control*	*Prenatal* (*900 units*) *and postnatal* (*450 units*) *Antiserum*	*Prenatal* (*900 units*) *and postnatal* (*900 units*) *Control*	*Prenatal* (*900 units*) *and postnatal* (*900 units*) *Antiserum*
	(Group I)		(Group II)		(Group III)		(Group IV)	
Number of mice:	8	8	7	8	6	6	3	3
Tissues								
Brain	144	132	149	147	159	137	130	136
	±6	±12	±9	±12	±7	±8	±10	±15
Submaxillary glands	1572	771[2]	1495	225[1]	1711	10[1]	1315	12[1]
	±151	±124	±141	±12	±168	±4	±94	±2
Heart	494	74[1]	467	10[1]	533	8[1]	467	0
	±45	±18	±38	±5	±57	±6	±51	
Spleen	117	3[1]	93	0	116	0	83	0
	±24	±2	±14		±29		±12	
Small intestine	180	48[1]	171	26[1]	201	4[1]	138	0
	±17	±13	±17	±9	±11	±4	±15	
Kidneys	164	114	173	40[2]	184	62[2]	183	12[2]
	±20	±23	±31	±12	±36	±21	±27	±7
Uterus (no. of mice)	271	206	249	23	241	38[2]	318	0
	±48 (2)	±0 (2)	±69 (2)	±23 (2)	±41 (3)	±24 (3)	(1)	(1)
Adrenal glands (μg/pair)	5.09	3.98	5.43	4.86	4.98	3.29	6.40	5.25
	±0.66	±0.47	±0.66	±0.49	±0.62	±0.42	±1.12	±0.83

[1] $P < 0.001$. [2] $P < 0.01$.

The concentrations of adrenaline were significantly decreased in the spleen (Groups I, II, III and IV), submaxillary glands (Groups II and III), heart (Groups I, II and III), small intestine (Groups III and IV) and uterus (Groups III and IV). (Klingman & Klingman, 1967*a*.)

of the actual duration of susceptibility of sympathetic postganglionic neurones is fragmentary. The period of susceptibility seems to be longer for the neurones that innervate the spleen and the heart than for neurones innervating the submaxillary glands and the uterus. Half the neurones innervating the spleen and 25 per cent of the neurones innervating the heart were destroyed during the earliest dose schedule (7–12 days), whereas innervation to other tissues apparently remained intact. The neurones that innervate the spleen and the heart were also susceptible postnatally. The postganglionic innervation of the submaxillary glands was affected during the later stages of gestation but maximum destruction was only achieved with postnatal treatment. This problem of susceptibility has not been studied systematically and many questions remain unanswered.

(5) The antiserum showed greater overall effectiveness near term.

(6) Maximum destruction of postganglionic sympathetic neurones was achieved by combining pre- and postnatal treatment with relatively large doses of antiserum, but even then residual cell populations persisted in ganglia (Table 3).

(7) Exposure of mice *in utero* to large doses of antiserum for three days resulted in more pronounced effects than did exposure to smaller doses for six days.

(8) With the doses used and the gestational periods investigated in these two studies, the central adrenergic neurones and the cells of the adrenal medulla were not affected by the prenatal antiserum treatment, as assessed by their catecholamine concentration and content. It must be emphasized that only the catecholamines of whole brain (minus the cerebellum) or the brainstem were measured. No attempts were made to measure the amines in specific brain areas; and thus, only large changes could be detected by such a gross sampling. We cannot rule out the possibility of a small change in large areas, or a substantial change in small areas, of central adrenergic representation.

Table 3 Total cell counts and S.E.M. of sympathetic ganglia from control and NGF-antiserum-treated mice

Ganglion	No. of mice	Control		No. of mice	NGF-antiserum treatment: Prenatal (Group I)		No. of mice	Postnatal (Group II)		No. of mice	Prenatal & postnatal (Group III)		No. of mice	Prenatal & postnatal (Group IV)	
Superior cervical (right)	5	14 248	±814	5	2630	±280	4	1965	±599	4	281	±17	3	467	±267
Superior cervical (left)	4	14 783	±681	5	3445	±328	4	2116	±806	4	257	±26	2	346	±82
Stellate (right)	4	18 556	±732	4	3547	±481	4	1487	±169	3	552	±98	3	865	±33
Stellate (left)	3	19 479	±1104	5	3320	±779	4	1528	±307	4	514	±57	3	944	±63
Superior mesenteric	3	25 175	±1964	4	7571	±1549	4	3358	±430	4	2053	±258	2	1924	±191
Coeliac	1	25 515		2	6559	±439	1	4030			—	—	1	1553	
Cardiac	2	10 888	±1944	2	2420	±62	2	452	±173	2	266	±21		—	—

Group I: prenatal: 900 units/g, subcutaneously, on 15th, 16th and 17th day of gestation. Group II: postnatal: 450 units/g, subcutaneously, on days 1–6. Group III: prenatal: same as Group I and postnatal: same as Group II. Group IV: prenatal: same as Group I and postnatal: 900 units/g, subcutaneously, on days 1–6. (Klingman & Klingman, 1967*a*.)

5-Hydroxytryptamine

Immunosympathectomy has a poorly understood effect on the peripheral levels of 5-hydroxytryptamine. We viewed our initial results on the peripheral tissue levels of 5-hydroxytryptamine in 1963–4 with scepticism. However, in 1965, Hamberger and co-workers published their observations on the increased 5-hydroxytryptamine fluorescence in mast cells and enterochromaffin cells of the intestinal mucosa from immunosympathectomized rats. Other tissues were not affected. A year later, Iversen and co-workers (1966) reported a 57 per cent increase in concentrations of intestinal 5-hydroxytryptamine in immunosympathectomized mice.

Our data (Klingman, 1969) showed significant elevations in the submaxillary glands, heart and caecum; and a trend toward increased amounts in several other tissues (uterus, lungs and portions of the small intestine). Clear-cut effects in the latter three tissues could not be obtained; the problem of the notoriously variable tissue levels frequently encountered with this amine was complicated by an occasional erratic observation. Since the biological function of this amine, and particularly of the peripherally located amine, is not known and is largely a matter of personal preference and interpretation, we felt that most would be gained by investigating whether the antiserum *per se* or the effects of sympathectomy were responsible for the increased levels of amine (Klingman & Klingman, 1969*b*). This was achieved by performing surgical unilateral and bilateral superior cervical ganglionectomies. Several weeks after ganglionectomy, the three amines, noradrenaline, adrenaline and 5-hydroxytryptamine were measured in the submaxillary glands (Table 4). The 5-hydroxytryptamine concentration and content of the denervated glands were significantly increased and this increase was of a similar magnitude to that seen in the submaxillary glands of immunosympathectomized rats.

Thompson and Campbell (Thompson, 1967; Thompson & Campbell, 1966; 1968) have investigated in greater detail intestinal 5-hydroxytryptamine after immunosympathectomy. The mucosal amine concentrations of the stomach and the small intestine (except upper duodenum) were markedly increased in

Table 4 Effects of immunosympathectomy and unilateral superior cervical ganglionectomy on the weight and on the content of 5-hydroxytryptamine, noradrenaline and adrenaline of the submaxillary glands of rats

	Control (2 lobes)	*Immunosympathectomy (2 lobes)*	*Percentage of control value*	*Control (1 lobe)*	*Ganglionectomy (1 lobe)*	*Percentage of control value*
Number of rats	17	17	—	16	16	—
Body weight, g ±S.E.M.	460 ±29	415 ±22	90.2	281 ±14	281 ±14	—
Tissue weight, mg ±S.E.M.	659 ±30	473 ±23	71.8[1]	235 ±8	216 ±7	91.9
Ratio of tissue weight/body weight, mg/g ± S.E.M.	1.49 ±0.07	1.17 ±0.06	78.5[2]	0.83 ±0.02	0.77 ±0.02	92.8[4]
5-Hydroxytryptamine, μg/tissue ±S.E.M.	0.85 ±0.09	1.19 ±0.14	140.0[4]	0.25 ±0.02	0.39 ±0.05	156.0[3]
5-Hydroxytryptamine, μg/g ± S.E.M.	1.29 ±0.13	2.51 ±0.29	194.6[1]	1.07 ±0.08	1.85 ±0.26	172.9[2]
Noradrenaline, μg/g ±S.E.M.	1.94 ±0.26(7)[5]	0.03 ±0.01(7)[5]	1.5[1]	1.91 ±0.09	0.06 ±0.02	3.1[1]
Adrenaline, μg/g ±S.E.M.	0.20 ±0.03(7)[5]	0.07 ±0.01(7)[5]	35.0[2]	0.13 ±0.02	0.05 ±0.02	38.5[3]

[1] $P < 0.001$. [2] $P < 0.01$. [3] $P < 0.02$. [4] $P < 0.05$. [5] Number of rats ( ).

(Klingman, 1969; Klingman & Klingman, 1969*b*.)

immunosympathectomized mice, while those of the colon, rectum and upper duodenum showed only statistically insignificant increases (Thompson & Campbell, 1966). Immunosympathectomy did not increase the argentaffin cell population of the gastrointestinal mucosa; and Thompson concluded that the increased amounts of amine were due to an increased 5-hydroxytryptamine concentration per cell (Thompson, 1967). Subsequently, Thompson & Campbell (1968) found the increased amine levels in portions of the intestine of immunosympathectomized mice to be associated with the particulate-bound fraction.

Ganglionic cholinesterases

The persistence of small numbers of sympathetic ganglionic cells in rats and mice treated with NGF-antiserum has not been satisfactorily explained. When larger numbers, such as 15–25 per cent in the superior cervical ganglion, escape destruction by the antiserum, a variety of contributing factors are probably responsible, such as failure to select a maximally effective dose schedule (i.e. time period of greatest susceptibility, adequate and repeated doses) and the species specificity of certain antisera. However, even when these conditions are satisfied, a few hundred or even a thousand cells survive. This was demonstrated in our studies of pre- and postnatal antiserum treatment; doubling the postnatal dose subsequently to prenatal treatment did not decrease the number of surviving cells (Klingman & Klingman, 1967*a*; see Table 3).

The percentage of surviving cells in sympathetic ganglia of rats and mice was similar in size to the cell population designated as cholinergic sympathetic cells in cat superior cervical and stellate ganglia. We, therefore, tentatively postulated that the cells persisting after immunosympathectomy were the cholinergic sympathetic cells. After the first few control ganglia from rats had been examined, it became obvious that the distribution of acetylcholinesterase in the postganglionic cell bodies differed from that in cats in the proportion of cells with marked, moderate and slight acetylcholinesterase activity (Holmstedt & Sjöqvist, 1959; Fredricsson & Sjöqvist, 1962; Sjöqvist, 1963*a*, *b*). In cat stellate ganglia, cells with marked acetylcholinesterase activity were identified by Sjöqvist (1963*a*) as cholinergic sympathetic

Table 5 Distribution of acetylcholinesterase (AChE) in sympathetic ganglia of control and immunosympathectomized rats

Ganglion cells	*Ganglion number*	GANGLION *Superior cervical*	*Stellate*	*Thoracic chain*	*Superior mesenteric*	*Coeliac*	*Cardiac (abdominal)*
CONTROL:							
Total number	1	35 551	38 464	7 748	15 580	15 908	14 980
	2	32 184			15 021		12 716
With marked	1	10 619	7 271	2 032	2 720	2 760	3 048
AChE activity	2	8 838			2 515		4 332
With slight	1	2 203	1 449	432	1 344	976	724
AChE activity	2	2 968			1 508		648
With moderate	1	22 741	29 760	5 284	11 516	12 172	11 208
AChE activity[1]	2	20 378			10 998		7 736
IMMUNOSYMPATHECTOMY:							
Total number	1	2 759	4 116	436	7 800	2 294	752
	2	2 548			5 902		694
With marked	1	1 340	337	196	288	412	124
AChE activity	2	1 206			348		151
With slight	1	332	103	48	580	316	204
AChE activity	2	203			432		140
With moderate	1	1 087	3 679	192	6 932	1 566	424
AChE activity[1]	2	1 139			5 122		303

[1] This category of cells was not counted. The 'counts' listed were obtained by difference, from other counts. (Klingman, 1967; 1970.)

cells. In contrast to sympathetic ganglia from rats (Klingman, 1967; 1970), cells with slight acetylcholinesterase activity predominate in cat ganglia, and cells with marked acetylcholinesterase activity are rare in the abdominal sympathetic ganglionic complexes of the cat.

After immunosympathectomy in rats the persisting cells of the superior cervical, stellate, thoracic chain, superior mesenteric, coeliac and cardiac ganglia represented random cell populations in terms of intracellular acetylcholinesterase activity (Table 5). Cells of each of the three types were destroyed and cells of each type survived the antiserum treatment. Cells with marked acetylcholinesterase activity did not show a unique capacity for survival (Klingman, 1967; 1970).

The activities of acetyl- and pseudocholinesterases were measured quantitatively by a differential assay (Klingman, Klingman & Poliszczuk, 1968) in the superior cervical, stellate, thoracic chain, superior mesenteric, coeliac and cardiac ganglia from immunosympathectomized rats and their control littermates (Klingman & Klingman, 1967*b*; Klingman & Klingman, 1969*a*). The specific activity (per g wet weight) of acetylcholinesterase was reduced to 14 per cent in superior cervical (right and left), 31 per cent in stellate (right and left), 47 per cent in thoracic chain, 19 per cent in cardiac, 34 per cent in coeliac and 56 per cent in superior mesenteric ganglia.

The specific activity of the pseudocholinesterases was reduced to 31 per cent in superior cervical, 35 per cent in stellate, 48 per cent in thoracic chain, 35 per cent in cardiac, 57 per cent in coeliac and 53 per cent in superior mesenteric ganglia. The activities of acetyl- and pseudocholinesterases in the cervical sympathetic trunk were 27 and 40 per cent of control values, respectively (Table 6).

In the superior cervical ganglion, the reduction of acetylcholinesterase activity after immunosympathectomy was greater than was to be anticipated from previous studies of residual cell populations (Levi-Montalcini & Angeletti, 1962; Klingman & Klingman, 1965; Levi-Montalcini & Angeletti, 1966; Klingman, 1967; Klingman & Klingman, 1967*a*, *b*) and from cell counts made in the study. Less than 10 per cent of the cells persisted in superior cervical ganglia (Klingman & Klingman, 1969*a*). By

Table 6 Total cholinesterase (*ChE*), acetylcholinesterase (*AChE*) and pseudocholinesterase (*PChE*) activities (μmol of substrate hydrolysed/min/g ± S.E.M.) of sympathetic ganglia of control (C) and immunosympathectomized (IM) rats

Ganglia	*Treatment*	*Number of ganglia*	*Wet weight mg*	*Total ChE*	*AChE*	*PChE*
Superior cervical, right	C	6	2.06 ± 0.21	28.8 ± 3.3	18.5 ± 2.1	8.6 ± 1.2
	IM	6	0.48 ± 0.04[1]	5.5 ± 0.9[1]	2.4 ± 0.5[1]	2.8 ± 0.5[2]
Superior cervical, left	C	7	1.86 ± 0.15	38.5 ± 5.5	23.6 ± 3.5	11.8 ± 1.2
	IM	7	0.44 ± 0.02[1]	7.7 ± 0.9[1]	3.7 ± 0.7[1]	3.6 ± 0.7[1]
Stellate, right	C	5	2.53 ± 0.14	32.2 ± 4.3	20.0 ± 4.2	9.2 ± 0.9
	IM	5	1.21 ± 0.19[1]	10.1 ± 1.9[2]	5.9 ± 1.6[3]	3.3 ± 0.2[1]
Stellate, left	C	6	2.50 ± 0.16	37.0 ± 2.8	21.4 ± 1.8	10.7 ± 1.1
	IM	6	1.48 ± 0.18[1]	12.0 ± 1.5[1]	6.5 ± 0.7[1]	3.7 ± 0.5[2]
Thoracic chain[5]	C	5	2.48 ± 0.38	16.0 ± 2.6	8.7 ± 1.2	6.4 ± 1.1
	IM	5	1.13 ± 0.11[1]	7.7 ± 1.1[3]	4.1 ± 0.9[3]	3.1 ± 0.6[4]
Superior mesenteric	C	5	2.28 ± 0.21	32.5 ± 7.4	18.2 ± 4.1	10.5 ± 1.5
	IM	4	1.71 ± 0.39	17.8 ± 5.1	10.2 ± 3.0	5.6 ± 2.1
Coeliac	C	3	2.09 ± 0.11	20.0 ± 3.3	13.1 ± 2.1	5.6 ± 0.9
	IM	3	0.78 ± 0.12[2]	8.0 ± 2.5[4]	4.4 ± 2.1[4]	3.2 ± 0.1[4]
Cardiac	C	4	2.34 ± 0.56	13.4 ± 3.0	7.0 ± 2.0	6.2 ± 1.5
	IM	4	1.08 ± 0.21	3.6 ± 0.2[3]	1.3 ± 0.3[4]	2.2 ± 0.3[4]
Cervical sympathetic trunks	C	6	1.50 ± 0.16[6]	11.0 ± 2.5	7.4 ± 1.8	3.0 ± 0.6
	IM	6	1.36 ± 0.20[6]	3.5 ± 1.1[3]	2.0 ± 0.7[3]	1.2 ± 0.3[4]

[1] $P < 0.001$. [2] $P < 0.01$. [3] $P < 0.02$. [4] $P < 0.05$.

[5] Three ganglia from the right and left thoracic chain caudally to the stellate ganglion were pooled; the thoracic sympathetic trunk was included.

[6] Weight of the sample.

(Klingman & Klingman, 1967*b*; 1969*a*.)

means of axotomy and decentralization, we verified that approximately half the acetylcholinesterase activity in superior cervical ganglia from control rats is associated with the postganglionic, and the other half with the preganglionic, elements. If the NGF-antiserum had destroyed 90 per cent of the postganglionic neurones without affecting preganglionic elements, over half of the acetylcholinesterase activity should be present in superior cervical ganglia from immunosympathectomized rats. However, only 13–15 per cent of the enzyme activity was demonstrable. This suggested that not only the postganglionic but also the preganglionic elements were affected by the antiserum treatment. The reduction of the acetyl- and pseudocholinesterase activities in the cervical sympathetic trunks of immunosympathectomized rats strongly supports this conclusion.

This effect on the preganglionic neurones was not unexpected. We have consistently noted thinner cervical sympathetic trunks in rats treated with NGF-antiserum by comparison with their control littermates. Berk and co-workers (1965) also mentioned a paucity of preganglionic fibres in immunosympathectomized rats, but they did not state the extent of the reduction. From the residual enzyme activity in other sympathetic ganglia, such as the stellate, cardiac and coeliac, it may be deduced that the preganglionic elements of these ganglia have been similarly affected. It would be more difficult to provide experimental proof, since these ganglia are less uniform and less accessible than is the superior cervical ganglion.

According to Dr Levi-Montalcini (personal communication) and Levi-Montalcini & Angeletti (1960), the preganglionic sympathetic cells from NGF-treated chick embryos with highly hypertrophied and hyperplastic sympathetic ganglia were not increased in size or number. Consequently, a direct effect of the NGF antiserum on the preganglionic sympathetic neurones seems unlikely and we have tentatively interpreted this effect as an example of a retrograde transneuronal degeneration resulting from the absence of over 90 per cent of the postganglionic neurones (Klingman & Klingman, 1967*b*; 1969*a*).

Table 7 (*a* and *b*) is a synthesis of the results from our studies of the superior cervical ganglion of immunosympathectomized rats and their control littermates. It represents an attempt to

Table 7*a* Tissue weight, cell population, action potential and dopa decarboxylase and monoamine oxidase activities of superior cervical ganglia from control and immunosympathectomized rats

Treatment	*Weight of ganglion pair mg*	*Number of cells in ganglion*	*Action potential: peak-to-peak amplitude μV*
Number of rats	7	4	10
Control	4.6 ± 0.3	39 206 ± 499	587 ± 53
Immunosympathectomy	1.3 ± 0.2	4 643 ± 341	78 ± 12
Percentage of control value	28.3	11.8	13.3

Treatment	*Dopamine decarboxylase activity: μmol dopamine formed/h/ganglion*	*Monoamine oxidase activity: nmol indoleacetic acid formed/h/ganglion pair*	
		No ADH[1]	*ADH*[1]
Number of rats	8	5	7
Control	0.175 ± 0.015	5.6 ± 1.9	71.6 ± 10.6
Immunosympathectomy	0.008 ± 0.006	0.3 ± 0.1	6.2 ± 1.8
Percentage of control value	4.6	5.4	8.7

[1] Assayed with and without exogenous aldehyde dehydrogenase.
The results from immunosympathectomized rats are statistically different from those of the controls (Klingman, 1964; 1965*a*; 1965*b*; 1966; Klingman & Klingman, 1965.)

correlate anatomical integrity (cell populations; intact compared to immunosympathectomy) with physiological function (action potential) and biochemical parameters (activities of monoamine oxidase, dopa decarboxylase, catechol-*O*-methyltransferase, acetylcholinesterase, pseudocholinesterase, noradrenaline and adrenaline concentration and content). It is reassuring that one can take fragments of results from eight studies, done during a six-year period with different batches of rats and antiserum and other variables, and obtain such a picture of uniformity. At the same time this composite table represents a challenge. There are many missing data and links that need to be added before we can understand the functioning of a relatively simple neuronal unit, the sympathetic ganglion.

Table 7*b* The noradrenaline and adrenaline content, and catechol-*O*-methyltransferase (*COMT*), total cholinesterase (*ChE*), acetylcholinesterase (*AChE*) and pseudocholinesterase (*PChE*) activities of superior cervical ganglia from control and immunosympathectomized rats

Treatment	*Noradrenaline* μg/g[2]	*Adrenaline* μg/g[2]	*COMT activity: μmol normetadrenaline formed/h/g supernatant protein*[1,2]	*μmol substrate hydrolysed/min/g* *ChE*	*AChE*	*PChE*
Number of rats	7	7	10	6	6	6
Control	13.9 ± 1.5	2.3 ± 1.1	3.71 ± 0.63	28.8 ± 3.3	18.5 ± 2.1	8.6 ± 1.2
Immunosympathectomy	6.9 ± 2.1	2.9 ± 0.6	2.93 ± 0.58	5.5 ± 0.9	2.4 ± 0.5	2.8 ± 0.5
Percentage of control value	49.6	126.1	79.0	19.1	13.0	32.6

Treatment	*Noradrenaline (ng/ganglion pair)*	*Adrenaline (ng/ganglion pair)*	*COMT activity: nmol normetadrenaline formed/h/ganglia*[1,2]	*nmol substrate hydrolysed/min/ganglia*[2] *ChE*	*AChE*	*PChE*
Number of rats	7	7	10	6	6	6
Control	62.5 ± 6.0	1.1 ± 0.5	10.00 ± 1.99	58.6 ± 6.3	37.4 ± 4.1	17.0 ± 1.9
Immunosympathectomy	7.4 ± 1.2	3.1 ± 0.4	4.39 ± 1.11	2.6 ± 0.4	1.1 ± 0.2	1.2 ± 0.2
Percentage of control value	11.8	281.8	43.9	4.4	2.9	7.1

[1] Pooled sympathetic ganglia.

The results from immunosympathectomized rats are statistically different from those of the controls, except for *COMT* activity: μmol normetadrenaline formed/h/g supernatant protein and adrenaline, μg/g (Klingman & Klingman, 1965; 1967*b*; 1969*a*; and [2] unpublished observations).

Acknowledgements

The research was supported by the following grants: (G.I.K.): AM-05694 from the National Institute of Arthritis and Metabolic Diseases, USPHS, (1962–8), NS–08349 from the National Institute of Neurological Diseases and Stroke, USPHS, (1968 to present) and Career Development Award K3-GM-5352, NIH, Division of General Medical Sciences, USPHS, (1962–7); (J.D.K.): NB-03697 from the National Institute of Neurological Diseases and Blindness, USPHS and NS-03697 from the National Institute of Neurological Diseases and Stroke, USPHS.

References

Armin, J., Grant, R. T., Thompson, R. H. S. & Tickner, A. (1953). *J. Physiol., Lond.* **121**, 603.

Axelrod, J., Albers, W. & Clements, C. D. (1959). *J. Neurochem.* **5**, 68.

Berk, L., Filipe, I. & Zaimis, E. (1965). *J. Physiol., Lond.* **177**, 1P.

Bueker, E. D. (1948*a*). *Anat. Rec.* **100**, 735.

Bueker, E. D. (1948*b*). *Anat. Rec.* **102**, 369.

Burn, J. H., Philpot, F. J. & Trendelenburg, U. (1954). *Br. J. Pharmac.* **9**, 423.

Burn, J. H. & Robinson, J. (1953). *J. Physiol., Lond.* **120**, 224.

Carpi, A. & Oliverio, A. (1964). *Int. J. Neuro-pharmacol.* **3**, 427.

Cohen, S. (1960). *Proc. natn. Acad. Sci. U.S.A.* **46**, 302.

Crain, S. M. & Wiegand, R. G. (1961). *Proc. Soc. exp. Biol Med.* **107**, 663.

Fredricsson, B. & Sjöqvist, F. (1962). *Acta. morph. neerl.-scand.* **5**, 140.

Håkanson, R. & Owman, C. (1965). *J. Neurochem.* **12**, 417.

Hamberger, B., Levi-Montalcini, R., Norberg, K.-A. & Sjöqvist, F. (1965). *Int. J. Neuro-pharmacol.* **4**, 91.

Holmstedt, B. & Sjöqvist, F. (1959). *Acta physiol. scand.* **47**, 284.

Iversen, L. L., Glowinski, J. & Axelrod, J. (1965). *Nature, Lond.* **206**, 1222.

Iversen, L. L., Glowinski, J. & Axelrod, J. (1966). *J. Pharmac. exp. Ther.* **151**, 273.

Klingman, G. I. (1964). *Fed. Proc.* **23**, 455.

Klingman, G. I. (1965*a*). *J. Pharmac. exp. Ther.* **148**, 14.

Klingman, G. I. (1965*b*). *Pharmacologist* **7**, 157.

Klingman, G. I. (1966*a*). *Biochem. Pharmac.* **15**, 1729.

Klingman, G. I. (1966*b*). *Int. J. Neuro-pharmacol.* **5**, 163.

Klingman, G. I. (1967). In *First Int. Meeting of Neurochemistry. Abstracts of Communications*, Strasbourg, France. p. 116.

Klingman, G. I. (1969). *Biochem. Pharmac.* **18**, 2061.

Klingman, G. I. (1970). *J. Pharmac. exp. Ther.* **173**, 205.
Klingman, G. I. & Klingman, J. D. (1965). *Life Sci.* **4**, 2171.
Klingman, G. I. & Klingman, J. D. (1967*a*). *Int. J. Neuro-pharmacol.* **6**, 501.
Klingman, G. I. & Klingman, J. D. (1967*b*). *Fed. Proc.* **26**, 618.
Klingman, G. I. & Klingman, J. D. (1969*a*). *J. Neurochem.* **16**, 261.
Klingman, G. I. & Klingman, J. D. (1969*b*). *Biochem. Pharmac.* **18**, 2069.
Klingman, G. I., Klingman, J. D. & Poliszczuk, A. (1968). *J. Neurochem.* **15**, 1121.
Levi-Montalcini, R. & Angeletti, P. U. (1960). In *Regional Neurochemistry, Proc. Fourth Int. Neurochemical Symp.*, p. 362. Ed. by Kety, S. S. & Elkes, J. New York: Pergamon Press.
Levi-Montalcini, R. & Angeletti, P. U. (1961). *Q. Rev. Biol.* **36**, 99.
Levi-Montalcini, R. & Angeletti, P. U. (1962). *Int. J. Neuro-pharmacol.* **1**, 161.
Levi-Montalcini, R. & Angeletti, P. U. (1966). *Pharmac. Rev.* **18**, 619.
Machado, C. R. S., Machado, A. B. M. & Wragg, L. E. (1969). *Endocrinology* **85**, 846.
Machado, C. R. S., Wragg, L. E. & Machado, A. B. M. (1969). *Science, N.Y.* **164**, 442.
Mueller, R. A., Thoenen, H. & Axelrod, J. (1969). *Science, N.Y.* **163**, 468.
Nagatsu, T., Rust, L. A. & De Quattro, V. (1969). *Biochem. Pharmac.* **18**, 1441.
Potter, L. T., Cooper, T., Willman, V. L. & Wolfe, D. E. (1965). *Circulation Res.* **16**, 468.
Sjöqvist, F. (1963*a*). *Acta physiol. scand.* **57**, 339.
Sjöqvist, F. (1963*b*). *Acta physiol. scand.* **57**, 352.
Sjöqvist, F., Titus, E., Michaelson, I. A., Taylor, P. Jr. & Richardson, K. C. (1965). *Life Sci.* **4**, 1125.
Snyder, S. H., Fischer, J. & Axelrod, J. (1965). *Biochem. Pharmac.* **14**, 363.
Thompson, J. H. (1967). *Archs Path.* **83**, 415.
Thompson, J. H. & Campbell, L. B. (1966). *J. Pharm. Pharmac.* **18** (Suppl.), 753.
Thompson, J. H. & Campbell, L. B. (1968). *Biochem. Pharmac.* **17**, 175.
Visscher, M. B., Lee, Y. C. P. & Azuma, T. (1965). *Proc. Soc. exp. Biol. Med.* **119**, 1232.
Wragg, L. E., Machado, C. R. S. & Machado, A. B. M. (1968). *Anat. Rec.* **160**, 453.
Zaimis, E., Berk, L. & Callingham, B. A. (1965). *Nature, Lond.* **206**, 1220.

Immunosympathectomy: A Method for Studying the Neural Control of Adipose Tissue Metabolism

GEORGE STEINER and EDOUARD SCHÖNBAUM

Departments of Medicine, Physiology and Pharmacology, University of Toronto, Canada

For many years our group has been interested in examining the role of the sympathetic nervous system in regulating adipose tissue metabolism. We have felt that if this study is to have any functional meaning we must aim to learn the physiological effects of the sympathetic nervous system in the whole animal. With this aim in mind the following general plan was chosen. The basic metabolic behaviour of the tissue under study was to be examined first. Secondly, the effect of chronic sympathetic hyperactivity on the tissue's metabolism was to be explored. In order to do this, we had to find a physiological method of producing chronic sympathetic hyperactivity. Thirdly, we wanted to determine whether an interruption of the sympathetic nerve supply to adipose tissue would prevent the changes previously observed. In undertaking this third phase of the project we examined several techniques by which the sympathetic nervous system could be interrupted. One of these techniques was immunosympathectomy. Our purpose in this paper will be to review our studies; to indicate the role played by immunosympathectomy in assisting us to come to our conclusions; and to point out that, from the physiological viewpoint, one cannot describe the function of the sympathetic nervous system either by any methods used *in vitro* or by examining the influence of injected noradrenaline.

Brown and white adipose tissue

We chose to concentrate our studies on adipose tissue since its pattern of metabolism *in vitro* is profoundly affected by added catecholamines (Himms-Hagen, 1967; Steiner & Cahill, 1966; Schönbaum, Steiner & Sellers, 1970). We undertook to explore two different forms of adipose tissue, white and brown. The former is the tissue usually thought of as adipose tissue. It consists of well-described unilocular cells containing 80–5 per cent lipid, of which close to 99 per cent is triglyceride (Jeanrenaud, 1965). Brown adipose tissue, by contrast, is a peculiar form of adipose tissue whose lipid is stored in multilocular cells containing 62 per cent lipid, of which 95 per cent is triglyceride and 5 per cent phospholipid (Steiner & Cahill, 1964). This tissue is found in all neonatal mammals and persists into adulthood in hibernators and certain rodents (for general reviews see Lindberg, 1970; Smith & Horwitz, 1969). It is capable of producing heat and this has been shown to be of considerable importance, at least in the newborn and in the hibernator during arousal.

The two tissues differ in some of their metabolic behaviour. Although noradrenaline stimulates lipolysis in both tissues, its effect on glucose utilization *in vitro* by white adipose tissue differs from that in brown adipose tissue (Steiner & Cahill, 1966). These effects are summarized in Table 1. Adding noradrenaline to the incubation flasks leads to an increase in the recovery of glucose-^{14}C in glyceride glycerol in white adipose tissue, but does not alter the recovery of label in glyceride glycerol of brown adipose tissue. It does not alter the recovery of ^{14}C in white adipose tissue fatty acids, but it decreases this in brown adipose tissue. The presence of noradrenaline leads to an increase in the production of $^{14}CO_2$ from glucose by white adipose tissue and a decrease in that produced by brown adipose tissue. These effects of noradrenaline on glucose metabolism are probably a consequence of the elevated intracellular concentration of free fatty acids. In part, the differences between the effects of this on glucose utilization by the two tissues may result from the presence of glycerol kinase in brown but not in white adipose tissue. The biochemical basis of these differences is more fully described elsewhere (Steiner & Cahill, 1966; Schönbaum *et al.*, 1970).

Table 1 The effect of noradrenaline on glucose utilization

	Recovery of ^{14}C *as percentage of control*	
	Brown adipose tissue	*White adipose tissue*
CO_2	60 ± 10	192 ± 22
Total lipid	58 ± 8	211 ± 37
Glyceride glycerol	100 ± 2	266 ± 24
Fatty acid	15 ± 15	102 ± 40

Slices of rat brown or epididymal white adipose tissue were incubated in Krebs-Ringer bicarbonate buffer with 4 per cent human serum albumin and [U-^{14}C] glucose (5 mM) for 90 min at 37°C under O_2:CO_2 (95:5). Noradrenaline (10^{-4}M) was added to half the flasks. Recovery of ^{14}C was measured in the end products listed. Data were calculated as percentage of control and expressed as mean ± S.E.M. (Adapted from Steiner and Cahill, 1966.)

Despite the differences in response to noradrenaline the tissues have a similar response to insulin (Steiner & Cahill, 1966). In both tissues there is an increase in the conversion of glucose to CO_2, total lipids, fatty acids, glyceride glycerol and glycogen (Table 2). This was shown to be a consequence of an increase in the tissue's uptake of glucose.

Table 2 The effect of insulin on glucose utilization by brown adipose tissue

	Glucose recovery μmol/mg N	
	Control	*Insulin*
CO_2	116 ± 9	492 ± 66
Total lipids	98 ± 2	489 ± 22
Fatty acids	43 ± 6	298 ± 63
Glyceride glycerol	55 ± 6	174 ± 16
Glycogen	18 ± 2	291 ± 40

Rat brown adipose tissue slices incubated as in Table 1. Insulin (10 mU/ml) was added to half the flasks. Data expressed as μmoles glucose recovered/mg N ± S.E.M. (Adapted from Steiner and Cahill, 1966.)

Cold-acclimatization: a method of producing sympathetic hyperactivity

Although studies *in vitro* in which hormones are added to incubating tissues provide much information, they do not allow one to examine the physiological role of the sympathetic neurotransmitter, noradrenaline. To do this one must explore the metabolic effects of noradrenaline released from sympathetic nerve endings. Although this can be done by isolating and electrically stimulating a nerve supplying a particular fat pad (Correll, 1963), we chose not to use this technique. Such a stimulus is too acute, it may not be specific for sympathetic fibres and it may have to be so large as to raise the possibility of non-specific effects. We preferred to use a situation in which the total sympathetic activity is increased and in which this is of long duration and otherwise compatible with normal life. We therefore chose as a model the cold-acclimatized rat (Schönbaum *et al.*, 1970). Cold-acclimatization is a state of homeostatic balance which is achieved in the rat that has lived at 4°C for four weeks. By this time the rat produces heat at a rate equal to the heat loss, and sufficient to maintain its body temperature at 37°C. It does so without shivering and hence this form of thermogenesis is called non-shivering thermogenesis. It has been well demonstrated that this state is associated with sympathetic hyperactivity. Leduc (1961) showed that noradrenaline turnover is increased in cold-acclimatized rats. Shum, Johnson & Flattery (1969) have also demonstrated that the excretion of noradrenaline and its metabolites is increased in rats acclimatized to cold (Fig. 1). Interestingly, they also found that adrenaline excretion is not markedly changed in cold-acclimatization, which suggested that this model was ideally suited for our studies.

Cold-acclimatization and brown adipose tissue metabolism

We next examined the changes in composition and metabolism of brown and white adipose tissue occurring as a result of cold-acclimatization. The metabolic behaviour of both adipose tissues was studied *in vivo* and *in vitro*. The fate of [U-^{14}C] glucose, injected intravenously, was followed in rats acclimatized to cold and to room temperature, and adipose tissue was excised from the two groups of rats and incubated in flasks containing Krebs-Ringer bicarbonate buffer with albumin and [U-^{14}C] glucose.

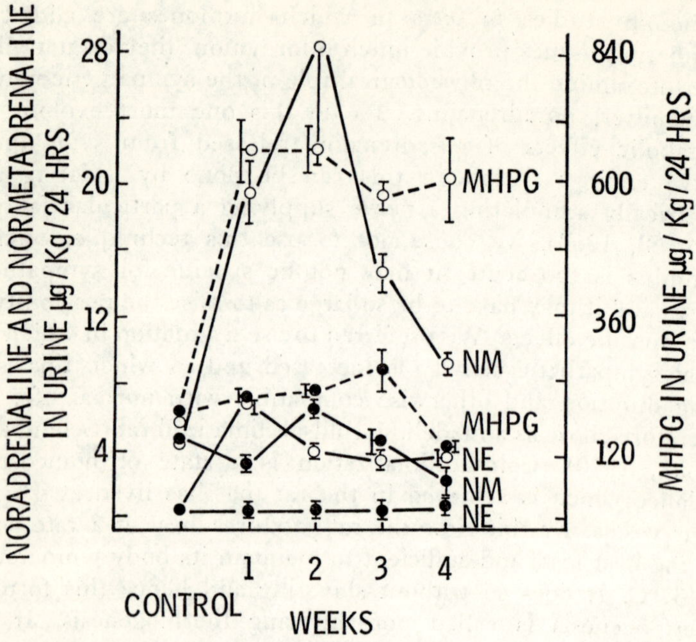

Fig. 1 Influence of cold exposure (4°C) on excretion of noradrenaline (NE), normetadrenaline (NM) and 3-methoxy-4-hydroxyphenylglycol (MHPG). ○, rats exposed to 4°C. ●, rats kept at 30°C. Points are means of four values. Standard errors are plotted for weeks 1, 2, 3 and 4. (From Shum, Johnson & Flattery, 1969.)

Acclimatization to cold produced a slight decrease in the relative lipid content of white adipose tissue. However, it did not change the way in which the tissue metabolized glucose (Table 3) (Steiner & Cahill, 1964; Steiner, Schönbaum, Johnson & Sellers, 1968). By contrast, cold-acclimatization led to: (*a*) a striking enlargement of the rat's interscapular brown fat pad; (*b*) a decrease in its relative content of lipid; and (*c*) a profound change in its utilization of glucose *in vivo* (Steiner & Cahill, 1964; Steiner *et al.*, 1968; Steiner, Johnson, Sellers & Schönbaum, 1969). These results, summarized in Table 4, show that increased amounts of the injected glucose were recovered in brown adipose tissue lipids. The metabolic behaviour of brown adipose tissue excised from cold-acclimatized rats and incubated *in vitro* was similar to that observed *in vivo* (Steiner & Cahill,

Table 3 The effect of cold exposure on white adipose tissue metabolism *in vivo*

	Rats at room temperature	*Cold-acclimatized rats*	*P*
Percentage composition:			
lipid	91 ± 2.0	82 ± 3.0	0.02
lipid free dry weight	5 ± 0.2	10 ± 0.5	0.001
water	4 ± 2.0	10 ± 3.0	0.05
Glucose incorporated into total lipids	34.7 ± 5.0	30.7 ± 6.5	ns

[U-^{14}C] glucose injected intravenously, epididymal fat pad removed 1 hour later and ^{14}C recovery measured. Data expressed as (d.p.m. recovered in total lipid/mg N ÷ d.p.m. glucose injected) (100/g body weight). All values given as mean ± S.E.M.

Table 4 *In vivo* response of brown fat to cold

	Rats at room temperature	*Cold-acclimatized rats*
Percentage composition:		
lipid	62 ± 1	27 ± 2
water	27 ± 1	52 ± 2
lipid free dry weight	11 ± 1	20 ± 1
Glucose recovered in tissue lipids	27 ± 6	60 ± 15

[U-^{14}C] glucose injected as in Table 3. Data expressed as (d.p.m. recovered/mg N ÷ d.p.m. glucose injected) (100/g body weight). Values are means ± S.E.M.

1964). The recovery of glucose in tissue fatty acids, glyceride glycerol and CO_2 was increased (Table 5). These data are consistent with an increase in the turnover of brown adipose tissue lipid in cold-acclimatized rats. At first glance, the observations also suggest that the metabolism of brown adipose tissue is profoundly affected by the sympathetic nerve supply. Furthermore, one could conclude, by comparing Tables 1 and 5, that the addition of noradrenaline to normal tissue *in vitro* is not a valid model for studying the influence of sympathetic hyperactivity.

Table 5 Cold acclimatization and brown fat metabolism *in vitro*

	Tissue from	
	Rats at room temperature	*Cold-acclimatized rats*
Glucose recovered in:		
total lipids	70 ± 10	340 ± 35
fatty acids	40 ± 5	230 ± 20
glyceride glycerol	29 ± 6	110 ± 15
CO_2	90 ± 10	115 ± 10

Slices of brown adipose tissue taken from rats acclimatized to room temperature or to 4°C and incubated as described in Table 1. Data given as in Table 1.

Although these conclusions may be valid, they cannot be made until it is demonstrated that, in the absence of an intact sympathetic nerve supply to brown adipose tissue, none of these changes occur. We therefore sought ways to interrupt the sympathetic nerve supply to this tissue. No use was made of drugs which interfere with sympathetic function partly because they may be non-specific and partly because animals treated with them die soon after exposure to 4°C (Schönbaum *et al.*, 1970). Two other techniques were used: (1) immunosympathectomy (Steiner *et al.*, 1968; Steiner, 1972), and (2) surgical interruption of the nerves supplying the brown adipose tissue on one side of the rat (Steiner *et al.*, 1969; Steiner, Loveland & Schönbaum, 1970).

Effect of immunosympathectomy on adaptation to cold

Before the metabolic consequences of interrupting the sympathetic nerve supply can be studied it is necessary to know the role of the sympathetic innervation in brown adipose tissue. Furthermore, as immunosympathectomy produces widespread destruction of the sympathetic nervous system, its effects on the whole animal and its ability to survive in the cold must be examined. The results of such examinations have been reviewed in detail by Schönbaum (1972). The changes in catecholamine excretion which occur as normal rats acclimatize to cold have already been described in Fig. 1. Immunosympathectomized rats survive as well as intact rats at 4°C. After four weeks in the cold, rats previously shown to be adequately immunosympathectomized excrete as much noradrenaline as do intact rats (Schönbaum *et al.*, 1966). However, there is evidence that the sympathetic reserve of these rats is limited. Firstly, the time course of changes in noradrenaline excretion (Table 6) after

Table 6 Effect of immunosympathectomy on cold acclimatization and noradrenaline excretion

Exposure time	*Urinary noradrenaline* (μg/kg/day) *Intact rats*	*Immunosympathectomized rats*
0 days (control)	0.82 ± 0.10	0.14 ± 0.08
1 day	2.29 ± 0.44	1.99 ± 0.25
2 days	5.74 ± 0.90	3.55 ± 0.50
2 weeks	3.10 ± 0.26	2.56 ± 0.74
3 weeks	2.80 ± 0.38	2.02 ± 0.23
4 weeks	2.56 ± 0.40	2.91 ± 0.31

Rats were kept at 28°C for one week (control period) and then placed at 4°C. Data given as mean ± S.E.M. (From Shum, Johnson and Flattery, 1971.)

placing rats at 4°C shows that the increase occurs more slowly in immunosympathectomized rats than in intact ones (Shum, Johnson & Flattery, 1971). Normetadrenaline follows a pattern similar to that of noradrenaline, while adrenaline and metadrenaline do not change greatly. The second line of evidence indicating the limited sympathetic reserve in immunosympathectomized rats lies in the observation that they excrete much less of the metabolite 3-methoxy-4-hydroxyphenylglycol (MHPG) than do intact rats. This is so even after living at 4°C for four weeks (Table 7). It suggests that the rat attempts to preserve its active catecholamine supply, in face of a limited reserve, by decreasing the catabolism of noradrenaline (Shum *et al.*, 1971). Thirdly, if the cold-acclimatized rats are acutely stressed by shaving and re-exposure to cold, the immunosympathectomized

Table 7 Effect of immunosympathectomy on cold acclimatization and 3-methoxy-4-hydroxyphenylglycol (MHPG) excretion

Exposure time	*Urinary MHPG (μg/kg/day)* *Intact rats*	*Immunosympathectomized rats*
0 days (control)	187.85 ± 18.86	61.79 ± 10.49
1 day	530.73 ± 63.63	90.72 ± 11.80
2 days	411.37 ± 59.61	124.45 ± 24.16
2 weeks	471.81 ± 43.08	111.67 ± 11.91
3 weeks	424.39 ± 36.37	112.09 ± 13.52
4 weeks	388.26 ± 27.24	127.03 ± 11.29

Conditions as in Table 6. (From Shum, Johnson and Flattery, 1971.)

rats are not so well able to increase their catecholamine output (Fig 2) (Schönbaum, Johnson & Sellers, 1966). Thus, immunosympathectomy impairs, but does not obliterate, the ability of the rat's sympathetic nervous system to respond to cold. This is fortuitous since the partial ability to respond is probably the factor chiefly responsible for the survival of these animals.

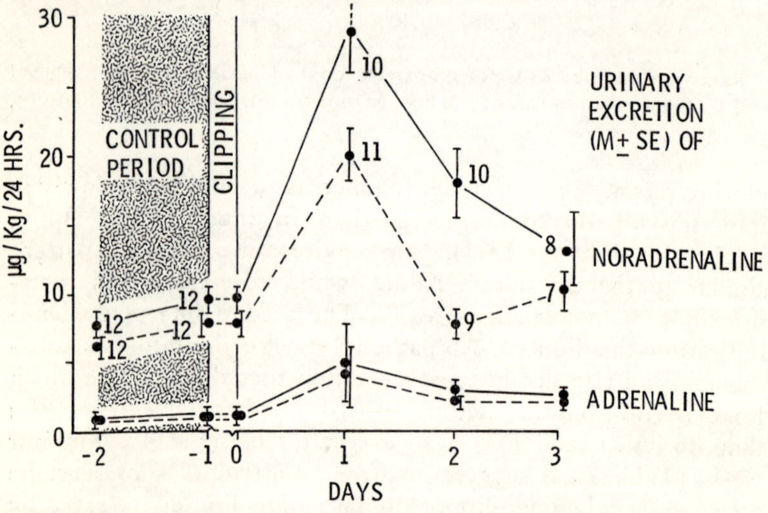

Fig. 2 Rats acclimatized to 4°C. Effect of severe cold stress on free noradrenaline and adrenaline excretion of normal (—) and immunosympathectomized (- - -) rats. Number of surviving rats is indicated at each point. (From Schönbaum, Johnson & Sellers, 1966.)

Sympathetic innervation of brown fat and effects of denervation

When examining the effect of the sympathetic nervous system on brown adipose tissue metabolism, one must understand both the nature of the nerve supply to the tissue and the effect of surgical or immunological sympathectomy. Brown adipose tissue has sympathetic nerves which end both on its blood vessels and on its fat cells (Wirsén & Hamberger, 1967; Napolitano & Fawcett, 1958; Bargmann, Hehn & Lindner, 1968; Derry, Schönbaum & Steiner, 1969). In this respect it differs from white adipose tissue, in which no sympathetic nerves have been observed to end on fat cells. Chemical analyses, kindly performed by Dr K. V. Flattery, showed that interruption of the sympathetic nervous system decreased the noradrenaline content of the interscapular brown fat pad (Table 8). This effect was

Table 8 Noradrenaline content of brown adipose tissue

		Noradrenaline (ng/g wet weight)
Immunosympathectomized rats:	whole pad	62 ± 7
Control rats:	whole pad	170 ± 46
P		<0.02
Normal rats:	denervated side	30 ± 7
	intact side	73 ± 4
P		<0.001

Estimations were kindly performed by Dr K. V. Flattery.

produced both by surgical denervation and by immunosympathectomy. The effects of surgical or immunological sympathectomy on the tissue's nerve supply were examined in greater detail (Derry *et al.*, 1969) using the fluorescence microscopic technique developed by Falck & Owman (1965). Denervation of the rat interscapular brown fat pad, either by immunosympathectomy or by surgical section of the nerves, as they enter the brown fat pad, produced the same histochemical picture. The nerves supplying the blood vessels were disrupted, while those supplying the fat cells were unchanged (Derry *et al.*, 1969).

These findings led us to postulate the existence of sympathetic ganglion cells, or related structures, which are resistant to immunosympathectomy and are located distal to the site of nerve section, that is, within the fat pad itself (Schönbaum *et al.*, 1970). For simplicity these will be referred to as 'ganglia' or as 'ganglion-like structures'. From the observations described above, we could not exclude the possibility that the denervation was incomplete. Recently Cottle and Cottle (1970) described large ganglion-like structures in brown adipose tissue, using fluorescence microscopy. Recent studies from our laboratories have further strengthened the ganglion concept by providing functional evidence for their existence (Steiner, Evans, Murthy & Schönbaum, 1970; Steiner, 1972). They demonstrated: (*a*) that when the nicotinic ganglionic stimulant, dimethylphenylpiperazinium iodide (DMPP) is added to incubated brown fat pad slices a metabolic response occurs which is typical of noradrenaline; (*b*) that DMPP has no effect on brown fat cells freed from all stromal elements, and (*c*) that DMPP has no effect on brown adipose tissue slices taken from rats pre-treated with reserpine (i.e. noradrenaline-depleted rats) (Table 9).

Thus immunosympathectomy destroys a portion, but not all

Table 9 Effect of dimethyl-4-phenylpiperazinium (DMPP) on brown adipose tissue

	Percentage of control	
Condition of incubation	*Fatty acid release*	*Glucose recovered in fatty acids*
Noradrenaline (10^{-6}M)[1]	900 ± 100	31 ± 7
DMPP (1 μg/ml)[2]	551 ± 90	45 ± 8
DMPP (1 μg/ml)[3]	—	125 + 10
DMPP (1 μg/ml) + 'reserpinized' tissue[4]	23 ± 25	110 ± 18

Brown adipose tissue was incubated as described in Table 1.

[1, 2] Slices from normal rats were incubated with noradrenaline (10^{-6}M) or DMPP (1 μg/ml).

[3] Isolated cells from normal rats (prepared with collagenase) were incubated with DMPP (1 μg/ml). Such cells respond to noradrenaline as in [1].

[4] Slices from rats pretreated with reserpine (5 mg/kg) were incubated with DMPP (1 μg/ml). Such tissue responds to noradrenaline as in [1].

All tissues are compared to corresponding controls, and data are expressed as percentages of control ± S.E.M.

of brown adipose tissue's sympathetic nerve supply. The resistant portion appears to be a series of short postganglionic neurones originating from ganglia located in the fat pad itself. Two possibilities may account for the resistance of these ganglia to NGF-antiserum. They may develop after the antibodies disappear from the body, or, they may develop before birth, before the antiserum is given. The possible importance of this to neonatal thermogenesis could be great.

Metabolic consequences of denervation and brown adipose tissue

The effects of sympathetic deprivation on the metabolic behaviour and response to cold of brown adipose tissue were next studied. Immunosympathectomized and intact rats were housed for four weeks at room temperature or at 4°C. The composition of their brown and white adipose tissues was examined and the fate of intravenously injected [U-^{14}C] glucose was followed (Steiner *et al.*, 1968). In rats kept at room temperature, immunosympathectomy did not affect either tissue. In the intact tissues cold-acclimatization produced the changes already described (Tables 3 and 4). Immunosympathectomy did not influence white adipose tissue from cold-acclimatized rats. However, immunosympathectomy partially inhibited the response of brown adipose tissue to cold (Table 10). In particular it decreased the extent to which brown adipose tissue became depleted of lipid, but it did not affect the utilization of [U-^{14}C] glucose (Steiner *et al.*, 1968). This suggested that the sympathetic nervous system may be responsible for part, but not all, of the tissue's response to cold. However, the variation between animals was too large to allow more definite conclusions to be drawn.

We therefore sought a technique which would allow each rat to serve as its own control. This was achieved by avulsing the nerves entering the brown fat pad on one side of the body. The contralateral side was left intact and served as a control (Steiner *et al.*, 1970). Although unilateral surgical denervation has some advantages it is not without its limitations. The procedure is traumatic; it cannot be restricted selectively to sympathetic fibres; and the nerves may regenerate after six weeks. However, within these limitations it has proved to be exceedingly useful.

Table 10 Effect of immunosympathectomy on the response of brown adipose tissue to cold

	ROOM TEMPERATURE		COLD-ACCLIMATIZED		P			
	Intact rats	*Immuno-sympathec-tomized*	*Intact rats*	*Immuno-sympathec-tomized*				
	(1)	(2)	(3)	(4)	1 *vs* 2	1 *vs* 3	3 *vs* 4	2 *vs* 4
Percentage composition:								
lipid	62 ± 1	49 ± 2	27 ± 2	36 ± 2	<0.01	<0.05	<0.01	<0.01
lipid free dry weight	11 ± 1	11 ± 1	20 ± 1	18 ± 1	ns	<0.01	<0.01	<0.01
tissue water	27 ± 1	38 ± 1	52 ± 2	46 ± 2	<0.01	<0.01	<0.05	<0.01
Glucose incorporated in total lipids	27 ± 6	23 ± 9	60 ± 15	62 ± 18	ns	0.05	ns	0.05

[U-^{14}C] glucose injected intravenously, tissue removed 1 hour later and ^{14}C recovery measured. Data expressed as [d.p.m. recovered in total lipid/mg N ÷ d.p.m. glucose injected (100/g body weight)]. All values given as mean ± S.E.M.

The composition of denervated brown adipose tissue and of contralateral intact tissue was identical in room-temperature rats. However, the compositions differed in cold-acclimatized rats (Fig. 3). Both showed reduced lipids but the extent of depletion was greater on the intact side than on the denervated side.

The recovery of intravenously administered [U-^{14}C] glucose was also examined. Cold-acclimatization produced the changes described previously (Steiner & Cahill, 1964; Steiner *et al.*, 1968).

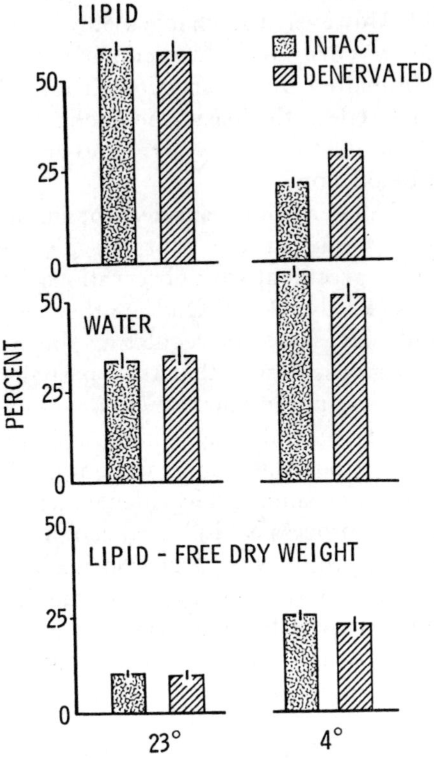

Fig. 3 Effect of denervation and cold acclimatization on rat brown adipose tissue composition. Brown adipose tissue on one side was denervated; that on the other was left intact. Rats were then housed at 23 or 4°C for four weeks. Each tissue was analysed separately. Bars represent means ± S.E.M. of analyses from 18 rats. (From Steiner, Loveland & Schönbaum, 1970.)

Denervation partially impaired, but did not obliterate, these changes (Table 11). Thus surgical denervation and immunosympathectomy produced similar effects. The findings again indicate that the sympathetic nervous system plays a partial role in mediating the response of brown adipose tissue to cold.

It has already been indicated that if brown adipose tissue is excised from cold-acclimatized rats and incubated *in vitro*, its metabolism resembles that observed *in vivo* (Tables 4 and 5). Such studies were now repeated with both intact and denervated tissues (Steiner *et al.*, 1970). The usual changes were observed in response to cold. However, the changes observed in the utilization of glucose *in vitro* by cold-acclimatized brown adipose tissue were not impaired by denervation (Table 12). As such *in vitro* experiments reflect the basic metabolic behaviour of the fat cells, they allow one to divorce it from other influences on the tissue, such as blood flow.

The failure of denervation, surgical or immunological, to influence adipose tissue in the 'unstressed' animal at room temperature are in agreement with observations frequently made with other tissues (Brody, 1972). On the other hand, the sympathetic nerves did play a role in regulating the response to the stress of cold. The observation that they partially regulated an *in vivo* process but did not impair the *in vitro* response of brown adipose tissue raises several interesting possibilities. It would appear that the long postganglionic neurones, affected by both immunosympathectomy and surgical denervation, regulated an *in vivo* process. This process could have been blood flow through the tissue. This suggestion would be consistent with the well-known influence of blood flow on lipid mobilization (Scow, 1965). It would also parallel our histochemical findings: that surgical denervation and immunosympathectomy both interrupted the sympathetic nerve supply to brown adipose tissue blood vessels but not to adipocytes. Whether it is another humoral factor or whether it is the sympathetic ganglia and short postganglionic neurones in the brown fat pad, that may be responsible for the basic behaviour of the brown fat cell, is now being studied. It is interesting to speculate about the development of these immunosympathectomy-resistant ganglia in a tissue responsible for thermogenesis in the newborn.

Table 11 The effect of surgical denervation on brown fat metabolism *in vivo*

	Acclimatization temperature °C	*Brown fat* *Intact*	*Brown fat* *Denervated*	*Difference*	*P*
Glucose label in total	23	7.2 ± 1.2	5.3 ± 0.6	-1.9 ± 0.6	<0.02
lipids	4	118 ± 12.2	75 ± 13.3	-43 ± 28	<0.02
P		<0.01	<0.01		
Fatty acid specific	23	5.2 ± 2.3	1.6 ± 0.4	-3.6 ± 2.2	ns
activity, d.p.m./mg	4	1217 ± 200	657 ± 167	-560 ± 204	<0.02
P		<0.01	<0.01		

See Table 10 for details of glucose administration and units. (From Steiner, Loveland & Schönbaum, 1970.)

Table 12 *In vitro* metabolism of denervated and intact brown fat from room temperature and cold-acclimatized rats

	ROOM TEMPERATURE-ACCLIMATIZED		COLD-ACCLIMATIZED	
Glucose recovery in	*Intact tissue*	*Denervated tissue*	*Intact tissue*	*Denervated tissue*
CO_2	86 ± 12	85 ± 10	123 ± 27	147 ± 26
Total lipid	69 ± 9	73 ± 8	254 ± 32	397 ± 36
Fatty acid	33 ± 5	39 ± 7	151 ± 22	253 ± 26
Glyceride glycerol	35 ± 5	31 ± 4	103 ± 12	144 ± 13

Brown adipose tissue was taken from rats acclimatized to room temperature or to cold. In each rat one side had been denervated five weeks previously and the other was intact. All incubations were done as in Table 1. Data expressed as μmol glucose recovered/mg N ± S.E.M.

Conclusions

The studies we have described demonstrate several features which must be considered in examining the influence of the sympathetic nervous system on the metabolic behaviour of a tissue. One can be led astray by only examining the effect of adding noradrenaline to the tissue. *In vitro* experiments alone are inadequate to allow one to describe the influence of the sympathetic nervous system on the physiological behaviour of a tissue. In order to establish this, one should first explore the effect of a situation naturally producing sympathetic hyperactivity; and one should then examine the effect of sympathetic deprivation on any changes observed. Several methods should be used to produce the sympathetic deprivation, as no single one is free of limitations. Immunosympathectomy has proved an invaluable technique because it is specific to the sympathetic nervous system, is of long duration and entails minimal risk to the animal.

Acknowledgements

We wish to acknowledge the invaluable assistance and inspiration of the many people who, over the years, have helped us in this work. Although it is impossible to mention all of them, we should particularly like to express our appreciation to Dr E. A. Sellers.

This work has been variously supported by grants from the

Medical Research Council of Canada, the Defense Research Board of Canada, the Playfair Foundation and Geigy (Canada) Ltd.

References

Bargmann, W., Hehn, G. V. & Lindner, E. (1968). *Z. Zellforsch. mikrosk. Anat.* **85**, 601.

Brody, M. J. (1972). In *Immunosympathectomy*. Ed. by Steiner, G. & Schönbaum, E. Amsterdam: Elsevier Publishing Co. (in the press).

Correll, J. W. (1963). *Science, N.Y.* **140**, 387.

Cottle, M. K. W. & Cottle, W. H. (1970). *J. Histochem. Cytochem.* **18**, 116.

Derry, D. M., Schönbaum, E. & Steiner, G. (1969). *Can. J. Physiol. Pharmac.* **47**, 57.

Falck, B. & Owman, C. (1965). *Acta Univ. lund.* **117**, 1.

Himms-Hagen, J. (1967). *Pharmac. Rev.* **19**, 367.

Jeanrenaud, B. (1965). In *Handbook of Physiology, Section V: Adipose Tissue*, p. 169. Ed. by Renold, A. E. & Cahill, G. F. Jr. Washington: Am. Physiol. Soc.

Leduc, J. (1961). *Acta physiol. scand.* **53**, Suppl. 183.

Lindberg, O. (1970). *Brown Adipose Tissue*. New York: American Elsevier Publishing Co.

Napolitano, L. & Fawcett, D. W. (1958). *J. biophys. biochem. Cytol.* **4**, 685.

Schönbaum, E. (1972). In *Immunosympathectomy*. Ed. by Steiner, G. & Schönbaum, E. Amsterdam: Elsevier Publishing Co. (in the press).

Schönbaum, E., Johnson, G. E. & Sellers, E. A. (1966). *Am. J. Physiol.* **211**, 647.

Schönbaum, E., Steiner, G. & Sellers, E. A. (1970). In *Brown Adipose Tissue*, p. 179. Ed. by Lindberg, O. New York: American Elsevier Publishing Co.

Scow, R. O. (1965). In *Handbook of Physiology, Section V: Adipose Tissue*, p. 437. Ed. by Renold, A. E. & Cahill, G. F. Jr. Washington: Am. Physiol. Soc.

Shum, A., Johnson, G. E. & Flattery, K. V. (1969). *Am. J. Physiol.* **216**, 1164.

Shum, A., Johnson, G. E. & Flattery, K. V. (1971). *Am. J. Physiol.* (in the Press).

Smith, R. E. & Horwitz, B. A. (1969). *Physiol. Rev.* **49**, 330.

Steiner, G. (1972). In *Immunosympathectomy*. Ed. by Steiner, G. & Schönbaum, E. Amsterdam: Elsevier Publishing Co. (in the press).

Steiner, G. & Cahill, G. F. Jr. (1964). *Am. J. Physiol.* **207**, 840.

Steiner, G. & Cahill, G. F. Jr. (1966). *Am. J. Physiol.* **211**, 1325.

Steiner, G., Evans, S., Murthy, V. K. & Schönbaum, E. (1970). *Fedn. Proc. Fedn. Am. Socs exp. Biol.* **29**, 267.

Steiner, G., Johnson, G. E., Sellers, E. A. & Schönbaum, E. (1969). *Fedn. Proc. Fedn. Am. Socs exp. Biol.* **28**, 1017.
Steiner, G., Loveland, M. & Schönbaum, E. (1970). *Am. J. Physiol.* **218**, 566.
Steiner, G., Schönbaum, E., Johnson, G. E. & Sellers, E. A. (1968). *Can. J. Physiol. Pharmac.* **46**, 453.
Wirsén, C. & Hamberger, B. (1967). *Nature, Lond.* **214**, 625.

Monoamine Metabolism in Immunosympathectomized Animals

M. SANDLER, P. M. CEASAR, G. G. S. COLLINS and C. R. J. RUTHVEN

Bernhard Baron Memorial Research Laboratories and Institute of Obstetrics and Gynaecology, Queen Charlotte's Maternity Hospital, London, UK

Our knowledge of the contribution of the sympathetic nervous system to total monoamine production is, at best, approximate. It therefore seemed that a study of monoamine metabolism in the immunosympathectomized animal might be a useful approach to obtaining further information about this contribution. Although the urinary output of noradrenaline is decreased after immunosympathectomy (Brody, 1964; Carpi & Oliverio, 1964; Schönbaum, Johnson & Sellers, 1965, 1966), catecholamines *per se* contribute only about 1–5 per cent of the urinary output of catecholamine metabolites (von Euler, 1956) and little is known of the effect of sympathectomy on total catecholamine metabolism.

Using rats treated with antiserum to nerve growth factor (NGF) we have investigated the effect of immunological sympathectomy on the daily excretion of a variety of monoamines or related compounds in the urine. In addition to catecholamine metabolites, we measured the output of 5-hydroxytryptamine (5-HT) and its deaminated metabolites 5-hydroxyindoleacetic acid (5-HIAA) and 5-hydroxytryptophol (5-HTOH). These 5-hydroxyindole metabolites were measured because 5-HT concentration increases have been found in the gastrointestinal tract (Hamberger, Levi-Montalcini, Norberg & Sjöqvist, 1965; Iversen, Glowinski & Axelrod, 1966; Thompson & Campbell, 1968), submaxillary glands, heart and caecum (Klingman, 1969) of immunosympathectomized animals. Studies on monoamine oxidase (MAO) activity in tissues of mice treated with NGF-antiserum have also been made.

Methods

Urine was collected from histologically-proven immunosympathectomized rats (kindly put at our disposal by Professor Eleanor Zaimis, Royal Free Hospital School of Medicine, London). Total 4-hydroxy-3-methoxyphenylglycol (HMPG), 4-hydroxy-3-methoxymandelic acid (VMA), normetadrenaline and metadrenaline were assayed in 24-hour urine collections from these animals by methods previously described (Ceasar, Ruthven & Sandler, 1969). Free homovanillic acid (HVA) was determined by the method of Sato (1965), free dopamine by the method of Sourkes & Murphy (1961) and free 5-HT and 5-HIAA as described by Oates (1961) and Contractor (1966) respectively.

Free plus conjugated 5-HTOH was measured as follows. Two 24-hour samples of urine were combined and divided into two equal portions, to one of which was added 100 μg 5-HTOH as an internal standard. The urines were hydrolysed overnight with a β-glucuronidase sulphatase preparation (Suc d'*Helix pomatia*, Industrie Biologique Française, Gennevilliers, Seine, France).

After centrifugation, the pH of the supernatants was adjusted to 7 with 0.1 N-NaOH and they were applied to a Sephadex G-15 column (1 × 35 cm) equilibrated with 0.2 M-ammonium acetate. The effluent included inorganic salts and aliphatic compounds present in rat urine. The column was then eluted with 75 ml 0.2 M-ammonium acetate, pH 7.0. The first 40 ml contained 5-hydroxytryptophan, 5-HT and 5-HIAA and were discarded. The remaining 35 ml, in which 5-HTOH was present, were collected and applied to a Sephadex G-10 column (2 g, 1 cm bore). The effluent was discarded, the column washed with water (10 ml) and 50 per cent aqueous methanol (2.5 ml), and 5-HTOH was eluted from the column with 75 per cent aqueous methanol (25 ml in 5 × 5 ml fractions).

A 1 ml sample of each fraction was diluted with 0.5 ml concentrated HCl and the relative fluorescence intensity of the samples determined within 15 minutes on an Aminco-Bowman spectrophotofluorometer, set for excitation at 295 nm and fluorescence at 535 nm (uncorrected wavelengths). One drop of a saturated solution of potassium persulphate in water was then added to the samples and five minutes later the fluorescence intensity reading was made to determine the blank values. The sums of the appropriate sets of five individual readings gave total test, total test-plus-internal standard, and total blank readings, respectively. The concentration of endogenous 5-HTOH was calculated from the difference between test and blank and the net reading due to internal standard.

Immunosympathectomized mice used for the measurement of tissue MAO activity were prepared by subcutaneous injection of newborn mice with 'Wellcome' NGF-antiserum for the first five days after birth. The animals were killed three months later. Subcellular fractions of the extracted tissues were prepared as described by Ceasar, Collins & Sandler (1970). MAO activity of the fractions was assayed by the method of Kraml (1965), using half quantities of reagents.

Results and discussion

Catecholamine metabolism

The urinary output of HMPG, the major *O*-methylated, oxidatively deaminated metabolite of noradrenaline in the rat (Kopin, Axelrod & Gordon, 1961), was significantly reduced after immunosympathectomy (Fig. 1). In contrast, the corresponding acidic metabolite of noradrenaline, VMA, was not reduced and, in fact, its excretion in μg/kg/24 hours was significantly increased ($P<0.05$).

It is possible that HMPG and VMA are formed in different tissue compartments, so that the amounts of HMPG may reflect intraneuronal metabolism of noradrenaline to a greater degree than may those of VMA. On the other hand, noradrenaline released from the adrenal glands might be preferentially metabolized to VMA rather than to the alcohol. The adrenal noradrenaline concentration is raised in immunosympathectomized animals (Carpi & Oliverio, 1964; Berk, Filipe & Zaimis, 1965; Visscher, Lee & Azuma, 1965) and the turnover of adrenal medullary catecholamines is reportedly doubled in immunosympathectomized mice (Iversen *et al.*, 1966).

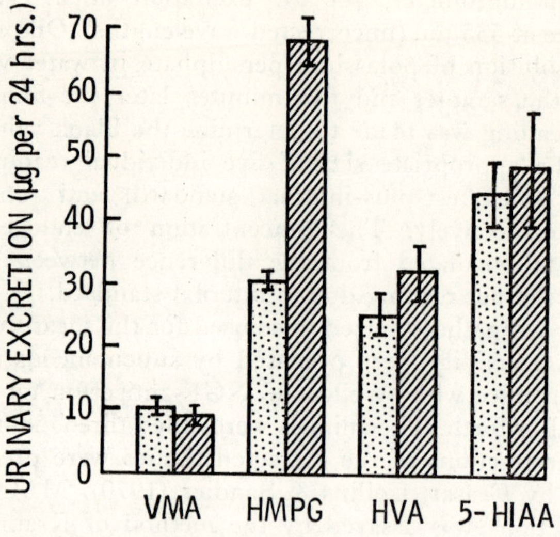

Fig. 1 Excretion of 4-hydroxy-3-methoxymandelic acid (VMA), 4-hydroxy-3-methoxyphenylglycol (HMPG)[1], homovanillic acid (HVA) and 5-hydroxyindoleacetic acid (5-HIAA) in the urine of immunosympathectomized (dots) and control (stripes) rats. [1] $P < 0.001$.

An increased turnover of noradrenaline in the adrenal gland may also be largely responsible for the unchanged concentration of normetadrenaline in the urine of immunosympathectomized rats (Fig. 2). Levels of metadrenaline in these animals also remained unchanged. The tendency for a greater proportion of noradrenaline secreted directly into the blood stream to undergo *O*-methylation compared with that metabolized within the cell (Kopin & Gordon, 1962, 1963), may account for a proportionally large contribution to the normetadrenaline output. It is probably relevant that the increased metabolism of radioactive noradrenaline in tissues of immunosympathectomized animals largely results in an increase in labelled normetadrenaline and acid metabolites (Iversen *et al.*, 1966; Sjöqvist, Taylor & Titus, 1967), so that any circulating noradrenaline released by the adrenal medulla and taken up by immunosympathectomized tissues might perhaps tend to undergo *O*-methylation rather than binding within a tissue.

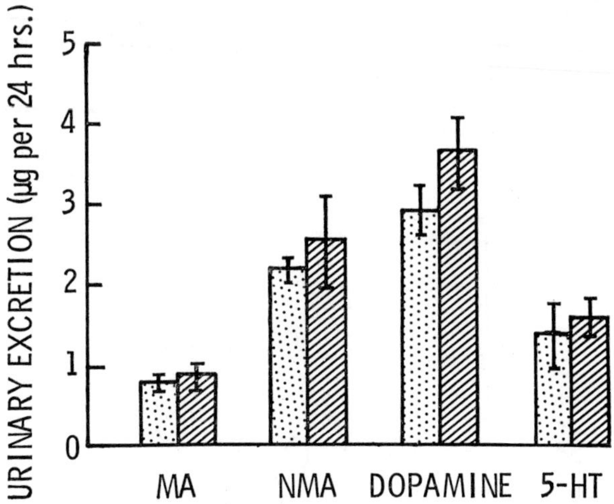

Fig. 2 Excretion of metadrenaline (MA), normetadrenaline (NMA), dopamine and 5-hydroxytryptamine (5-HT) in the urine of immunosympathectomized (dots) and control (stripes) rats.

Urinary normetadrenaline levels are a finer gauge of small increases in catecholamine overproduction in such pathological conditions as phaeochromocytoma than are corresponding concentrations of oxidatively deaminated metabolites. This finding seems to stem from the direct access of amine from tumour tissue to the circulation, where it is predominantly inactivated by catechol-*O*-methyltransferase (see Sandler & Ruthven, 1966, for fuller discussion of this point). Thus the experimental counterpart of the noradrenaline disposition pattern in this pathological state is provided by intravenous catecholamine injection, which gives a similar pattern, different from that encountered in neuroblastoma. The pattern in the latter results from degradation within the tissue and is similar to that found in the normal or immunosympathectomized state. This tissue degradation pattern appears to be dominated by oxidative deamination, an interpretation supported by the observation that HMPG output (Ceasar *et al.*, 1970) also reflects noradrenaline overproduction after adrenalectomy (von Euler, Franksson & Hellström, 1954; Imms & Jones, 1967) more faithfully than normetradrenaline, which is unchanged (Fig. 3). The human counterpart is provided by the careful experiments on a number of *Project Mercury* pilots (Weil-Malherbe, Smith & Bowles, 1968), where small stress changes at normal excretion levels were mirrored by oxidatively deaminated metabolites rather than metadrenalines.

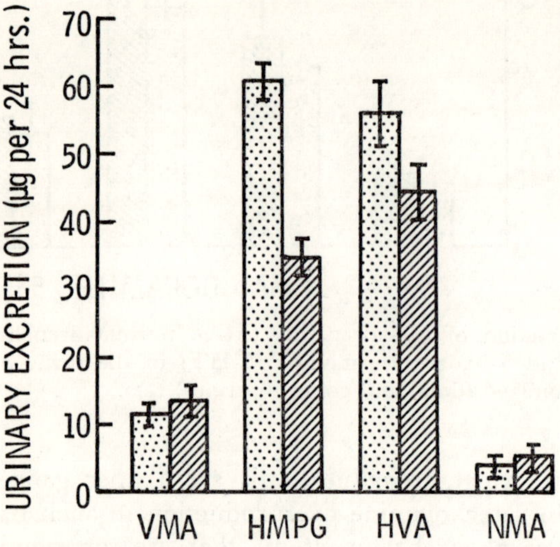

Fig. 3 Excretion of 4-hydroxy-3-methoxymandelic acid (VMA), 4-hydroxy-3-methoxyphenylglycol (HMPG)[1], homovanillic acid (HVA)[2] and normetadrenaline (NMA) in the urine of adrenalectomized (dots) and control (stripes) rats. [1] $P < 0.001$; [2] $P < 0.05$.

Neither the urinary excretion of free dopamine (Fig. 2) nor of one of its major metabolites, HVA (Fig. 1), was significantly altered in the urine of immunosympathectomized rats, indicating that only a small proportion of the amine arises directly from the sympathetic nervous system. Intraneuronal dopamine is presumably converted largely to noradrenaline by dopamine β-hydroxylase in the synaptic vesicles; dopamine and its metabolites in the urine presumably derive from other sites in the body. The increased daily output of HVA in the urine of adrenalectomized rats (Fig. 3) may, however, point to a greater production of dopamine as a result of an increase in turnover and synthesis of noradrenaline in the heart (Landsberg & Axelrod, 1968; Landsberg, de Champlain & Axelrod, 1969; Westfall & Osada, 1969) and, brain (Javoy, Glowinski & Kordon, 1968) of the adrenalectomized animal.

5-Hydroxytryptamine metabolism

Daily 5-HT (Fig. 2) and 5-HIAA (Fig. 1) excretion was unchanged in immunosympathectomized rats despite reports of increased levels of the monoamine in tissues of immunosympathectomized animals (Hamberger *et al.*, 1965; Iversen *et al.*, 1966; Thompson & Campbell, 1968; Klingman, 1969). The output of 5-HTOH in terms of body weight, however, was depressed (Fig. 4). Since the excretion of the quantitatively more

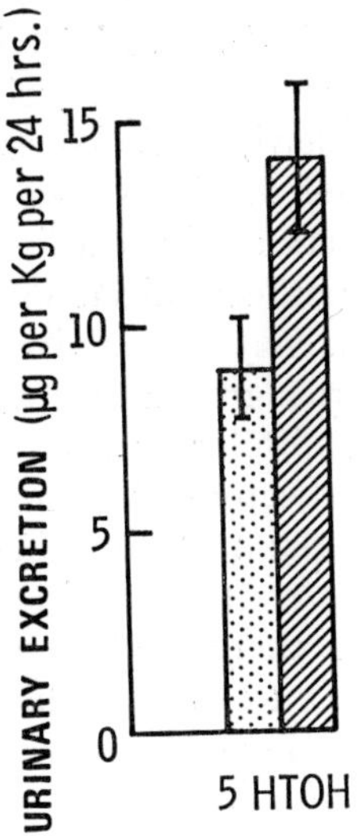

Fig. 4 Excretion of 5-hydroxytryptophol (5-HTOH)[1] in the urine of immunosympathectomized (dots) and control (stripes) rats. [1] $P = 0.05$.

important deaminated metabolite, 5-HIAA, was unaltered, a reduction in MAO activity is unlikely to have been responsible for the increased tissue levels of 5-HT in these animals; nor do MAO inhibitors further increase the 5-HT concentration

(Klingman, 1969). Whatever the explanation, it would be interesting to investigate other alcoholic metabolites of monoamines, such as 4-hydroxy-3-methoxyphenylethanol (from dopamine), after immunosympathectomy.

Recent studies suggest a link between raised tissue levels of 5-HT and reduced ability of stores to discharge their 5-HT content resulting from impairment of sympathetic nervous control (Klingman & Klingman, 1969). If gastric enterochromaffin cells receive an adrenergic innervation (Håkanson, Lilja & Owman, 1969) might not other likely constituents of enterochromaffin cells, such as kallikrein and prostaglandins (Sandler, Williams & Karim, 1969), be similarly affected by sympathectomy? The problem obviously deserves further investigation.

The activity of enzymes involved in monoamine metabolism

Previous investigations of MAO activity in tissues of immunosympathectomized animals have not yielded consistent results Levi-Montalcini & Angeletti, 1962; Iversen *et al.*, 1966; Klingman, 1966). Using 'Wellcome' NGF-antiserum we have observed significant reductions in cardiac and hepatic MAO activity in immunosympathectomized mice (Fig. 5); however, paradoxical increases in enzyme activity were detected in the submaxillary gland and, to a greater extent, in the small intestine.

Jarrott (1971), using a similar preparation of NGF-antiserum to attain immunosympathectomy in mice, did not detect any change in submaxillary gland or intestinal MAO activity; but neither did he observe any alteration in cardiac MAO activity. Thus it seems likely that there are important strain differences in the response of MAO to NGF-antiserum, a factor which could help to explain the inconsistent results of earlier studies of MAO activity in immunosympathectomized animals.

An analysis of subcellular enzymic activity showed that only 'microsomal' MAO activity was significantly reduced in the hearts of immunosympathectomized mice (Table 1) whereas in the liver a decrease in activity was observed in all three fractions studied. The considerable portion of cardiac MAO activity present in the 'microsomal' fraction may just conceivably be associated with noradrenaline storage particles (Stjärne, Roth & Giarman, 1968; de Champlain, Mueller & Axelrod, 1969),

Table 1 MAO activity of immunosympathectomized and control mouse tissues. Activity expressed in terms of μg 4-hydroxyquinoline formed/min/g wet weight of tissue ± S.E.M.

Tissue	*Number of animals*	*Mitochondrial fraction*	*Microsomal fraction*	*Supernatant fraction*	*Sum of fractions*
Control	5	6.51 ± 0.52	3.77 ± 0.31[1]	0.71 ± 0.06	10.99 ± 0.35[1]
Heart					
Immunosymp.	5	4.97 ± 0.83	2.09 ± 0.22	1.24 ± 0.30	8.31 ± 0.49
Control	5	22.43 ± 0.37[2]	11.31 ± 1.82[3]	4.04 ± 0.34[1]	37.78 ± 2.25[1]
Liver					
Immunosymp.	5	14.59 ± 2.03	6.01 ± 1.18	1.79 ± 0.30	22.47 ± 2.05

[1] $P < 0.005$. [2] $P < 0.01$. [3] $P < 0.05$.

although it is perhaps more likely to be derived from stripped-off outer membranes of mitochondria, where the enzyme is located (Schnaitman, Erwin & Greenawalt, 1967). Hepatic MAO is predominantly mitochondrial in origin (Cotzias & Dole, 1951; Hawkins, 1952; Ostwald & Strittmatter, 1963; Baudhuin, Beaufay, Rahman-Li, Sellinger, Wattiaux, Jacques & de Duve, 1964; de Champlain *et al.*, 1969).

Catechol-*O*-methyltransferase activity in the tissues of immunosympathectomized mice does not differ significantly from that of control mice (Iversen *et al.*, 1966; Jarrott, 1971).

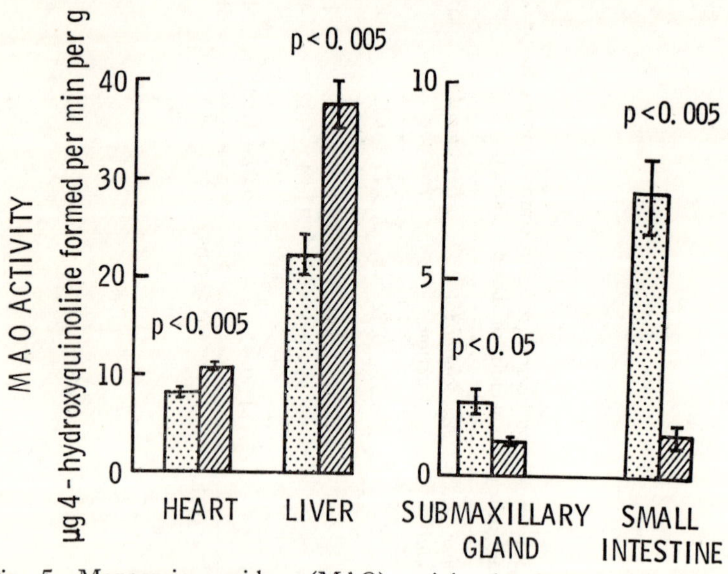

Fig. 5 Monoamine oxidase (MAO) activity in tissues of immunosympathectomized (dots) and control (stripes) mice.

Conclusions

The assay of HMPG, the alcohol deriving from the oxidative deamination of noradrenaline and adrenaline, appears to provide a good pointer to alterations in catecholamine production in the rat. Thus a decreased output was observed after immunosympathectomy in the absence of convincing changes in the excretion of other metabolites; conversely the noradrenaline overproduction brought about by adrenalectomy results in an elevated HMPG output. Changes in 5-hydroxyindole metabolism resulting from immunosympathectomy were equivocal. Alterations in MAO activity stemming from such treatment were complex, varying from tissue to tissue.

References

Baudhuin, P., Beaufay, H., Rahman-Li, Y., Sellinger, O. Z., Wattiaux, R., Jacques, P. & de Duve, C. (1964). *Biochem. J.* **92**, 179.

Berk, L., Filipe, I. & Zaimis, E. (1965). *J. Physiol., Lond.* **177**, 1P.

Brody, M. J. (1964). *Circulation Res.* **15**, 161.

Carpi, A. & Oliverio, A. (1964). *Int. J. Neuropharmacol.* **3**, 427.

Ceasar, P. M. Ruthven, C. R. J. & Sandler, M. (1969). *Br. J. Pharmac.* **36**, 70.

Ceasar, P. M., Ruthven, C. R. J. & Sandler, M. (1969). *Br. J. Pharmac.* **19**, 921.

Contractor, S. F. (1966). *Biochem. Pharmac.* **15**, 1701.

Cotzias, G. C. & Dole, V. P. (1951). *Proc. Soc. exp. Biol. Med.* **78**, 157.

de Champlain, J., Mueller, R. A. & Axelrod, J. (1969) *J. Pharmac. exp. Ther.* **166**, 339.

Håkanson, B., Lilja, B. & Owman, C. (1969). *Histochemie* **18**, 74.

Hamberger, B., Levi-Montalcini, R., Norberg, K.-A. & Sjöqvist, F. (1965). *Int. J. Neuropharmacol.* **4**, 91.

Hawkins, J. (1952). *Biochem. J.* **50**, 577.

Imms, F. J. & Jones, M. T. (1967). *J. Endocr.* **38**, xvii.

Iversen, L. L., Glowinski, J. & Axelrod, J. (1966). *J. Pharmac. exp. Ther.* **151**, 273.

Jarrott, B. (1971). *J. Neurochem.* **18**, 7.

Javoy, F., Glowinski, J. & Kordon, C. (1968). *Eur. J. Pharmac.* **4**, 103.

Klingman, G. I. (1966). *Biochem. Pharmac.* **15**, 1729.

Klingman, G. I. (1969). *Biochem. Pharmac.* **18**, 2061.

Klingman, G. I. & Klingman, J. D. (1969). *Biochem. Pharmac.* **18**, 2069.

Kopin, I. J., Axelrod, J. & Gordon, E. (1961). *J. biol. Chem.* **236**, 2109.

Kopin, I. J. & Gordon, E. (1962). *J. Pharmac exp. Ther.* **138**, 351.

Kopin, I. J. & Gordon, E. (1963). *J. Pharmac. exp. Ther.* **140**, 207.

Kraml, M. (1965). *Biochem. Pharmac.* **14**, 1684.

Landsberg, L. & Axelrod, J. (1968). *Circulation Res.* **22**, 559.

Landsberg, L., de Champlain, J. & Axelrod, J. (1969). *J. Pharmac. exp. Ther.* **165**, 102.

Levi-Montalcini, R. & Angeletti, P. U. (1962). *Int. J. Neuropharmacol.* **1**, 161.

Oates, J. A. (1961). In *Methods in Medical Research*, vol. 9, p. 169. Ed. by Quastel, J. H. Chicago: Year Book Publishers.

Ostwald, E. O. & Strittmatter, C. F. (1963). *Proc. Soc. exp. Biol. Med.* **114**, 668.

Sandler, M. & Ruthven, C. R. J. (1966). In *Recent Results in Cancer Research. II. Neuroblastomas. Biochemical Studies*, p. 55. Ed. by Bohuon, C. Berlin: Springer.

Sandler, M., Williams, E. D. & Karim, S. M. M. (1969). In *Prostaglandins, Peptides and Amines*, p. 3. Ed. by Mantegazza, P. & Horton, E. W. London: Academic Press.

Sato, T. L. (1965). *J. Lab. clin. Med.* **66**, 517.

Schnaitman, C., Erwin, V. G. & Greenawalt, J. W. (1967). *J. cell Biol.* **32**, 719.

Schönbaum, E., Johnson, G. E. & Sellers, E. A. (1965). *Acta physiol. pharmac. néerl.* **13**, 368.

Schönbaum, E., Johnson, G. E. & Sellers, E. A. (1966). *Am. J. Physiol.* **211**, 647.

Sourkes, T. L. & Murphy, G. F. (1961). In *Methods in Medical Research*, vol. 9, p. 147. Ed. by Quastel, J. H. Chicago: Year Book Publishers.

Sjöqvist, F., Taylor, P. W. & Titus, E. (1967). *Acta physiol. scand.* **69**, 13.

Stjärne, L., Roth, R. H. & Giarman, N. J. (1968). *Biochem. Pharmac.* **17**, 2008.

Thompson, J. H. & Campbell, L. B. (1968). *Biochem. Pharmac.* **17**, 175.

Visscher, M. B., Lee, Y. C. P. & Azuma, T. (1965). *Proc. Soc. exp. Biol. Med.* **119**, 1232.

von Euler, U. S. (1956). *Noradrenaline*. Springfield, Illinois: Thomas.

von Euler, U. S., Franksson, C. & Hellström, J. (1954). *Acta physiol. scand.* **31**, 1.

Weil-Malherbe, H., Smith, E. R. & Bowles, G. R. (1968). *J. appl. Physiol.* **24**, 146.

Westfall, T. C. & Osada, H. (1969). *J. Pharmac. exp. Ther.* **167**, 300.

Early Effect of Antiserum to the Nerve Growth Factor on Ganglion Metabolism and Synaptic Transmission

MARTIN G. LARRABEE

Thomas C. Jenkins Department of Biophysics, Johns Hopkins University, Baltimore, Md, USA

This paper deals with a group of metabolic and functional changes which occur in sympathetic ganglia of mice during the first few days after an intact animal has received an injection of antiserum to the nerve growth factor. These changes follow the earliest morphological alterations which have been observed by electron microscopy during the first few hours after treatment with antiserum (Sabatini, Pellegrino de Iraldi & De Robertis, 1965; Levi-Montalcini & Angeletti, 1968; Levi-Montalcini, Caramia & Angeletti, 1969), and lead to the ultimate destruction of the ganglion cells. The experimental observations come from the doctoral dissertation of Dr David C. Halstead. They are reported in greater detail elsewhere, together with some additional experiments (Halstead, 1971; Halstead & Larrabee, 1972).

Methods

The experiments were conducted on mice, which received a single injection of NGF-antiserum or of control serum (0.1 ml per g body weight) at seven to ten days of age. Both superior cervical ganglia were later excised, after periods varying from three hours to many days, and were tested in various ways. The measurements included (*a*) dry weight, (*b*) rate of incorporation of labelled precursors into RNA and protein, (*c*) rate of oxidation of [U-^{14}C] glucose to labelled CO_2 and (*d*) synaptic transmission through the ganglion (method of Larrabee, Klingman & Leicht, 1963). During the tests of metabolism and transmission, the excised preparations were kept at 37°C in a complex culture medium (CMRL 1066, Grand Island Biological Co., cat. no. 153G). To each ml of the medium was added 10 µl of a solution of penicillin, streptomycin and fungazone (Grand Island Biological Co., cat. no. 524) and enough HCl to adjust the pH to 7.2–7.4 after equilibration with 5 per cent CO_2–95 per cent O_2. The antiserum, produced in a horse, was donated by the Wellcome Research Laboratories through the kind arrangements of Dr D. Caird Edwards.

The age of seven to ten days was chosen for injection of the antiserum as a compromise between the newborn, in which the antiserum is believed to be most effective, and older animals, in which the ganglia seemed mechanically stronger and the electrical measurements could be made more reproducibly and with more confidence. The only systematic age study that was available when we were designing these experiments concerned NGF rather than its antiserum. It had been shown that fibre outgrowth nearly as great as with ganglia from the newborn, could be obtained from ganglia from mice as old as seven to ten days, but that the growth response subsequently declined, so that no growth was obtained at 17 days of age (Brown, Partlow & Larrabee, unpublished, illustrated in Halstead & Larrabee, 1972). Some further justification for using mice seven to ten days old was found in the course of the present experiments: effects of antiserum on ganglionic RNA metabolism in a few mice injected at two to three days were identical with those after injection at seven to ten days.

Results

Effects on ganglion weight and metabolism

Results are summarized in Fig 1. All measured variables were reduced within 12 hours of the injection of antiserum and declined further as time progressed. Other studies on the dry weight of the ganglia, extending over periods longer than those shown in Fig 1, indicated that the maximal depression was reached

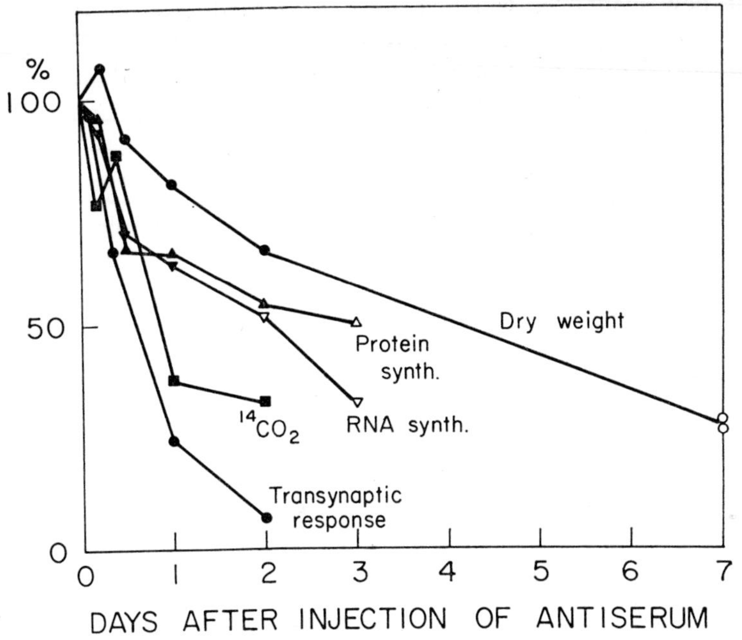

Fig. 1 Effects on the superior cervical ganglion of the mouse of a single injection of NGF-antiserum at 7–10 days of age. Filled points indicate means of three or more determinations; unfilled points are for single determinations. Each measure is expressed as the percentage of the value found in ganglia excised from control littermates at the same age as excision of the ganglia from the animals that had received the antiserum (Halstead & Larrabee, 1972).

in about one week, after which the weights increased for several weeks, at a rate suggesting that the surviving cells grew nearly normally (Fig. 2). In rank order, the metabolic effects were on the average greatest on the rate of oxidation of glucose, less on labelling of RNA and protein, and least on the dry weight. This raises the possibility that an effect initiated by the antiserum early in the sequence of events is an inhibition of glucose oxidation. The consequent loss of energy production could then account for all the other metabolic effects. An alternative possibility is that the antiserum might act primarily by modifying RNA metabolism. However, this now seems unlikely, in view of new evidence, which I have presented elsewhere in this symposium (p. 76), showing that the growth factor itself can act independently of nucleic acid metabolism (Partlow, 1969; Partlow & Larrabee, 1971).

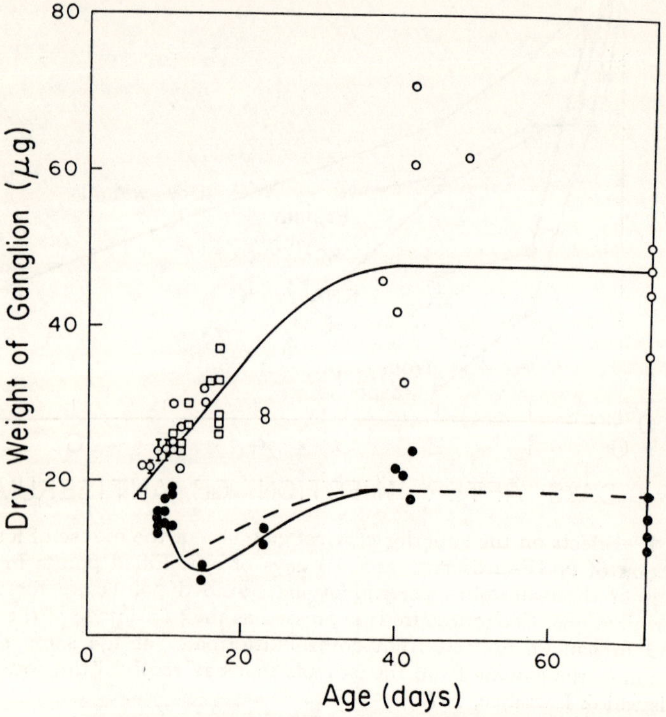

Fig. 2 Dry weights of superior cervical ganglia from mice following a single injection of NGF-antiserum (●), control serum (○) or no injection (□); (Φ) mean ± S.E.M. for several animals. All other points are averages of two ganglia from the same animal. The two solid lines were fitted by eye. Ordinates for the dashed line are 0.4 times those of the control line (Halstead, 1971; Halstead & Larrabee, 1972).

Effects on transmission

The transynaptic response was the variable affected most rapidly among those we have studied (Fig. 1). This response was measured by the amplitude of the action potential recorded from the postganglionic nerve, in response to a maximal stimulus to the preganglionic nerve (Fig. 3). Reduction of ganglionic transmission has been observed in rats several months after injection of antiserum, but the time course of development of the effect does not seem to have been studied previously (Klingman & Klingman, 1965). In our experiments the transmitted response was reduced on the average by more than 30 per cent within 12 hours of the administration of the antiserum and was almost abolished within two days. A similar decline was observed in other experiments in which transmission was tested with a ganglion still with its natural circulation, *in situ* in an anaesthetized animal. These measurements were made *in situ* to avoid any damage that might be associated with excision of the preparations, which seemed more delicate in treated animals than in the controls.

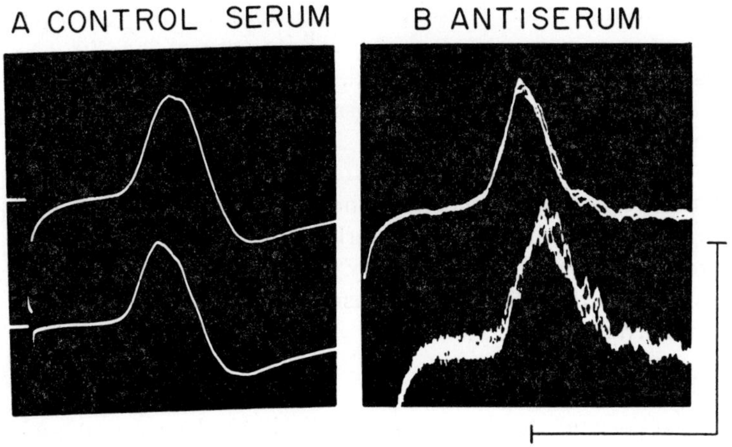

Fig. 3 Depression of the transynaptic response of superior cervical ganglia, excised from mice one day after a single injection of control serum or of NGF-antiserum. The amplification was greater for the preparations from the treated mouse than for those from the control mouse, by a factor of ten in the upper record and 40 in the lower. Several responses, photographed while stimulating five times per second, are superimposed in each record. Upper and lower records are from the right and left ganglia respectively. Mouse A received control serum at 8 days of age; mouse B received antiserum at 7 days. Calibrations at lower right; 10 mV for A; 1 mV for B, upper: 0.25 mV for B, lower; 10 ms for all (Halstead, 1971; Halstead & Larrabee, 1972).

Two studies were made in an attempt to localize the site of the blockade of ganglionic transmission. (*a*) The compound action potential of the cervical sympathetic trunk, which contains the preganglionic fibres, was found to be reduced to about half the control value two days after injection of antiserum. This is reminiscent of the reduction in the diameter of this nerve trunk which has been observed two or more months after treatment with antiserum (Berk, Filipe & Zaimis, 1965; Zaimis, 1967), and suggests that the antiserum may affect sympathetic preganglionic neurones as well as the ganglion cells. However, it also seems possible that the cervical trunk may contain axons of ganglion cells whose bodies are located in the superior cervical or other ganglia. Thus the findings cannot be considered unequivocal evidence of an effect on preganglionic neurones. (*b*) The discharge of impulses over the postganglionic nerve, in response to the addition of acetylcholine to the fluid bathing an excised ganglion, was reduced to about half its control amplitude two days after antiserum was injected. Thus many cells had already become less sensitive to the transmitter or possibly had already been destroyed.

It is not clear whether these effects on the cervical trunk and on the response to acetylcholine, when taken together, are sufficient to account for the nearly complete loss of the transmitted response. Thus there may be some additional effect, for example on the release of transmitter. No evidence on this point is available.

Discussion

These experiments demonstrate a variety of profound effects on sympathetic ganglia in mice receiving antiserum at ages older than those usually used in such studies. In addition it has been shown that even in one-day-old mice, many ganglion cells have already matured to the point at which they are innervated by preganglionic fibres and can respond to incoming impulses by discharging impulses over the postganglionic nerve fibres (Fig. 4). Thus synaptically excitable cells are clearly affected by the antiserum. This raises the question of what particular 'maturation' processes can later occur to reduce the response of the ganglion cells to NGF and to its antiserum. For example, the outgrowth of fibres from mouse ganglia exposed to the growth factor is reduced if the ganglia are excised as late as the tenth day after birth and is absent at the 17th day (Brown *et al.*, unpublished, illustrated in Halstead & Larrabee, 1972). Moreover, the ability of the antiserum to cause degeneration of sympathetic ganglia is also reduced with increasing age (Levi-Montalcini & Angeletti, 1966; Angeletti, Levi-Montalcini & Caramia, 1971). To discover the nature of the changes causing these losses in effectiveness is a challenging problem. In view of the synaptic excitability of cells which may have been affected by the antiserum it is unlikely that the answer lies in changes coincident with the cessation of mitosis.

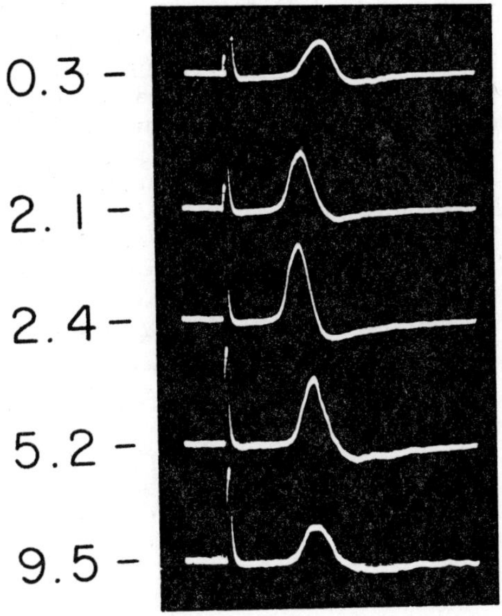

Fig. 4 Transynaptic response of a ganglion that was excised from a mouse 1–1½ days after birth. Numbers at left indicate the time in hours after mounting the ganglion on the electrodes and raising the temperature to 37°C (Toschi & Larrabee, unpublished observations).

Acknowledgements

Investigations reported in this paper were supported by research grant no. NS-00702 from the National Institute of Neurological

Diseases and Stroke and by training grant no. 5T1-GM-716 from the National Institute of General Medical Sciences.

References

Angeletti, P. U., Levi-Montalcini, R. & Caramia, F. (1971). *Brain Res.* **27**, 343.

Berk, L., Filipe, I. & Zaimis, E. (1965). *J. Physiol., Lond.* **177**, 1P.

Halstead, D. C. (1971). Doctoral Dissertation. Johns Hopkins University, Baltimore, Maryland, U.S.A.

Halstead, D. C. & Larrabee, M. G. (1972). In *Immunosympathectomy*, Ed. by G. Steiner & E. Schönbaum, Amsterdam: Elsevier (in the press).

Klingman, G. I. & Klingman, J. D. (1965). *Life Sci.* **4**, 2171.

Larrabee, M. G., Klingman, J. D. & Leicht, W. S. (1963). *J. Neurochem.* **10**, 549.

Levi-Montalcini, R. & Angeletti, P. U. (1966). *Pharmac. Rev.* **18**, 619.

Levi-Montalcini, R. & Angeletti, P. U. (1968). *Physiol. Rev.* **48**, 534.

Levi-Montalcini, R., Caramia, F. & Angeletti, P. U. (1969). *Brain Res.* **12**, 54.

Partlow, L. M. (1969). Doctoral Dissertation. Johns Hopkins University, Baltimore, Maryland, U.S.A.

Partlow, L. M. & Larrabee, M. G. (1971). *J. Neurochem.* **18**, 2101.

Sabatini, M. T., Pellegrino de Iraldi, A. & De Robertis, E. (1965). *Exp. Neurol.* **12**, 370.

Zaimis, E. (1967). In *The Scientific Basis of Medicine Annual Reviews*, p. 59. London: Athlone Press.

The Usefulness of the Immunosympathectomized Animal in Pharmacological Studies

ELEANOR ZAIMIS

Department of Pharmacology, Royal Free Hospital School of Medicine, University of London, UK

Experimental exclusion of the peripheral sympathetic nervous system has so far been achieved either by surgical means or through the use of pharmacologically active substances. Complete surgical sympathectomy, however, is a very difficult operation. With drugs, on the other hand, the possibility of the blocking agent producing additional pharmacological effects cannot be ruled out.

Levi-Montalcini and her co-workers (for references see Levi-Montalcini, 1964) discovered that the growth and maintenance of sympathetic nerve cells are controlled by a specific protein referred to as the 'nerve growth factor' (NGF). By injecting purified NGF into rabbits, Stanley Cohen (1960) prepared an antiserum to it. Together with Professor Levi-Montalcini (Levi-Montalcini & Cohen, 1960) he demonstrated that the administration of this antiserum to newborn mice resulted in a rapid and extensive destruction of the nerve cells of the sympathetic ganglia. Thus, the discovery made by Levi-Montalcini and her co-workers has made available to the research worker a laboratory animal devoid of its sympathetic nervous system but in all other respects normal.

In a field like pharmacology, in which one is attempting to assess the mechanism of action of drugs in relation to highly complex, and still inadequately understood, structures, the immunosympathectomized animal provides ideal material on which to test current theories concerning the role of the sympathetic nervous system and the way in which structures innervated by it can be affected by drugs. Thus, the opportunity to make use of these animals in pharmacological studies was to be welcomed. Using a generous supply of NGF-antiserum provided by Professors R. Levi-Montalcini and P. U. Angeletti, Dr R. K. Richards and Dr D. C. Edwards, we were able to treat newborn rats. The treatment resulted in almost complete destruction of the paravertebral ganglia, and severe atrophy of the coeliac ganglion, but had a very limited effect on the mesenteric ganglion (Zaimis, Berk & Callingham, 1965). In the treated animals there was a good correlation between the degree of destruction of the sympathetic ganglia and the biochemical changes in tissues supplied with adrenergic neurones by these ganglia. For example, the noradrenaline content of the heart and spleen was almost zero, that of the small intestine was about 25 per cent of normal, while the vas deferens contained 65 per cent of the amount found in the controls. Finally, these results correlated well with the loss of the capacity of various tissues to take up noradrenaline. In the treated animals, the uptake of [^{3}H] noradrenaline was less than 14 per cent of that of the controls in the heart, spleen, lungs and kidney; about 30 per cent in the small intestine and colon; unchanged in the uterus; and increased in the vas deferens. Assays of catecholamine content of the peripheral tissues and their uptake of tritiated noradrenaline were carried out by my colleagues Lucienne Papadaki and B. Large.

As a result of introducing immunosympathectomy into our pharmacological studies we have obtained a great deal of useful information. While it is obviously impossible to summarize several years' work in one article, the following examples may serve to indicate the usefulness of this experimental tool.

The following methods have been used to establish the degree of immunosympathectomy: (*a*) macroscopical and microscopical examination of sympathetic ganglia; (*b*) determination of catecholamine levels in peripheral organs; and (*c*) electrical stimulation of the cervical sympathetic trunk. The electrical stimulation of the cervical sympathetic trunk causes an immediate contraction of the inferior eyelid in the control rats, while no responses can be elicited in the immunosympathectomized animals, suggesting that the eyelid has been denervated. Similarly, Brody (this volume, p. 201) recorded very reduced potentials from the lumbar sympathetic nerves of immunosympathectomized rats; in addition, electrical stimulation produced no response in the vessels of the hind limbs.

Blood pressure, heart rate and pulse pressure

In the conscious immunosympathectomized rat the average blood pressure is between 130 and 145 mm Hg, almost exactly the same as that of the controls, but it is very labile. For example, the blood pressure falls rapidly when the rat moves about or becomes frightened; there is also a marked variation with respiration. Under chloralose anaesthesia the mean resting blood pressure in the immunosympathectomized rat is 70 mm Hg whereas that of the controls is 100 mm Hg. Moreover, blood pressure becomes very steady. In both anaesthetized and unanaesthetized animals the resting heart rate is almost 400 beats/min, which is similar to that found in the controls. Finally, there is no change in average pulse pressure. Fig. 1 shows the mean

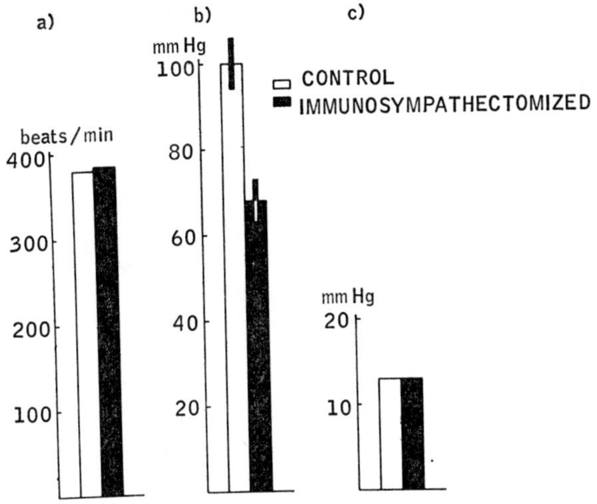

Fig. 1 Rats, anaesthetized with chloralose; two to five months old. The resting heart rate (*a*); blood pressure (*b*); and pulse pressure (*c*) in control and immunosympathectomized animals. The histograms show mean values obtained from 26 control and 11 treated rats.

resting heart rate, blood pressure and pulse pressure calculated from rats under chloralose anaesthesia—26 control and 11 immunosympathectomized animals.

Noradrenaline and adrenaline

Immunosympathectomy produces a striking increase in the responses of the cardiovascular system to injected adrenaline and noradrenaline. In the control vagotomized rats, under chloralose anaesthesia, the threshold dose of adrenaline and noradrenaline required to produce a barely detectable rise in blood pressure and heart rate was about 10 to 30 ng/animal. In the immunosympathectomized animals, the responses were markedly increased; doses of 10 and 30 ng of either adrenaline or noradrenaline produced pressor responses three to five times greater than those in the controls (Fig. 2). Furthermore, the response was considerably prolonged.

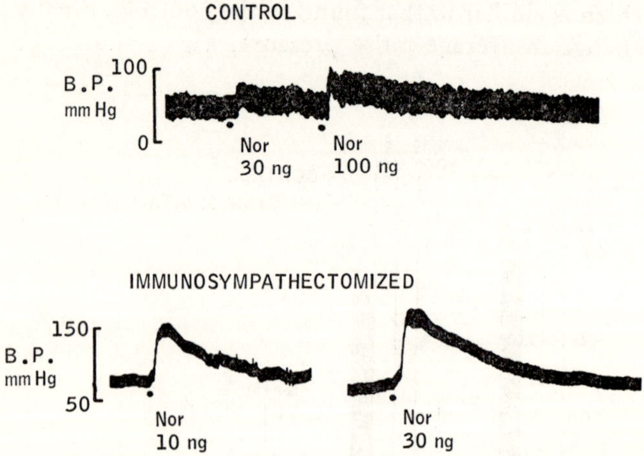

Fig. 2 In this and all the following figures the control and immunosympathectomized rats belonged to the same litters, or litters of the same age, and were studied between two and five months after birth.

Blood pressure (B.P.) responses to noradrenaline (Nor) are compared in a control and an immunosympathectomized rat.

The positive chronotropic and inotropic effects were also increased and prolonged after immunosympathectomy. Fig. 3

shows the effect of noradrenaline on the blood pressure and heart rate of a control and two immunosympathectomized rats, one treated at birth with Wellcome NGF-antiserum and the other with Abbott NGF-antiserum.

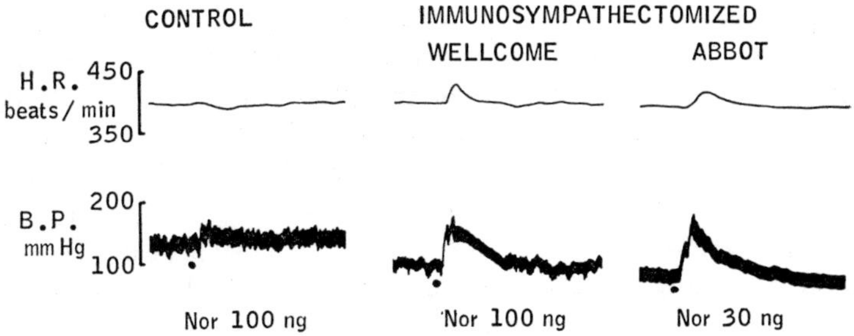

Fig. 3 Blood pressure (B.P.) and heart rate (H.R.) responses to noradrenaline (Nor) in a control and two immunosympathectomized rats—one treated at birth with Wellcome NGF-antiserum, the other with Abbott NGF-antiserum.

The results which Brody (this volume, p. 205) obtained by recording responses from the perfused hindquarters of immunosympathectomized and control rats, are only in part similar to those in the present study. For example, in his experiments the duration—but not the magnitude—of the constrictor responses produced by adrenaline and noradrenaline was increased in immunosympathectomized rats both before and after adrenal demedullation. These discrepancies may arise from differences in the preparations used and in the routes of drug administration.

Other pressor substances

Tyramine

The assumption that pharmacological effects of drugs acting on structures innervated by adrenergic nerves take place almost exclusively at nerve endings underlies a great many statements made during the past few years (for details see Zaimis, 1964*a*, 1968). For example, the hypothesis has been put forward that the cardiovascular effects of several sympathomimetic amines, such as tyramine, are indirect and depend on the release of noradrenaline from tissue stores. Studies of tyramine in our department, however, strongly suggest a direct action on the effector cells themselves.

Depletion of noradrenaline by immunosympathectomy does not reduce the cardiovascular effects of tyramine (Zaimis, 1966). A comparison of changes in blood pressure and heart rate in response to adrenaline, noradrenaline and tyramine in control and immunosympathectomized rats showed that the pressor as well as the chronotropic effects are greater and more prolonged for all three sympathomimetic amines in the immunosympathectomized animals; with tyramine the increase in the pressor effects was less than that with adrenaline and noradrenaline but the increase in heart rate was very marked (Fig. 4). After bilateral adrenalectomy the magnitude and duration of the chronotropic responses remained similar to those observed before adrenalectomy. It must be emphasized that when doses of tyramine, adrenaline and noradrenaline, equipotent in their effects on blood pressure, are administered, the increase in heart rate produced by tyramine is significantly greater than that produced by adrenaline and noradrenaline in both control and immunosympathectomized rats. We also studied the effect of tyramine in isolated perfused hearts removed from both control and NGF-antiserum-treated rats. Tyramine produced longer

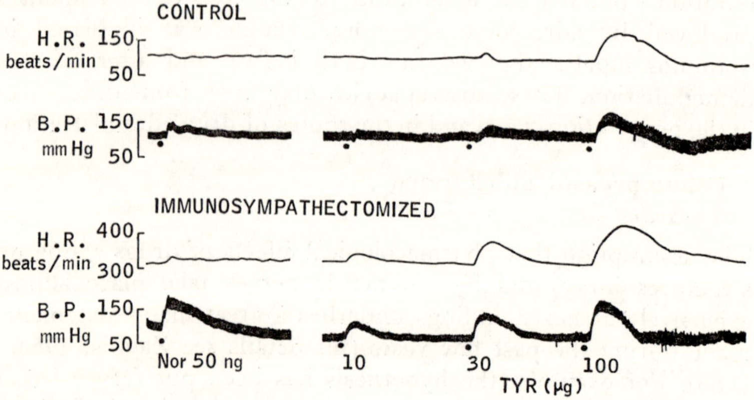

Fig. 4 Blood pressure (B.P.) and heart rate (H.R.) responses to noradrenaline (Nor) and tyramine (TYR) in a control and an immunosympathectomized rat.

chronotropic and inotropic responses in the hearts removed from the immunosympathectomized animals—hearts which contained neither sympathetic nerves nor catecholamines.

Many more authors have obtained results which are difficult to reconcile with the view that the action of tyramine is entirely the result of noradrenaline liberation from tissue stores (for details see Zaimis, 1964*a* and 1968).

Metaraminol

Tritiated noradrenaline, which is rapidly taken up and stored in sympathetically innervated tissues, can be released by sympathomimetic amines, apparently by exchange with the natural mediator (for references see Nash, Wolff & Ferguson, 1968). A good deal of recent biochemical work has indicated the ability of metaraminol to release noradrenaline (Crout, Alpers, Tatum

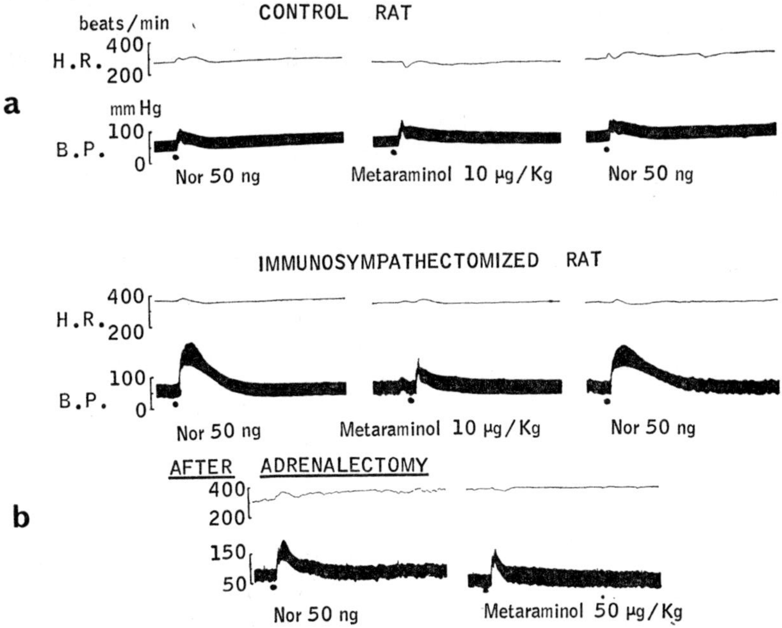

Fig. 5 Blood pressure (B.P.) and heart rate (H.R.) responses to noradrenaline (Nor) and metaraminol in (*a*) control rat; and (*b*) immunosympathectomized rat, before and after bilateral adrenalectomy.

& Shore, 1964; Shore, 1966). However, information derived from functional studies in both man and animals points to a predominantly direct action of this sympathomimetic amine (for details see Zaimis, 1968). A direct action is also supported by our more recent experimental results. E. Larbi and I (unpublished observations) have compared, in control and immunosympathectomized rats, the effects of metaraminol and noradrenaline on heart rate and blood pressure. As Fig. 5 shows, no differences were found. Since immunosympathectomy (and bilateral adrenalectomy) had no effect on the cardiovascular responses to metaraminol it was concluded that this pressor amine has a predominantly direct action.

Angiotensin

A number of investigators have suggested that the vasoconstrictor action of angiotensin is partially due to a release of catecholamines from adrenergic neurones (Beaulnes, 1963; Benelli, Della Bella & Gandini, 1964). Moreover, there is evidence for the release of medullary catecholamines from the suprarenal

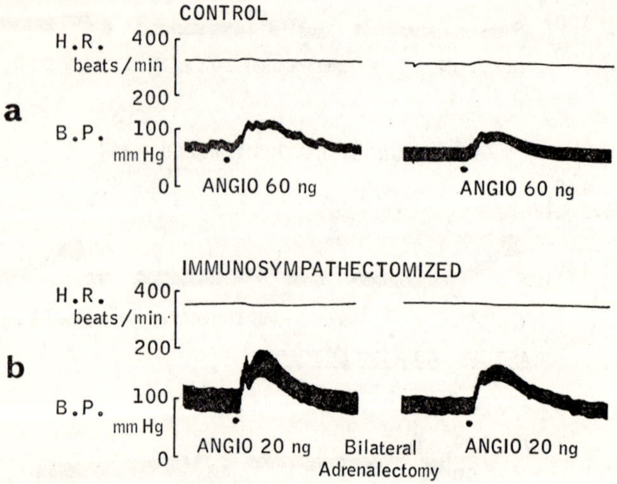

Fig. 6 Blood pressure (B.P.) and heart rate (H.R.) responses to angiotensin (ANGIO) before (left-hand panel) and after (right-hand panel) bilateral adrenalectomy in (*a*) control rat; and (*b*) immunosympathectomized rat.

gland (Feldberg & Lewis, 1964). But the contribution, if any, made by the released amines to the pressor action of angiotensin must be minimal; the powerful vasoconstrictor effect of angiotensin persists in the presence of ganglionic and α-adrenoceptor blocking drugs and is unchanged by immunosympathectomy and bilateral adrenalectomy. In the control rats, angiotensin in doses ranging from 30 ng to 60 ng produced a rise in blood pressure unaccompanied by any effect on heart rate. In the immunosympathectomized and adrenalectomized rats, the pressor response to angiotensin was not only present but increased; still with little effect on heart rate (Fig. 6).

Hypotensive drugs

Reserpine, guanethidine and α-methyldopa

The discovery that reserpine can influence the storage and uptake of the catecholamines understandably aroused a great deal of interest. But there is now an almost compulsive desire to demonstrate, for all drugs that affect structures innervated by sympathetic nerve fibres, an effect in terms of uptake or storage or metabolism of adrenergic transmitter. However, this avenue of enquiry does not seem to have been very successful, and there is still much to be learned about the mechanism of action of drugs such as reserpine, guanethidine and α-methyldopa (Zaimis, 1964*a*, *b*, 1965).

In order to discover the extent to which the absence of sympathetic innervation modifies the effects produced by the three hypotensive drugs, immunosympathectomized and normal adult rats were treated for four to six weeks with reserpine, guanethidine and α-methyldopa (Zaimis, 1966). In both groups of animals observations were made of: (*a*) the growth rate; (*b*) the resting blood pressure and heart rate; (*c*) the blood pressure and heart rate responses to adrenaline, noradrenaline and tyramine, injected intravenously.

The growth rate of both control and immunosympathectomized animals was not affected by either α-methyldopa or guanethidine. All the rats receiving reserpine, however, lost weight during the last two weeks of treatment, and the percentage loss was almost the same for both control and immunosympathectomized animals. At the end of the chosen period the animals were anaesthetized with chloralose, both vagi cut and their systemic *blood pressure* and *heart rate* recorded simultaneously on a Grass polygraph. In the guanethidine- and reserpine-treated control and immunosympathectomized rats the resting heart rate and blood pressure decreased significantly. The decrease in heart rate was almost the same in the two groups of animals. The overall decrease in blood pressure, however, was smaller in the immunosympathectomized animals, possibly because their resting blood pressure, under anaesthesia, is always lower than that of the normal rats (Fig. 1). Treatment with α-methyldopa made little difference to the resting blood pressure and heart rate in either normal or immunosympathectomized rats.

An overall comparison of changes in blood pressure and heart rate in response to adrenaline (30 ng), noradrenaline (30 ng) and tyramine (30 μg) in both control and immunosympathectomized animals showed that the responses to the three pressor agents were significantly altered by the treatment with reserpine, guanethidine or α-methyldopa but that the changes recorded were very similar in both control and immunosympathectomized animals. For example, noradrenaline and especially adrenaline produced larger rises in blood pressure in all the animals treated with any of the three drugs. The pressor response to tyramine was significantly increased in the α-methyldopa-treated rats, both control and immunosympathectomized. On the other hand, the chronotropic response to tyramine was increased in all the animals treated with guanethidine. A comparison between the groups of animals injected with saline and reserpine showed that in both control and immunosympathectomized rats the pressor responses to adrenaline and noradrenaline were potentiated while those to tyramine remained the same or were slightly reduced.

From these results it is obvious that the peripheral adrenergic neurone is not the only point of attack of reserpine, guanethidine and α-methyldopa. The fact that the three hypotensive drugs produced very similar effects in both normal and immunosympathectomized animals strongly suggests a direct action on the effector cells themselves.

That α-methyldopa has a direct action on the effector cells is also suggested by the results of Varma (1967) who found that the effect of α-methyldopa in hypertensive rats was unchanged by immunosympathectomy, and by those of Ayitey-Smith & Varma (1970) who demonstrated that α-methyldopa 'significantly decreased the blood pressure in control hypertensive; immunosympathectomized normotensive; and normal rats'.

Several groups of investigators (Carlsson & Lindqvist, 1962; Day & Rand, 1963) have suggested that foreign amines may replace noradrenaline in its storage sites and be released by nerve stimulation as 'false neurochemical transmitters'. For example, it was suggested that α-methyldopa causes a partial

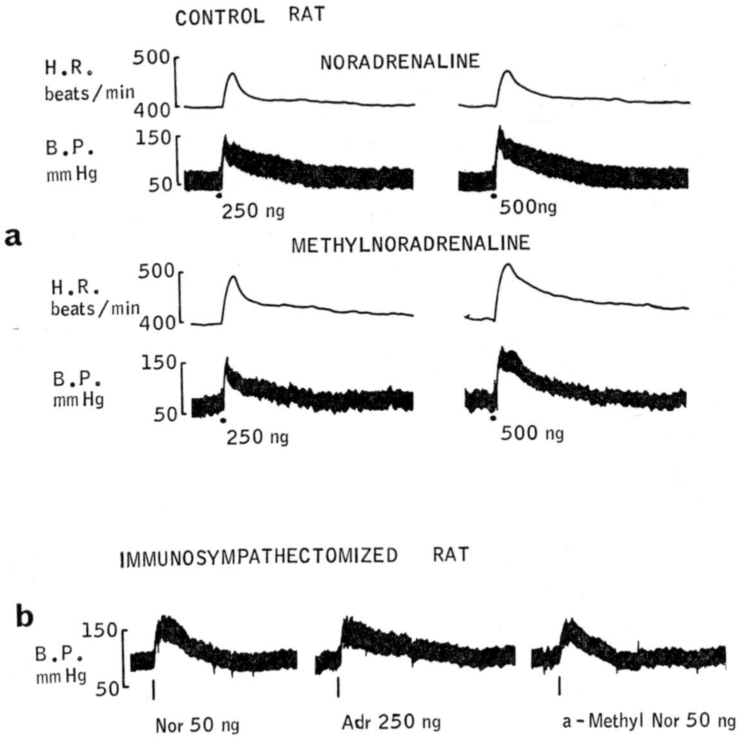

Fig. 7 Blood pressure (B.P.) and heart rate (H.R.) responses: (*a*) to noradrenaline and α-methylnoradrenaline in a control rat; and (*b*) to noradrenaline (Nor); adrenaline (Adr); and α-methylnoradrenaline (a-Methyl Nor) in an immunosympathectomized rat.

loss of sympathetic activity by acting as a precursor for α-methylnoradrenaline which may then function as a less efficient transmitter. It was Carlsson & Lindqvist (1962) who demonstrated that α-methylnoradrenaline could be formed from α-methyldopa in the body. However, the functional significance of the formation of α-methylnoradrenaline is questioned by many observations (for details see Goodman & Gilman, 1970), but mainly by the fact that the vasoconstrictor activity of α-methylnoradrenaline is as powerful as that of noradrenaline. Fig. 7*a* and *b* shows a comparison between α-methylnoradrenaline and noradrenaline and, in addition, demonstrates that α-methylnoradrenaline is active in both control and immunosympathectomized animals.

Clonidine

Clonidine, an imidazoline derivative, has been found effective in the treatment of moderately severe or severe hypertension (for references see Zaimis & Hanington, 1969). The hypotensive effect of this drug cannot, however, be fitted into any existing pharmacological or clinical pattern. Clonidine has neither a direct vasodilator effect, nor a ganglionic or postganglionic blocking action; it is free of α- and β-adrenoceptor blocking actions; it does not reduce the catecholamine content of the various tissues; and it is free of any veratrine-like action. On the other hand, this drug, on acute intravenous administration, has a direct vasoconstrictor action, which can be easily demonstrated in both man and animals (Ehringer, 1966; Zaimis, 1970). That clonidine has a direct vasoconstrictor effect was well demonstrated in experiments on immunosympathectomized rats. In these animals (Fig 8), the intravenous injection of clonidine produced a clear-cut rise in blood pressure, similar to that produced by either noradrenaline or adrenaline, and a reflex bradycardia. Heart rate and blood pressure changes, induced by either clonidine or the two catecholamines, were prevented by α-adrenoceptor blocking drugs, such as phentolamine or phenoxybenzamine. Taking all these factors into account, we concluded that results obtained in acute experiments probably have little relationship to changes occurring during the chronic administration of this drug in man. We were thus led to concentrate our attention on animal experiments in which the drug was administered chronically, in doses approximating to those given to man. In this way, we obtained much useful information relating to the drug's mechanism of action (Zaimis, 1970; Zaimis & Hanington, 1969; Larbi, 1970).

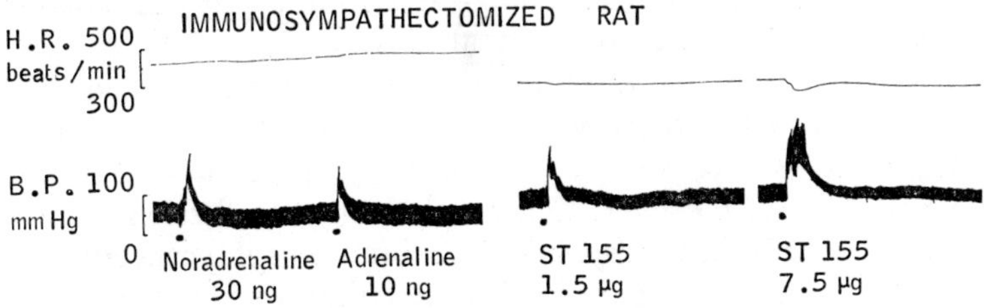

Fig. 8 Immunosympathectomized rat. A comparison of changes in blood pressure and heart rate in response to noradrenaline; adrenaline; and clonidine (ST 155).

It was found that clonidine, administered chronically to cats, reduces both the magnitude and the duration of vasoconstrictor and vasodilator responses elicited either by the electrical stimulation of the lumbar sympathetic chain, or by the close-arterial administration of vasoconstrictor and vasodilator drugs. Our conclusion, therefore, was that under the influence of clonidine, a change occurs in the smooth muscle which makes the vessels less capable of responding to, or of sustaining, either vasoconstriction or vasodilatation. The fact that clonidine has been found to affect both vasoconstrictor and vasodilator responses in animals, has been at the base of the suggestion that the drug should be given a trial in the treatment of migraine (Zaimis & Hanington, 1969). The encouraging clinical results obtained so far support this view and also the direct vascular effect of the drug.

The isolated perfused heart

In much work reported in recent years there is an underlying assumption that experiments on isolated muscle preparations are unlikely to produce results significantly different from those found in the intact animal. However, our pharmacological studies have demonstrated that the uniformity and predictability of responses present in the muscle studied *in vivo* are lost when the same muscle is studied *in vitro* (Zaimis, 1962; 1969; Maclagan, 1962).

In a recent study, the aim of which was to determine whether long-lasting perfusion of the heart alters its function and structure, my colleague, H. T. Toh, and I found that the isolation of the heart from the body is always accompanied, in every animal species studied, by an immediate and significant reduction in heart rate. One could be tempted to think that this decrease in heart rate was caused by the loss of sympathetic innervation. We have found, however, that an equivalent reduction in heart rate is present in hearts isolated from immunosympathectomized rats (Table 1). With the help of these animals we may therefore

Table 1

		Heart rate (beats/min) 'In vivo'	*Isolated*
Guinea-pigs		260	190
Chicks		400	165
Rats	Normal	490	290
	Immunosympathectomized	440	280

conclude that this decrease in heart rate is not related to the absence of sympathetic nervous influence but is the result of a change in the heart muscle after isolation and perfusion.

Conclusions

The possibilities which immunosympathectomized animals offer to pharmacological research have hardly begun to be exploited. The fact that NGF-antiserum has a very limited effect on the mesenteric ganglion and does not destroy about 25 per cent of the coeliac ganglion has been considered a disadvantage by some workers. Because of this, Burnstock and his colleagues (Burnstock, Evans, Gannon, Heath & James, 1971) have proposed another method of producing sympathectomy in rats: chronic treatment for six weeks with 25 or 30 mg/kg per day of guanethidine, injected intraperitoneally. This treatment results in widespread sympathectomy which persists over long periods. However, the assumption that sympathectomy by guanethidine is a 'simple' method producing an animal which is normal in other respects, but with its sympathetic system destroyed, is an over-simplification. Such very large doses of guanethidine administered for six weeks are likely to affect other organs and other tissues and to alter their responses to either natural transmitters or other drugs. The guanethidine-induced sympathectomy may be advantageous, as Burnstock and his colleagues conclude, when denervation of the male reproductive tract is required, but for cardiovascular studies immunosympathectomy has, to my mind, all possible advantages. While the heart and vessels are truly free of sympathetic innervation, the animals are in all other respects normal and their tissues are unaffected by any foreign pharmacologically active substances; their body temperature is practically the same as that of the untreated rats; they are active, eat, drink, clean themselves and breed normally; and their life span is similar to that of the controls. Such animals are a most valuable tool in cardiovascular research.

Acknowledgements

I wish to express my thanks to Mr R. Owen and Mr H. J. Fearn for their expert technical assistance; and to the Medical Research Council and the Palisades Foundation, Inc. of the U.S.A. for partially financing this research.

References

Ayitey-Smith, E. & Varma, D. R. (1970). *Br. J. Pharmac.* **40**, 186.
Beaulnes, A. (1963). *Biochem. Pharmac.* **12**, Suppl. 181.
Benelli, G., Della Bella, D. & Gandini, A. (1964). *Br. J. Pharmac.* **22**, 211.
Burnstock, G., Evans, Barbara, Gannon, B. J., Heath, J. W. & James, Vicki. (1971). *Br. J. Pharmac.* **43**, 295.
Carlsson, A. & Lindqvist, M. (1962). *Acta physiol. scand.* **54**, 83.
Cohen, S. (1960). *Proc. natn. Acad. Sci. U.S.A.* **46**, 302.
Crout, J. R., Alpers, H. S., Tatum, E. L. & Shore, P.A. (1964). *Science* **145**, 828.
Day, M. D. & Rand, M. J. (1963). *J. Pharm. Pharmac.* **15**, 221.

Ehringer, H. (1966). *Arzneimettel-Forsch.* **16**, 1165.
Feldberg, W. & Lewis, G. P. (1964). *J. Physiol., Lond.* **171**, 98.
Goodman, L. S. & Gilman, A. (Ed.) (1970). *The Pharmacological Basis of Therapeutics*, 4th ed. p. 578. New York: Macmillan Co.
Larbi, E. B. (1970). Ph.D. Thesis. University of London.
Levi-Montalcini, R. (1964). *Science* **143**, 105.
Levi-Montalcini, R. & Cohen, S. (1960). *Ann. N.Y. Acad. Sci.* **85**, 324.
Maclagan, J. (1962). *Br. J. Pharmac.* **18**, 204.
Nash, C. W., Wolff, S. A. & Ferguson, B. A. (1968). *Can. J. Physiol. Pharmac.* **46**, 35.
Shore, P. A. (1966). *Pharmac. Rev.* **18**, 561.
Varma, D. R. (1967). *J. Pharm. Pharmac.* **19**, 61.
Zaimis, E. (1962). In *Curare and Curare-Like Agents*, Ciba Foundation Study Group No. 12, p. 75. Ed. by de Reuck, A. V. S. London: Churchill.
Zaimis, E. (1964*a*). *Ann. Rev. Pharmac.* **4**, 365.
Zaimis, E. (1964*b*). In *Cardiomyopathies*, Ciba Foundation Symposium, p. 214. Ed. by Wolstenholme, G. E. W. & O'Connor, M. London: Churchill.
Zaimis, E. (1965). In *Evaluation of New Drugs in Man*. Proc. 2nd Int. Pharmac. Meeting, vol. 8, p. 57. London & New York: Pergamon Press.
Zaimis, E. (1966). In *Antihypertensive Therapy—Principles and Practice*, An International Symposium, p. 59. Ed. by Gross, F. Berlin: Springer Verlag.
Zaimis, E. (1968). *Anesthesiology* **29**, 732.
Zaimis, E. (1969). In *Disorders of Voluntary Muscle*, 2nd ed., p. 46. Ed. by Walton, J. N. London: Churchill.
Zaimis, E. (1970). In *Catapres in Hypertension*, p. 9. Ed. by Conolly, M. E. London: Butterworths.
Zaimis, E., Berk, L. & Callingham, B. A. (1965). *Nature, Lond.* **206**, 1220.
Zaimis, E. & Hanington, E. (1969). *Lancet* **ii** 298.

The Functional Status of the Cardiovascular System in Immunosympathectomized Rats

M. J. BRODY

Department of Pharmacology, College of Medicine, University of Iowa, Iowa City, USA

Extensive experience with surgical sympathectomy and with pharmacological denervation has made it abundantly clear that alterations in the functional status of the denervated organ or organism are not easily demonstrated unless responses to specific challenges are evaluated. The stimuli used to evoke these responses should ordinarily result in a marked activation of the sympathetic nervous system. The ease with which the cardiovascular system can be studied makes this system an excellent model in which to examine the functional deficits produced by sympathectomy.

When the antiserum to the nerve growth factor (NGF) was discovered and became available (Levi-Montalcini & Angeletti, 1966), our interest was immediately caught. The material appeared to be an extraordinary tool for producing, with great ease, an animal deprived from birth of its peripheral sympathetic nervous system. The potential applications of this tool to the physiology and pathophysiology of the sympathetic nervous system are, of course, numerous. Practically speaking, however, the utility of the NGF-antiserum depends in large part upon a demonstration that treatment with it produces functional deficits analogous to those produced by surgical or pharmacological denervation. The studies reviewed in this paper were undertaken to determine how the cardiovascular system in particular was affected by this unique type of sympathectomy.

Methods

Newborn rats were immunized with bovine antiserum developed to NGF isolated from mouse salivary glands. Treatment was begun at birth with daily injections for 14 days (Brody, 1964).

Heart rates were determined from ECG records taken under light ether anaesthesia. In unanaesthetized animals blood pressure was recorded either using a caudal plethysmograph or by measurements made from indwelling aortic catheters implanted chronically (Dorr & Brody, 1966). Vascular responses to sympathetic nerve stimulation or to drugs were measured in autoperfused hind-quarters (Brody, 1964). Recordings of electrical activity in sympathetic nerves were made as described in detail by Brody (1963). Responses of the heart were examined in several ways. Isolated atria were prepared and responses to drugs and to transmural stimulation through field electrodes were recorded (Brody, 1967). Cardiac output was measured in open-chest animals using an electromagnetic flowmeter probe on the aorta (Brody, 1967). Responses of the coronary circulation were measured with a modified Langendorf preparation from which outflow was determined under constant perfusion pressure (Brody, 1967).

Results and discussion

Blood pressure

A demonstrable effect of immunosympathectomy on arterial pressure appears to be dependent on the conditions under which the measurement is made, and on whether the adrenal medulla is intact or has been extirpated. In the conscious state arterial pressure has been reported to be the same in immunosympathectomized and control rats (Dorr & Brody, 1966; Varma, 1967; Willard & Fuller, 1969; Finch & Leach, 1970). However, it was found that the arterial pressure of conscious animals could not be recorded in immunosympathectomized rats by the usual method of tail plethysmography. Neither local warming of the tail nor whole-body warming was sufficient to allow arterial pressure to be transmitted through the tail of immunosympathectomized rats (Brody, 1964). Other investigators have not reported this difficulty. Direct measurements of arterial pressure with indwelling catheters in conscious animals show that mean, systolic and diastolic pressures are equivalent in normal and immunosympathectomized rats (Dorr & Brody, 1966).

Considerable differences in arterial pressure are found when recordings are made under anaesthesia. Anaesthetized immunosympathectomized rats usually (Zaimis, 1965*a*; 1966; Zaimis, Berk & Callingham, 1965), but not invariably (Brody, 1964; 1966), have significantly lower arterial pressures than anaesthetized control rats. The explanation for this difference between conscious and anaesthetized rats is not known, although it may be suggested that the sympathetic nervous system helps to sustain arterial pressure in the normal animal during anaesthesia but cannot be called upon in animals deprived of sympathetic innervation.

The adrenal medulla is relatively unaffected by treatment with NGF-antiserum. Adrenal discharge of catecholamines appears to help sustain arterial pressure. When the adrenal medulla is removed from immunosympathectomized animals, arterial pressure falls below that seen in immunosympathectomized animals with intact adrenals (Berti, Lentati & Usardi, 1965; Brody, 1966).

Heart rate

In the normal animal, heart rate is under the control of complex interactions between neurogenic, humoral and intrinsic chronotropic influences. Positive chronotropic influences include the effects of noradrenaline released from adrenergic nerve terminals and the effects of any other catecholamines circulating in the blood; while negative chronotropic effects result largely from the release of acetylcholine from cholinergic nerves associated with the parasympathetic branch of the autonomic nervous system. Interestingly, immunosympathectomy has little effect on resting heart rate (Brody, 1964; 1966; 1967; Dorr & Brody, 1966), an effect noted by others (Berti *et al.*, 1965; Chung, 1966; Wenzel, Carson & Chase, 1966; Zaimis, 1965*b*; 1967; Wekstein, 1965). As with blood pressure, it might be predicted that in the absence of functional sympathetic innervation, heart rate is sustained by the positive chronotropic action of catecholamines secreted by the intact adrenal medulla. This proves not to be the case, however, since adrenal-demedullated immunosympathectomized rats have normal heart rates (Brody, 1966). The rate of spontaneously beating atria isolated from immunosympathectomized rats was also normal (Brody, 1967). In contrast, the spontaneous rate of atria from animals treated with reserpine was reduced significantly (Brody, 1967).

Immunosympathectomy appears to be without any influence on the functioning of parasympathetic innervation to the heart. Electrical stimulation of the vagus nerve in anaesthetized animals reduces heart rates of immunosympathectomized and normal animals to an equivalent degree (Brody, 1967; Zaimis, 1965*b*). In isolated atria, the initial slowing of rate produced by field stimulation is the result of a cholinergic mechanism, presumably from the liberation of acetylcholine from cholinergic nerve endings. This slowing effect is the same in atrial tissue from control and immunosympathectomized rats (Brody, 1967).

Tests on the functional integrity of sympathetic innervation to the heart have been made, both in the intact animal and in isolated cardiac tissue. Electrical stimulation of the thoracic sympathetic chain in the normal rat elevates heart rate significantly. Conversely, the same stimulus reduces the heart rate of immunosympathectomized rats (Brody, 1967).

Although resting heart rates are not altered by immunosympathectomy, Zaimis (1965*b*; 1967) has found functional evidence for the absence of sympathetic innervation by the demonstration of typical denervation supersensitivity to the chronotropic effects of catecholamines. Chronotropic responses to adrenaline and noradrenaline were enhanced significantly in spontaneously beating atria from immunosympathectomized rats (Brody, 1967). The change in sensitivity appeared to be specific for the amines, since the chronotropic effects of barium chloride were unaltered (Brody, 1967).

Contractility

The basal inotropic state of the immunosympathectomized heart appears to be unaltered. Isometric tension developed by isolated atria, and the cardiac output of intact animals, were unchanged by immunosympathectomy (Brody, 1967). Although cardiac output is not necessarily an index of the inotropic state of the heart, the fact that arterial pressure, vascular resistance and cardiac output appear to be unchanged in immunosympathectomized animals (Brody, 1967) strongly suggests that the contractile state of the hearts of these animals is not impaired.

Vascular responses

A technique for autoperfusion of the rat hind-quarters was used to study the influence of immunosympathectomy on the control of reactivity of the vascular system (Brody, 1964; 1966). Electrical stimulation of the lumbar sympathetic chains in normal animals produces vasoconstrictor responses which are graded in proportion to the frequency of stimulation. In immunosympathectomized rats electrical stimulation of the small residual lumbar chains failed to elicit any vasoconstrictor response (Brody, 1964; 1966). Thus the residual sympathetic fibres which survive treatment with NGF-antiserum apparently have no vasomotor function. The ganglionic stimulant 1:1-dimethyl-4-phenylpiperazinium (DMPP), by activating adrenergic ganglionic synapses, produced vasoconstriction in the hind-limbs of normal rats but failed to exert any effect in the perfused hind-quarters of immunosympathectomized animals (Brody, 1964; 1966), thus providing additional evidence for the lack of functional integrity of the surviving sympathetic structures.

Responses to several vasoconstrictor agents, administered locally into the perfused hind-quarters, were tested. In two separate studies the major effect on responses to the catecholamines adrenaline and noradrenaline was an increase in the duration, as opposed to an increase in the magnitude, of vasoconstriction (Brody, 1964; 1966). Thus, typical denervation supersensitivity was noted in immunosympathectomized rats, but this was manifested most clearly by prolongation of the vasoconstrictor responses.

Zaimis (1965*b*; 1966; 1967) has studied the pressor effects of catecholamines in rats, recording the arterial pressure of the whole animal. In this case there is substantial denervation supersensitivity to adrenaline and noradrenaline. It may be presumed that the greater pressor effects noted were the result of a considerable participation of increased cardiac rather than vascular sensitivity, since the magnitude of vascular responses to these amines is not greatly altered (Brody, 1964; 1966).

Responses to angiotensin, vasopressin and barium chloride were not altered significantly in immunosympathectomized rats (Brody, 1966). The response to tyramine, on the other hand, although not abolished by immunosympathectomy, was reduced significantly (Brody, 1966). These data indicate that blood vessels of immunosympathectomized animals exhibit classical supersensitivity to directly acting catecholamines and reduced sensitivity to the indirectly acting amine, tyramine, and they further indicate that this altered sensitivity is specific for catecholamines, since vasoconstrictor responses to non-adrenergic vasoconstrictor agents were essentially unchanged.

The adrenal medulla appears to play an important role in immunosympathectomized rats in the maintenance of vasoconstrictor tone. Despite the fact that the innervation of blood vessels in the hind-quarters is non-functional, resistance to blood flow is slightly above normal (Brody, 1964) or normal (Brody, 1966), as shown by the pressure-flow relationships. When the adrenal medulla is removed chronically, resistance to blood flow in the hind-quarter vessels of immunosympathectomized rats falls significantly below normal (Brody, 1966). It appears that vasoconstrictor tone is maintained in the immunosympathectomized rat in part by the effect of catecholamines released from the adrenal medulla and circulating in the blood.

In summary, immunological sympathectomy deprives the cardiovascular system of regulation by sympathetic innervation. Adaptive processes, whose nature is largely unknown, appear to mask the functional deficits in sympathetic regulation, thus allowing the cardiovascular system to act in a relatively normal fashion. However, stimuli which would ordinarily result in sympathetic nervous activation of the heart and blood vessels are largely devoid of effect in immunosympathectomized rats, hence making this experimental model an excellent tool for future studies on the physiological and pathophysiological role of the sympathetic nervous system in the control of cardiovascular function.

Acknowledgements

Part of the work reported here was supported by USPHS Grant NB-04889 and by Grants-in-Aid from the Iowa and American Heart Associations.

References

Berti, F., Lentati, R. & Usardi, M. M. (1965). *Med. Pharmac. Exp.* **13**, 227.

Brody, M. J. (1963). *Proc. Soc. exp. Biol. Med.* **114**, 565.

Brody, M. J. (1964). *Circulation Res.* **15**, 161.

Brody, M. J. (1966). *Am. J. Physiol.* **211**, 198.

Brody, M. J. (1967). In *Factors Influencing Myocardial Contractility*, p. 479. Ed. by Tanz. R. D., Kavaler, F. & Roberts, J. New York: Academic Press Inc.

Chung, E. (1966). Ph.D. Thesis: University of Toronto.

Dorr, L. D. & Brody, M. J. (1966). *Proc. Soc. exp. Biol. Med.* **123**, 155.

Finch, L. & Leach, G. D. H. (1970). *Br. J. Pharmac.* **39**, 317.

Levi-Montalcini, R. & Angeletti, P. U. (1966). *Pharmac. Rev.* **18**, 619.

Varma, D. R. (1967). *J. Pharm. Pharmac.* **19**, 61.

Wekstein, D. R. (1965). *Am. J. Physiol.* **208**, 1259.

Wenzel, B. M., Carson, V. & Chase, K. (1966). *Percept. Mot. Skills Res. Exch.* **23**, 1009.

Willard, P. W. & Fuller, R. W. (1969). *Nature, Lond.* **223**, 417.

Zaimis, E. (1965*a*). *Proc. R. Soc. Med.* **58**, 1067.

Zaimis, E. (1965*b*). *J. Physiol., Lond.* **177**, 35P.

Zaimis, E. (1966). In *Antihypertensive Therapy—Principles and Practice, An International Symposium*, p. 59. Ed. by Gross, F. Berlin: Springer-Verlag.

Zaimis, E. (1967). In *The Scientific Basis of Medicine Annual Reviews*, p. 59. London: Athlone Press.

Zaimis, E., Berk, L. & Callingham, B. A. (1965). *Nature, Lond.* **206**, 1220.

Effects of Drugs on the Behaviour of Immunosympathectomized Mice

BERNICE M. WENZEL

Department of Physiology and Brain Research Institute, UCLA School of Medicine, Los Angeles, USA

The immunosympathectomized animal can be characterized by fewer neural cells in paravertebral sympathetic ganglia, lower concentrations of noradrenaline in organs normally innervated by neurones from these ganglia, increased amounts of chromaffin tissue in visceral organs, and altered levels of serotonin in the gut. These animals also behave differently from normal animals, especially in tests that include aversive stimuli (Wenzel, 1972). One way of studying possible relations between the somatic and behavioural effects of immunosympathectomy is through the use of drugs acting on adrenergic mechanisms. This paper presents results obtained with three such agents; reserpine, a drug that affects the tissue content of noradrenaline and serotonin both centrally and peripherally; DMPP (dimethylphenylpiperazinium iodide), a ganglionic stimulant; and nicotine, which is also a ganglion stimulant at low doses, but which also has central effects. Some preliminary work with mecamylamine and pentolinium, two ganglionic blocking agents with and without central effects, is discussed.

The animals used in all these experiments were Webster Swiss mice from the Department of Medical Microbiology and Immunology at UCLA. Most procedural details, of injecting the pups with nerve growth factor (NGF) antiserum and control substances, and of the behavioural testing, can be found in previous publications (Wenzel, 1968*a*, *b*; Wenzel & Jeffrey, 1967). At the end of each experiment, the mice were killed with sodium pentobarbitone or by cervical fracture and placed in buffered formalin solution, after removal of their backbones. The number of sympathetic ganglion cells in the immunosympathectomized groups averaged 10–15 per cent of normal; the injected controls showed a normal number. Results of all behavioural tests were treated by analysis of variance, with time scores normalized by transformation to logarithms.

Reserpine

Sixty-two Webster Swiss mice completed this experiment. They were divided as follows into four groups according to treatment during the first week of life: IS—14 (7 males, 7 females) had received NGF-antiserum to produce immunosympathectomy; GG—13 (3 males, 10 females) had been injected with gamma globulin; H—18 (8 males, 10 females) had been handled as if to be injected but were not injected; NH—17 (10 males, 7 females) had been left undisturbed (not handled). The mice had been individually housed since weaning.

Two tests from a former battery of tests (Wenzel, 1968*a*), shock-avoidance runway and food runway, were used and will be described briefly here. Both tests required the mouse to run down a 1.05 m runway from a start box to a goal box. In the shock-avoidance test the floor and walls of both the start box and the runway were electrified 4.24 seconds after the start box door had been opened on to the runway. If the mouse reached the goal box within that time, no shock was received because the goal box could not be electrified. But, if the mouse had remained in the start box after the door opened or was still in the runway, then a shock of approximately 0.25 mA was experienced. Time was measured automatically between the opening of the start box door and the arrival of the mouse in the goal box. The goal box of the food runway contained a small Perspex well in which liquid food (undiluted evaporated milk plus sugar water) was provided. In this runway, as in the shock-avoidance runway, time was recorded from the opening of the start box door until the mouse reached the goal box. The two runways were identical in all respects, except that the food runway was constructed entirely of wood, which was painted white, and the shock runway was built of galvanized steel with a 5 mm gap down the centre. For each runway, a test session consisted of five trials with no resting time between trials.

In addition to the time scores in the runway, three additional scores were obtained on each mouse at every test session after injection of reserpine. After the lid of the home pan was removed and before the animal was touched in any way, the mouse was rated on a four-point scale for ptosis and for activity. It was then nudged gently at the base of the tail and was rated on a four-point scale for responsiveness. At the end of the test session, each mouse was weighed and returned to the home pan.

The general procedure of the experiment was to administer reserpine (Serpasil, CIBA Co.) or reserpine vehicle as a placebo shortly after a pre-injection test session. Post-injection test sessions were held at standard intervals for 48 hours, or longer if performance had not returned to the pre-injection level. Each mouse received two injections, four weeks apart, of either reserpine or placebo. In association with the first injection, the mouse was tested either in the shock-avoidance runway or in the food-getting runway; in association with the second injection, the same mouse was tested in the other runway. Approximately half of the males and of the females in each treatment group were tested first with each runway. The body weight of all mice assigned to the food runway was reduced to approximately 80 per cent of free-feeding weight, as previously described. All injections were made between 0930 and 1030 hours about one hour after the pre-injection test session. Post-injection testing was done at the following intervals: $1\frac{1}{2}$, $4\frac{1}{2}$, $7\frac{1}{2}$, 11, 24, 30 and 48 hours. If pre-injection performance had not been reached, testing then continued at 24-hour intervals. The total experiment was run in three replications, approximately one-third of the group being tested each time. All treatment groups were represented in the first two replications, but only handled and not-handled groups were tested in the third. The subjects were six months old at the time of their first injection and had previously participated in experiments already described (Wenzel, 1968*a*).

The dosage of reserpine was 2.0 mg per kg body weight for animals being tested in the shock-avoidance runway and 1.5 mg per kg for mice running in the food runway. Equivalent volumes of the vehicle were administered to the control subjects. Injections were given subcutaneously in the dorsal pelvic area.

Because of the hypophagia experienced by many of the mice after injection of reserpine, any animal that fell below 80 per cent free-feeding body weight was force-fed with a solution of evaporated milk and sugar water until its weight reached the 80 per cent level. Such feeding was always done approximately one hour after completion of a test session and was never required earlier than 12 hours after the injection.

The mean running times for each group in each runway after injection of reserpine and of placebo are shown in Figs. 1 and 2.

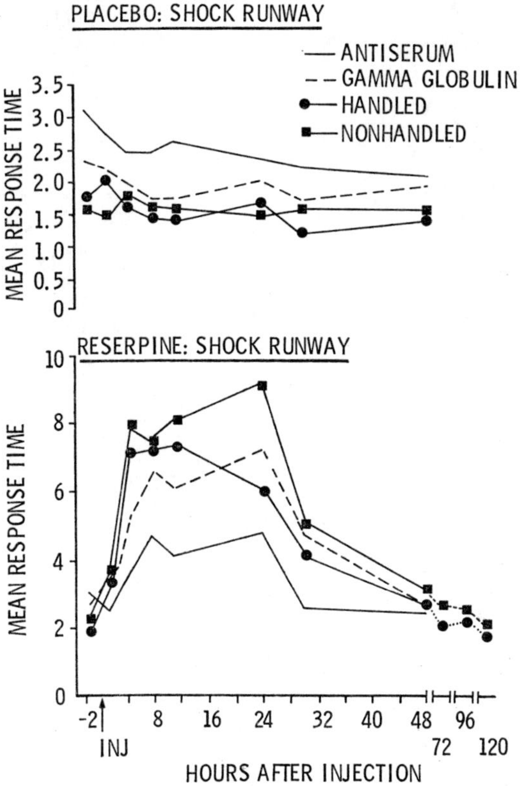

Fig. 1 Mean running time of each group in shock runway immediately before and at various times after injection of reserpine or placebo.

The most notable feature of the results is the lesser effect of reserpine on the immunosympathectomized mice than on those of the other groups when they were assigned to the shock-avoidance runway. The immunosympathectomized group differed significantly from the not-handled group at all post-injection testing times from $4\frac{1}{2}$ to 48 hours ($P<0.05$ at $4\frac{1}{2}$ hours; <0.025 or 0.005 at others), and from the handled group at $1\frac{1}{2}$, $7\frac{1}{2}$, 11 and 24 hours ($P<0.05$ at $1\frac{1}{2}$, <0.01 or 0.025 at others). Immunosympathectomized and γ-globulin-treated mice did not

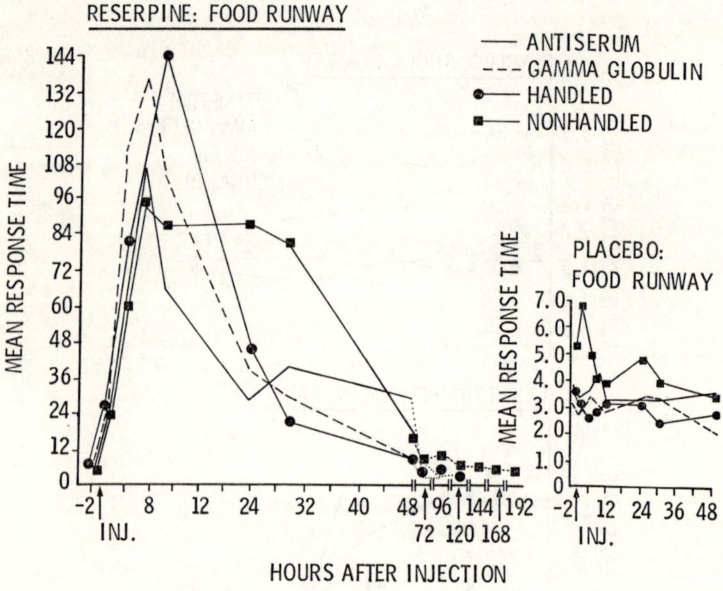

Fig. 2 Mean running time of each group in food runway immediately before and at various times after injection of reserpine or placebo.

differ significantly because of unusual variability in the γ-globulin-treated group; the trend is, however, consistent with the other control groups. When the same animals were running for food, no group differences appeared in spite of the fact that the dose of reserpine at that time was 25 per cent lower than during testing in shock-avoidance.

The same effect can be seen in Figs. 3 and 4, which show the mean group ratings for ptosis, motility and reactivity. The higher the ratings for ptosis, the more was ptosis present; the higher the ratings for activity, the more was motility reduced. In the part of the experiment in which the mice were being tested in the shock-avoidance runway, reserpine had a smaller effect on these ratings in the immunosympathectomized group, just as it did

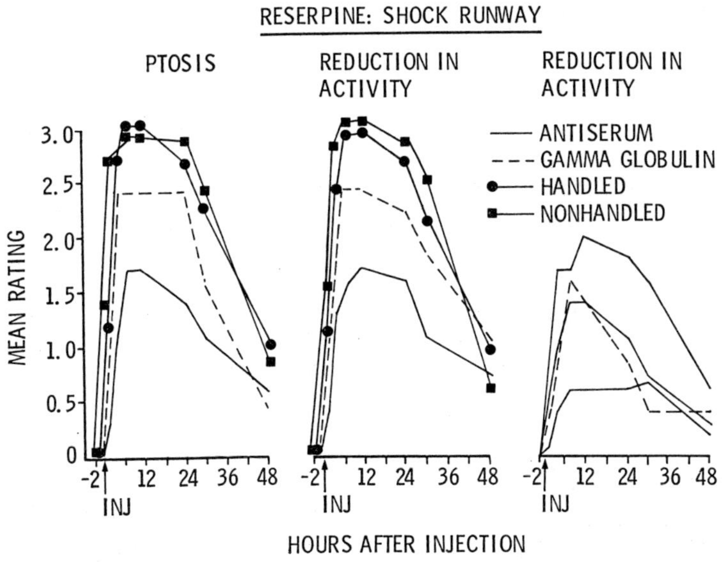

Fig. 3 Mean group ratings of ptosis, spontaneous activity and reactivity for each group at start of each testing session in shock runway immediately before and at various times after injection of reserpine.

on running time. Significant differences ($P<0.05$) occurred at 11, 24 and 30 hours after the injection for ptosis, and at 11 and 30 hours for motility. The differences in reactivity ratings were not significant although their direction was the same as was that for the other ratings. It should be remembered that the ratings were made immediately before each test session in the runway so that they reflect some long-term effect rather than any immediate energizing influence from the test session.

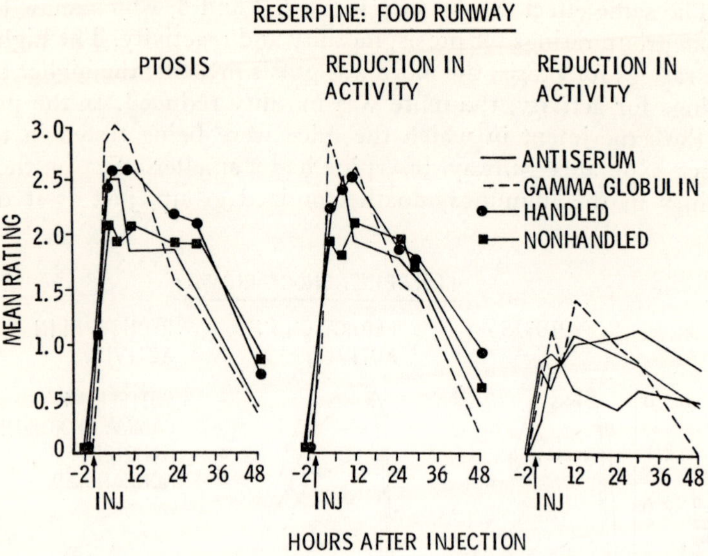

Fig. 4 Mean group ratings of ptosis, spontaneous activity and reactivity for each group at start of each testing session in food runway immediately before and at various times after injection of reserpine.

The superiority of the immunosympathectomized mice to those in the other groups in the shock-avoidance runway after reserpine is in sharp contrast to the same group's poorer performance in shock-avoidance following injection of placebo. As can be seen in Fig. 1, the immunosympathectomized group's response time was consistently slower than that of all other groups throughout the repeated testing that followed placebo injection. This finding agrees closely with that obtained during earlier testing (Wenzel, 1968*a*) when the mice were learning the tasks and approaching the asymptotic performance that had been reached by the time of the present experiment.

The general time-course of the reserpine effect for all groups was consistent with that usually described for this type of experiment. For example, data obtained from cats in my laboratory, in an experiment in which both the shock-avoidance and food-getting responses consisted of pressing a lever, showed the reserpine effect on the food-getting response as occurring relatively sharply; whereas the peak effect on the shock-avoidance response was spread over many hours (Wenzel, 1959).

DMPP and nicotine

Experiments have been completed with three tests: open field, water escape and non-discriminated avoidance. Preliminary data have been obtained in a shuttle-box avoidance task. All animals were housed in groups of two to five after weaning, according to sex and litter. The dosage of DMPP was 400 μg/kg body weight, and that of nicotine tartrate was 500 μg/kg (calculated as base). The solutions were adjusted so that comparable volumes would be injected in each case. Equivalent volumes of normal saline solution were injected into control subjects. All injections were subcutaneous in the dorsal pelvic region. During waiting periods between injections and testing, or between trials, the mice were kept in individual holding pans lined with clean paper towels.

Open field; water escape

These tests were administered to 136 mice in the following groups: immunosympathectomized 48 (25 males, 23 females) injected as described above; horse serum-treated—43 (25 males, 18 females) injected in the same manner with whole horse serum (HS) as control substance; not handled—45 (22 males, 23 females) left undisturbed (after continual findings of no difference between handled and non-handled control groups, the former control is no longer included). Each of these groups was divided into three subgroups for injection of saline (17 IS, 16 HS, 15 NH), DMPP (14 IS, 14 HS, 15 NH), or nicotine (14 IS, 15 HS, 16 NH). Males and females were assigned to these subgroups as evenly as possible. The mice were approximately three months old.

The apparatus and general procedure for both tests have been described previously (Wenzel & Jeffrey, 1967). The open field is a circular area, 0.6 m in diameter. Five minutes after injection the mouse was placed in the centre and locomotor activity was counted for three minutes. In this test, a loud clicking noise was presented during the second and third minutes because of the previously noted tendency of immunosympathectomized mice to overreact to auditory stimuli. It was thought that the noise might amplify possible differences between the immunosympathectomized subgroups and others.

Immediately after removal from the open field, the mouse was dropped into a sink (0.86 m long × 0.42 m wide) of water (0.18 m deep) at room temperature (20–25°C). It was placed in the water with its head pointed into the corner diagonally opposite an escape ramp, and time was taken until it had four feet on the ramp or three minutes had elapsed. In the latter case, it was guided to the ramp. Time was measured with an electric timer controlled by a hand switch. A second trial was given, commencing at a variable number of minutes after the first. One week later, each mouse was reinjected and given five additional water-escape trials. Three mice were injected at a time, one with each drug, and were tested in succession on each trial, beginning 10 minutes after injection. Intervals between trials varied slightly, therefore, as individual escape times varied.

The mean number of lines crossed on the floor of the open

Table 1 Open field test: mean numbers of lines crossed and standard deviations (S.D.) during first minute and the second and third minutes combined

	Mean		S.D.	
	Minute 1	*Minutes 2 & 3*	*Minute 1*	*Minutes 2 & 3*
Immunosympathectomized				
Saline solution	23	36	15	23
DMPP	24	31	14	16
Nicotine	18	23	15	24
Horse serum-treated				
Saline solution	22	29	13	15
DMPP	25	29	18	13
Nicotine	28	33	21	28
Not handled				
Saline solution	30	34	15	20
DMPP	26	24	14	17
Nicotine	23	17	19	21

field is shown in Table 1 for each subgroup during the first minute (silence) and during the second and third minutes combined (clicking noise). No main effect or interaction was significant and only the immunosympathectomized mice tended to show increased activity during the noise.

Fig. 5 presents the results for the subgroups for the first trial in water escape. Both drug and treatment effects were significant ($P<0.05$, $P = 0.01$, respectively) on Day 1, but only the drug effect reached significance on Day 2 (trial 1, $P<0.0005$; mean of trials 1–5, $P<0.05$). No drug-treatment interactions were significant at any time.

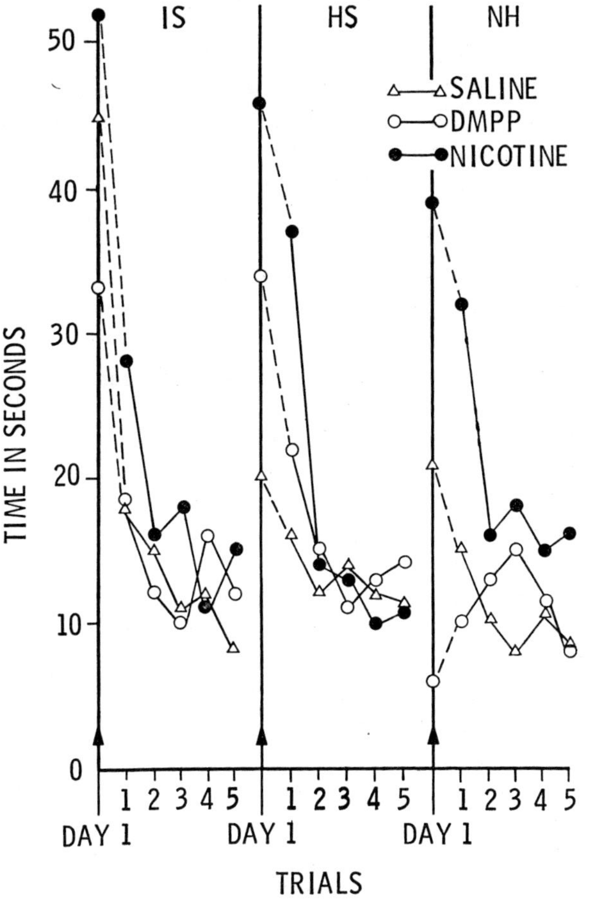

Fig. 5 Mean times for water escape in the first trial on Day 1 and five trials on Day 2.

The strongest effect in this experiment, shown in all three treated groups, was that of nicotine, which caused slower escape times, especially during the first 5–10 minutes after injection. From watching the mice, it was apparent that they were swimming aimlessly in all directions and were not necessarily swimming at a different speed. The immunosympathectomized group escaped very slowly because the deleterious effect of nicotine, which in their case was slight, added to their basically slower performance as exhibited after saline injection.

Non-discriminated avoidance

This experiment was conducted two to three months after that described above. The same animals were used. Thirteen had died of various causes between experiments, three died during the experimental period, and four were dropped because they did not learn the lever-pressing response well enough, leaving a total of 116 (61 males, 55 females).

Their task was to escape or delay an electric shock to their feet by depressing a lever that projected into a circular Perspex enclosure 0.145 m in diameter. Shock (about 280 μA) was delivered automatically through the floor of brass rods every 20 seconds and stayed on continuously until the lever was pressed. Pressing the lever in the absence of shock delayed the next shock for 20 seconds. It was possible, therefore, to prevent all but the first shock at the start of each session. A description of the apparatus and training procedure can be found in an earlier article (Wenzel, 1968*b*).

After ten minutes of exploration in the enclosure on one day, each mouse was individually trained on the next day, tested without injection on the following day in a 20-minute session, and then tested for seven more days in 20-minute sessions, each beginning five minutes after injection. Dosages were the same as those specified above. Two days with no injections or testing intervened between the third and fourth of the eight test days.

The two direct measures of performance were (*a*) the total number of responses made by each mouse in each session and (*b*) the total number of shocks received. The maximum number of shocks possible was 60 (one every 20 seconds for 20 minutes), if each shock was terminated immediately and no inter-shock responses were made. The more inter-shock responses, the better were the chances of minimizing the number of shocks. The response/shock ratio is a derived measure of performance. The higher this value, the more effective is the avoidance of shock.

Analysis of the ratios of responses to shocks, which are shown in Fig. 6 for the mean number of responses and shocks on the

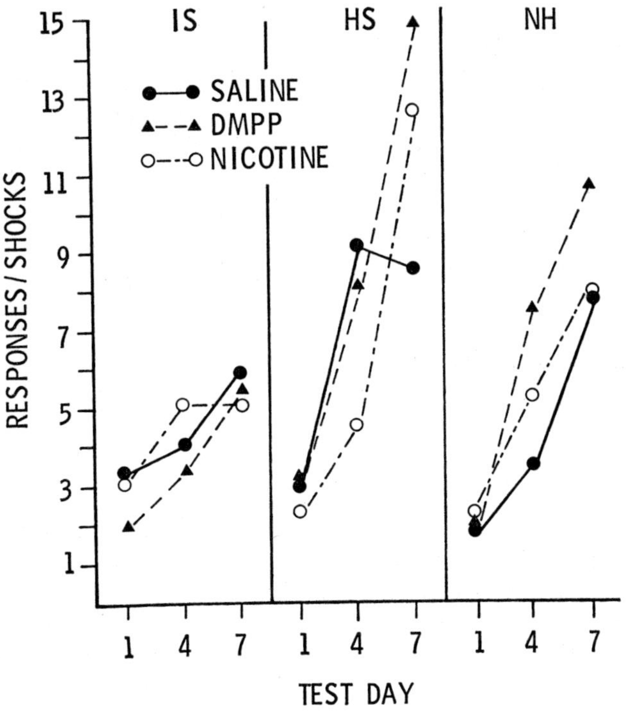

Fig. 6 Group ratios of mean responses to mean shocks on the first, fourth, and seventh days of testing with drugs.

first, fourth, and last days of testing with drugs, indicates significant differences due to treatment on the first and last days but no significant effects of drugs at any time. Although the immunosympathectomized group began with a slight superiority on Day

1, it soon fell behind as the performance of the two control groups steadily improved with practice. This difference is consistent with results obtained previously (Wenzel, 1968*b*). There is no suggestion in these data that DMPP had stimulated performance of the immunosympathectomized group as it tended to do in the control mice in later sessions.

Several trends emerged from these experiments. (1) Regardless of drugs, the immunosympathectomized mice generally performed more poorly than the two sets of control mice except in the open field test. These relationships are consistent with earlier results from my laboratory. (2) There was at least a tendency for nicotine to degrade performance. This effect was greater in the control groups than in the immunosympathectomized group. (3) At the dosage used, DMPP had relatively little and inconsistent effect. It was not generally facilitatory. (4) The horse serum-treated group showed somewhat different patterns from both of the other groups. This accords with previous findings, at least in the animals' lack of identity with uninjected controls.

Shuttle-box avoidance

Mice are being tested in this procedure (as described by Bovet, Bovet-Nitti & Oliverio, 1966) 15 minutes after injection of saline solution, DMPP, nicotine, mecamylamine or pentolinium. The animals' task here is to move from one compartment of the box to the other in order to escape foot shock or to avoid it. Avoidance is possible by running in response to the onset of a light, which precedes the onset of shock by 4.5 seconds. In the results so far obtained, DMPP is followed by faster response times in the not-handled group than occur after injection of normal saline, but no effect is seen for immunosympathectomized mice. The immunosympathectomized mice, on the other hand, are slowed by mecamylamine, in contrast to the other groups where it has no effect. A slight tendency is emerging for nicotine to facilitate response times in both control groups, which would agree with Bovet's finding of a large improvement after nicotine in Swiss mice. In sharp contrast, the immunosympathectomized mice so far are much slower after nicotine in this task. These results are mentioned only as a preliminary report.

Conclusions

The discrepant behaviour of the immunosympathectomized mice indicates discrepant reactions to pharmacological agents which can be attributed to their treatment with NGF-antiserum. The location and nature of these differences obviously cannot be identified on the basis of the data presented here. The most common hypothesis about reserpine-induced behavioural depression relates it to depletion of brain catecholamines. Morrison (1968), Morrison, Goodyear & Sellers (1969) and Olds & Domino (1969*a*, *b*) have presented evidence that the behavioural effects of nicotine are or can be centrally mediated. The fact that immunosympathectomized mice show behavioural reactions that are different from those of control mice to both reserpine and nicotine implies that their brain chemistry is altered or that altered feedback to central sites from peripheral effectors is significant. These possibilities await further study.

Acknowledgements

This research was supported by grant MH 08839 from the United States Public Health Service and a grant from the Committee for Research on Tobacco and Health, Education and Research Foundation of the American Medical Association. Thanks are expressed to CIBA Pharmaceutical Co. for supplying the reserpine vehicle, and to Dr R. K. Richards of Abbott Laboratories and Dr D. C. Edwards of Wellcome Research Laboratories for the NGF-antiserum. Bibliographic assistance was obtained from the Brain Information Service, UCLA, under contract NIH 70-2063. Computing assistance was provided by the Data Processing Laboratory of the UCLA Brain Research Institute under contract NIH NSO2501 and by the Health Sciences Computing Facility, UCLA, sponsored by NIH Special Research Grant RR-3. Phyllis Albritton, Theodore Baker, Irene Jones, Richard Josslin, Glenn Larrabee, Harold McCaffery and Kathryn Rosenberg provided technical services of various sorts.

References

Bovet, D., Bovet-Nitti, F. & Oliverio, A. (1966). *Psychopharmacologia* **10**, 1.

Morrison, C. F. (1968). *Br. J. Pharmac. Chemother.* 32, 28.

Morrison, C. F., Goodyear, J. M. & Sellers, C. M. (1969). *Psychopharmacologia* **15**, 341.

Olds, M. E. & Domino, E. F. (1969*a*). *J. Pharmac. exp. Ther.* **166**, 189.

Olds, M. E. & Domino, E. F. (1969*b*). *J. Pharmac. exp. Ther.* **170**, 157.

Wenzel, B. M. (1959). *J. comp. physiol. Psychol.* **53**, 673.

Wenzel, B. M. (1968*a*). *J. comp. physiol. Psychol.* **66**, 354.

Wenzel, B. M. (1968*b*). *Physiol. & Behav.* (*G.B.*) **3**, 907.

Wenzel, B. M. (1972). In *Immunosympathectomy*. Ed. by Steiner, G. & Schönbaum, E. Amsterdam: Elsevier Publishing Co. (in the press).

Wenzel, B. M. & Jeffrey, D. W. (1967). *Physiol. & Behav.* (*G.B.*) **2**, 193.

Hypothermia and Behaviour of Immunosympathectomized Mice

C. VAN-TOLLER* and R. M. TARPY

Department of Psychology, University of Durham, UK; Department of Psychology, Williams College, Williamstown, Massachusetts, USA*

One of the enigmas about immunosympathectomy is that its effects on behaviour do not parallel the extensive reduction in the peripheral sympathetic neural network. Although behavioural differences have been shown between immunosympathectomized and intact animals (Wenzel & Jeffrey, 1967; Wenzel, 1968) they have usually been small and inconsistent, and a number of conflicting and negative results have been reported (Wenzel & Jeffrey, 1967; Wenzel & Nagle, 1965; Van-Toller, 1970).

Ramey & Goldstein (1957) pointed out that sympathectomy both reduces the range of an animal's adaptive responses and limits its ability to cope with tasks requiring large energy expenditure. Thus one could suggest that the failure to observe large behavioural differences has been due to the fact that the immunosympathectomized animals have not been required to make responses outside their normal range. We therefore decided to investigate the effect of imposing additional stresses on immunosympathectomized animals.

A major function of the sympathetic nervous system is to maintain body temperature within certain limits. In a normal mammal, exposure to cold induces peripheral vasoconstriction which prevents heat loss. This mechanism is largely controlled by the sympathetic nervous system. Earlier workers (Cannon, 1927; Cannon, Querido, Britton & Bright, 1927; Sawyer & Schlossberg, 1933) showed that sympathectomized cats had deficiencies in thermoregulation. Cold stress was therefore chosen as the additional stressor.

Effect of cold stress on behavioural responses

The effect of cold stress on an alley escape response was studied. It had been previously found that immunosympathectomized mice did not differ significantly from controls in this task at room temperature (Van-Toller, 1970). The animals used were 24 male mice from a genetically heterogeneous strain maintained at the Department of Psychology of Durham University. Half the neonates in each litter were used as experimental subjects and the other half as controls. Injections of concentrated freeze-dried Wellcome NGF-antiserum were given daily to the experimental group for the first three days after birth. The volumes injected were 0.05 ml on days 1 and 2 and 0.1 ml on day 3. Equivalent volumes of normal horse serum were injected into the control mice. Thus, handling and the injection regimen were the same for each group.

The alley, shown in Fig 1, was 45 cm long, 3.5 cm wide and 5.3 cm deep, with a 6.25 cm start and goal section at each end. Mice could be restrained in either of the two end sections by grills over the entrance. The walls were made from opaque white plastic and the roof from clear Perspex. The grid floor was constructed from 0.125 cm stainless steel tubing spaced 0.75 cm apart. With the exception of the goal section, a 1.0 mA scrambled shock (unconditioned stimulus) could be delivered throughout the alley. Running speeds were recorded automatically by using pressure-sensitive floor sections which controlled timing mechanisms. Baffles were suspended above the midpoint of each section to ensure that the mouse would depress the section and thereby activate the switch. The conditioned stimulus was a 2.85-second train of white noise.

The experiment utilized a 2×2 design and two temperatures (low, 3.5°C; normal, 22.5°C). At 28 days of age one immunosympathectomized mouse and one control littermate were placed in plastic cages. On the following day, the boxes were allocated to one of the temperature conditions for two hours. The mice were then given five massed trials in the alley, at a temperature of 3.5°C. This procedure was repeated on three subsequent days.

When the mouse had been placed in the start section, a trial began when the conditioned stimulus (white noise) was switched on for 2.85 seconds and the grill drawn up. The shock began with the termination of the conditioned stimulus and remained on until the mouse activated the final pressure-sensitive section and entered the goal-box. When it did so, a grill was lowered behind it to prevent retracing. The mouse was then transferred by hand to the start-box and after four seconds the next trial began.

The mean speed for each group (100 × reciprocal mean total latency) for each of the four days is shown in Fig. 2. Analysis of the data revealed no significant differences between the groups

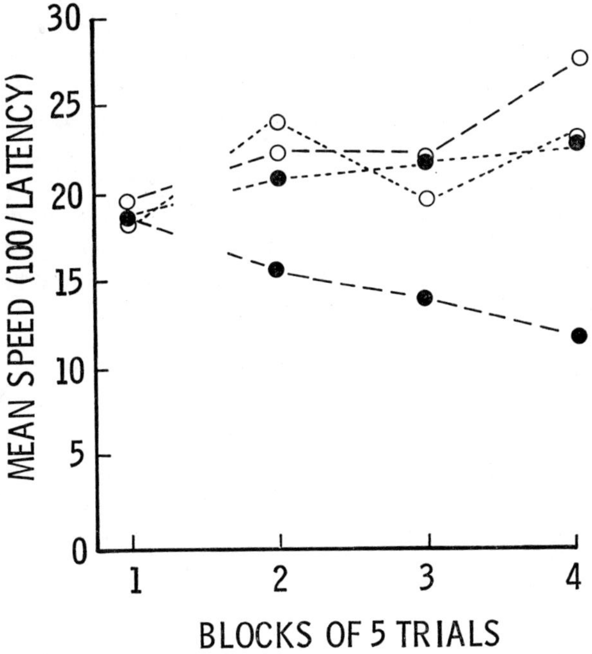

Fig. 2 Mean speed for each group over the four daily blocks of five trials. Absence of differences between groups on Block 1 are thought to be due to the mice gaining thermal insulation from their bedding material. The break between Blocks 1 and 2 indicates that the bedding was removed for subsequent trials.

For Figs. 2, 5: – – – – = Cold
- - - - - = Warm
○ = Normal Horse Serum (N.H.S.)
● = Immunosympathectomized (Immuno.)

for the main effects of treatment or temperature. However, the interaction between these two variables was significant (F = 4.37; df = 1/20; $P<0.05$), indicating that immunosympathectomized mice, detained at 3.5°C, ran significantly more slowly than the other three groups. Moreover, relative to the other groups, the immunosympathectomized-cold group showed a progressive decrement in performance. The results were significant in both trials (*a*) by treatment interaction (F = 5.54; df = 3/60; $P<0.001$), and (*b*) by temperature interaction (F = 16.04; df = 3/60; $P<0.001$).

On day 1 it was apparent that the mice were gaining considerable insulation from their bedding material. This was therefore removed before the temperature detention period on the following days of testing. Since the statistical analyses were based on data from all the blocks of trials, this procedure would, if anything, tend to reduce the levels of significance found.

The results of this experiment indicate that temperature is an important variable affecting the behaviour of immunosympathectomized mice. The decrement in performance was observed only after cold stress; no such decrement was found when the animals were detained at room temperature.

Combined effects of activity and body temperature on behavioural performance

The experiment described above showed that massive cold stress produced inferior performance in immunosympathectomized mice. One of the factors may have been a change in their level of activity. On the one hand, cold stress may have suppressed activity, therefore making successful performance less probable. Alternatively, the immunosympathectomized mice may have increased their activity in order to maintain body temperature. That is, a form of exercise may have taken place in order to attempt to compensate for the absence of the sympathetic nervous system. This inverse relationship between activity and temperature has been shown in another context, for rats, by Campbell (1964), Campbell & Lynch (1968) and Stevenson & Rixon (1957). Accordingly, immunosympathectomized mice and mice injected with normal horse serum were compared in terms of activity and body temperature.

Sixty-six male and female mice were used. They were injected and handled as described earlier. Three small identical running wheels were constructed from two circular plates and wire mesh. The wheels were 13 cm in diameter and 5.5 cm in width with 1.3 cm^2 mesh. Each balanced wheel operated a counter when rotated 90°. As shown in Fig. 3, the wheels could be either free to rotate or locked in position by a tight spring placed across the axle. Body temperatures were recorded using an S.T.C. thermistor (type number U23US) and a sensitive digital voltmeter.

This experiment had three variables. These factors, combined factorially in a 2 × 2 × 2 design, were NGF-antiserum and normal horse serum treatment; cold (3.5°C) and warm (22.5°C); wheel-free and wheel-locked. One immunosympathectomized and one control group was run in each of the four testing conditions: cold wheel-free (C-WF), cold wheel-locked (C-WL), warm wheel-free (W-WF) and warm wheel-locked (W-WL). There were eight mice in each group, except for the two C-WF groups which contained nine animals each.

After selection and weighing, the body temperature of the mouse was measured. The thermistor, lubricated with liquid paraffin, was inserted $\frac{1}{4}$ inch (controlled by a collar) into the rectum. The average time taken to make this measurement was 6 seconds. The mouse was then placed in the activity wheel and activity and/or body temperature was recorded hourly for the next four hours.

The mean body temperatures for the groups run in the cold condition are shown in Fig. 4. In the C-WF groups (left panel) analysis showed a significant overall decrease in temperature ($F = 11.0$; df = 4/64; $P < 0.001$). No differences between immunosympathectomized and control mice were found. In contrast, the C-WL groups (right panel, Fig. 4) indicate a significant difference between immunosympathectomized and control mice ($F = 14.3$; df = 1/14; $P < 0.001$) which increased with time ($F = 14.5$; df = 4/56; $P < 0.001$). Again there was an overall decrease in temperature during the testing session ($F = 27.3$; df = 4/56; $P < 0.001$).

Mean activity scores (transformed from revolutions to square root revolutions to normalize the data) are shown, for the two

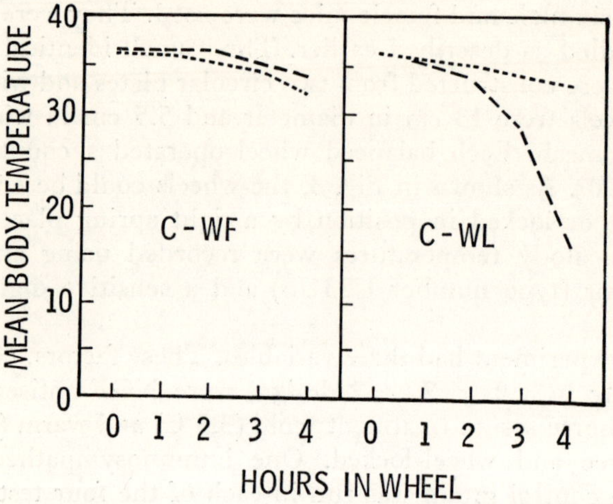

Fig. 4 Mean body temperature as a function of hours in the wheel for the cold-wheel free (left) and cold-wheel locked (right) conditions. Figs. 4 & 6: – – –, Immuno.; - - - -, N.H.S. (See Fig. 2).

C-WF groups, in the lower curves of Fig. 5. Analysis showed a significant decrease in activity for both groups over the course of the test (F=18.2; df=3/48; $P<0.001$). The overall activity for the immunosympathectomized mice did not differ significantly from the activity of the control mice; however, the hours by groups interaction was also significant (F=7.3; df=3/48; $P<0.001$). This shows that the immunosympathectomized mice remained significantly more active during the test compared to the control group, whose activity declined considerably.

In summary, these results showed that a temperature difference occurred only in the wheel-locked situation where the mean temperature of the immunosympathectomized mice dropped significantly below that of the control mice. No temperature difference between the groups was observed in the wheel-free situation, but the immunosympathectomized group was significantly more active, suggesting that vigorous exercise was responsible for maintaining body temperature.

Mean body temperatures for the groups run at room temperature are shown in Fig. 6. In the W-WF condition (left panel) no difference was found between the immunosympathectomized

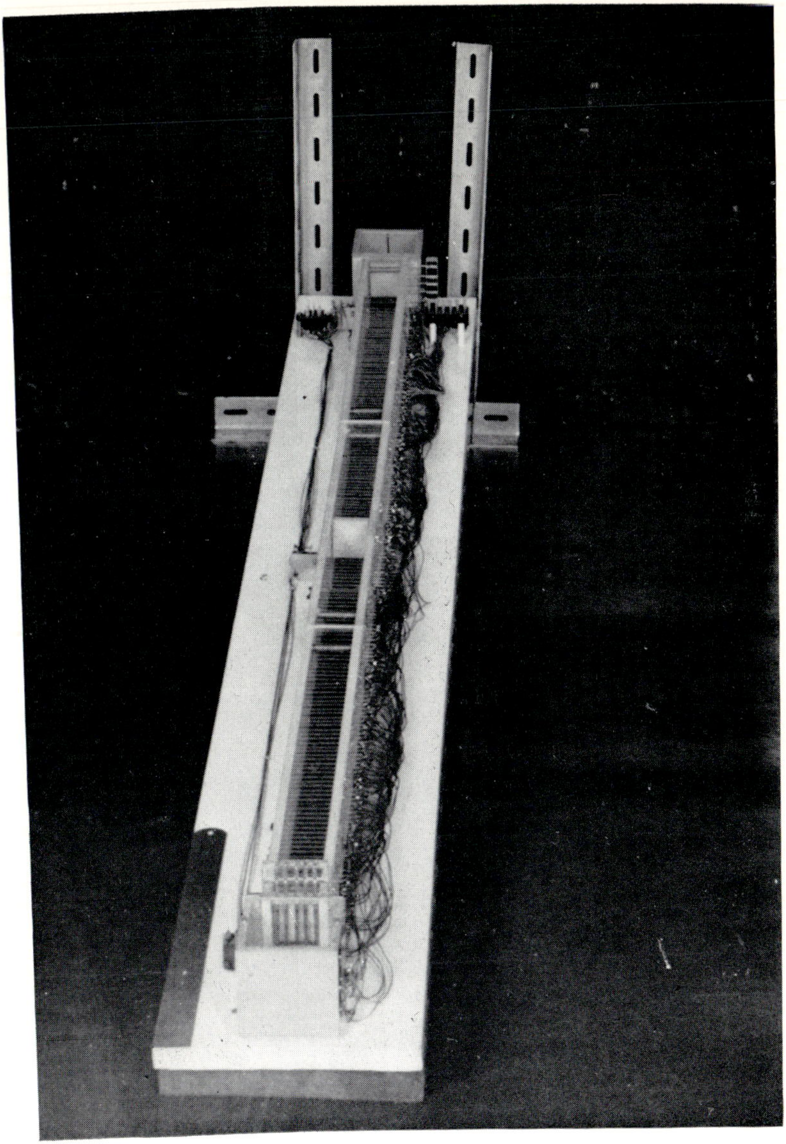

Fig. 1 Overhead view of alley.

Plate XXXIV

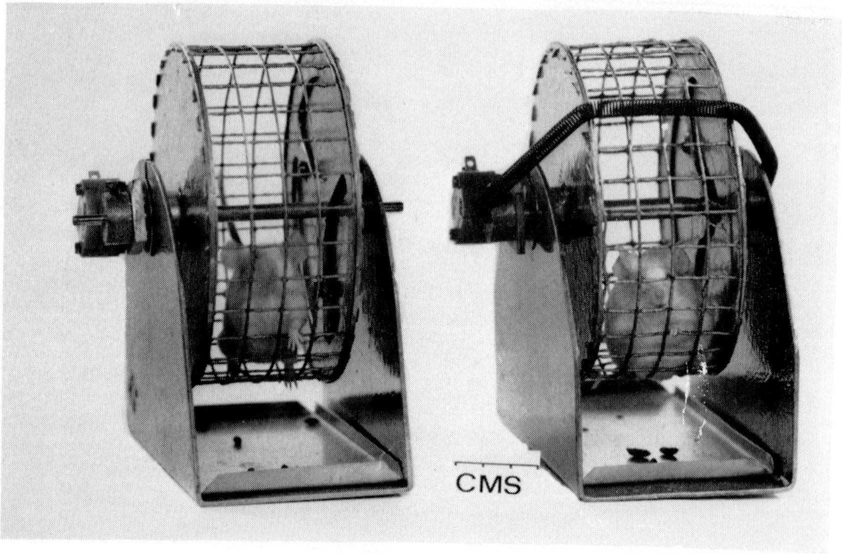

Fig. 3 Activity wheel in the free and locked position.

and control groups. For the W-WL condition, however, there was a significant difference between the immunosympathectomized and control mice ($F = 6.11$; $df = 1/14$; $P<0.001$). Both the main effect of hours ($F = 20.3$; $df = 4/56$; $P<0.001$), and the groups by hours interaction ($F = 3.0$; $df = 4/56$; $P<0.001$) were also significant.

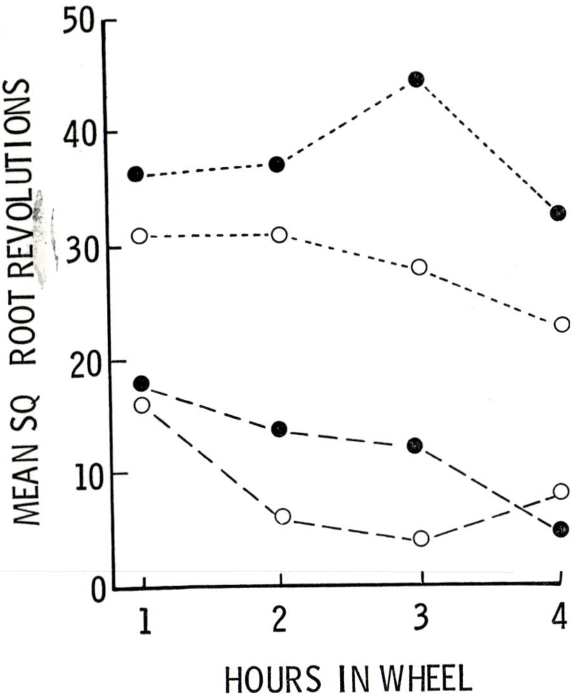

Fig. 5 Mean square root revolutions as a function of hours in the wheel for the wheel-free groups.

Activity, as indicated in the upper curves of Fig. 5, was both higher and more variable under warm than under cold conditions. No difference between immunosympathectomized and control mice was found although the F was nearly significant. The scores of the immunosympathectomized mice were consistently above those of the control group.

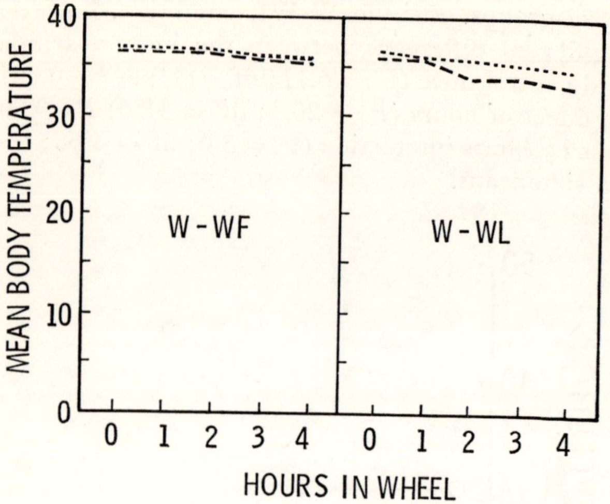

Fig. 6 Mean body temperature as a function of hours in the wheel for the warm-wheel free (left) and warm-wheel locked (right) conditions.

With some qualification the results obtained under temperatures of either 22.5°C or 3.5°C were the same. No temperature difference between the immunosympathectomized and control mice was observed when the mice were free to run vigorously. However, when the extent of activity was reduced (in the wheel-locked condition), immunosympathectomized mice were significantly colder than the control mice. Furthermore, the immunosympathectomized mice were uniformly more active than were the control animals, although not significantly so in the warm condition.

Discussion

The main findings from these experiments are: (*a*) cold stress produces a decrement in the performance of immunosympathectomized mice in an alley escape task; (*b*) the body temperature of immunosympathectomized mice decreases more rapidly than that of the control mice when the range of gross locomotor activity is restricted. This effect was found even at room temperature, although it was more pronounced at low temperature; (*c*) immunosympathectomized mice were consistently more active when allowed to turn a running wheel; in this situation, the mean body temperature of immunosympathectomized mice did not differ from that of control mice.

We feel that immunosympathectomized mice are more active than control mice in order to help maintain their body temperature. In the immunosympathectomized mice, the almost total lack of peripheral sympathetic nervous network, and thus the reduction in ability to vasoconstrict, makes locomotor activity a relatively more important means of homeostatic temperature control. That is, activity compensates for the lack of the physiological mechanisms normally present. To maintain the vital 'inner-core' temperature, the immunosympathectomized mice engage in activity. That animals may become active in order to raise their body temperature has been shown by Campbell & Lynch (1968). In their experiments, however, activity was induced by food deprivation.

The reduced ability of immunosympathectomized mice to thermoregulate could account for some discrepancies in the literature. For example, in one study, Wenzel & Jeffrey (1967) found that immunosympathectomized mice were inferior to controls in acquiring a water escape response when given trials spaced 15 minutes apart. In contrast, in a later experiment (Wenzel, 1968), when the trials were given five seconds apart, the immunosympathectomized mice were no longer inferior. It is possible that in the first study hypothermia was induced in the immunosympathectomized mice by condensation and drying during the long interval between trials. In the massed trials, the sustained muscular activity may have served to counteract any large and differential drop in body temperature. We are currently testing this idea. Another example involving hypothermia has been described by Stone (1970). He concluded that what was previously held to be a state of stress-induced catalepsy in rats was a function of the hypothermia arising from the temperature of the water rather than the stress of forced swimming. Prevention of the hypothermia by using warm water eliminated the catalepsy.

Two studies (Berti, Lentati & Usardi, 1965; Schönbaum, Johnson & Sellers, 1966) have reported no temperature differences between immunosympathectomized and control rats;

moreover, immunosympathectomized rats were able to withstand long periods at a low temperature. In these studies, no reference was made to the behaviour of the cold-stressed rats and therefore the contribution of activity to thermoregulation is not known. Two points, however, can be made: (*a*) the rat is a much larger animal than the mouse, with different metabolic requirements, and (*b*) the rat has a relatively smaller surface area than the mouse, and this would be a critical variable.

Our first experiment showed a performance decrement in the immunosympathectomized mice following cold stress; the second experiment showed that immunosympathectomized mice were more active in the cold. It is therefore plausible to suggest that immunosympathectomy influences the performance of an aversively motivated task by causing other changes in behaviour associated with thermoregulation. That is, 'apparent' learning deficiencies in immunosympathectomized mice subjected to cold stress may be produced by activity which competes with the alley task. Further support for this idea would be gained if a situation were used in which increased activity facilitates a response by making it more probable. In such a case, the performance of immunosympathectomized mice should be superior to that of the controls. Our preliminary studies suggest that better performance can be obtained from immunosympathectomized mice, in a situation where movement is reinforced by presenting short intervals of infra-red heat to hypothermic mice. The immunosympathectomized mice turned on the heat lamp a significantly greater number of times than the control mice. Although the results are preliminary they suggest that activity in immunosympathectomized mice plays an important role in determining behavioural performance.

Acknowledgements

R.M.T. was a Durham University Fellow while on sabbatical leave during the academic year 1970–71 from Williams College.

The authors would like to thank Dr D. C. Edwards of the Wellcome Research Laboratories, Beckenham, England, for generously supplying the NGF-antiserum used in these studies.

References

Berti, F., Lentati, R. & Usardi, M. M. (1965). *Med. Pharmac. Exp.* **13**, 227.

Campbell, B. A. (1964). In *Thirst.* Ed. by Wayner, M. J. New York: Pergamon Press.

Campbell, B. A. & Lynch, G. S. (1968). *J. comp. physiol. Psychol.* **65**, 492.

Cannon, W. B. (1927). *Boston med. surg. J.* **147**, 514.

Cannon, W. B., Querido, A., Britton, S. W. & Bright, E. M. (1927). *Am. J. Physiol.* **79**, 466.

Ramey, E. R. & Goldstein, M. S. (1957). *Physiol. Rev.* **37**, 155.

Sawyer, M. E. M. & Schlossberg, T. (1933). *Am. J. Physiol.* **104**, 172.

Schönbaum, E., Johnson, G. E. & Sellers, E. A. (1966). *Am. J. Physiol.* **211**, 647.

Stevenson, J. A. F. & Rixon, R. H. (1957). *Yale J. Biol. Med.* 6, 575.

Stone, E. (1970). *Life Sci.* **9**, 877.

Van-Toller, C. (1970). Ph.D. Thesis: University of Durham.

Wenzel, B. M. (1968). *J. comp. physiol. Psychol.* **66**, 354.

Wenzel, B. M. & Jeffrey, D. W. (1967). *Physiol. & Behav.* (*G.B.*) **2**, 193.

Wenzel, B. M. & Nagle, B. (1965). *Expl Neurol.* **12**, 399.

SECTION III

Problems in the Assay of NGF and its Antiserum

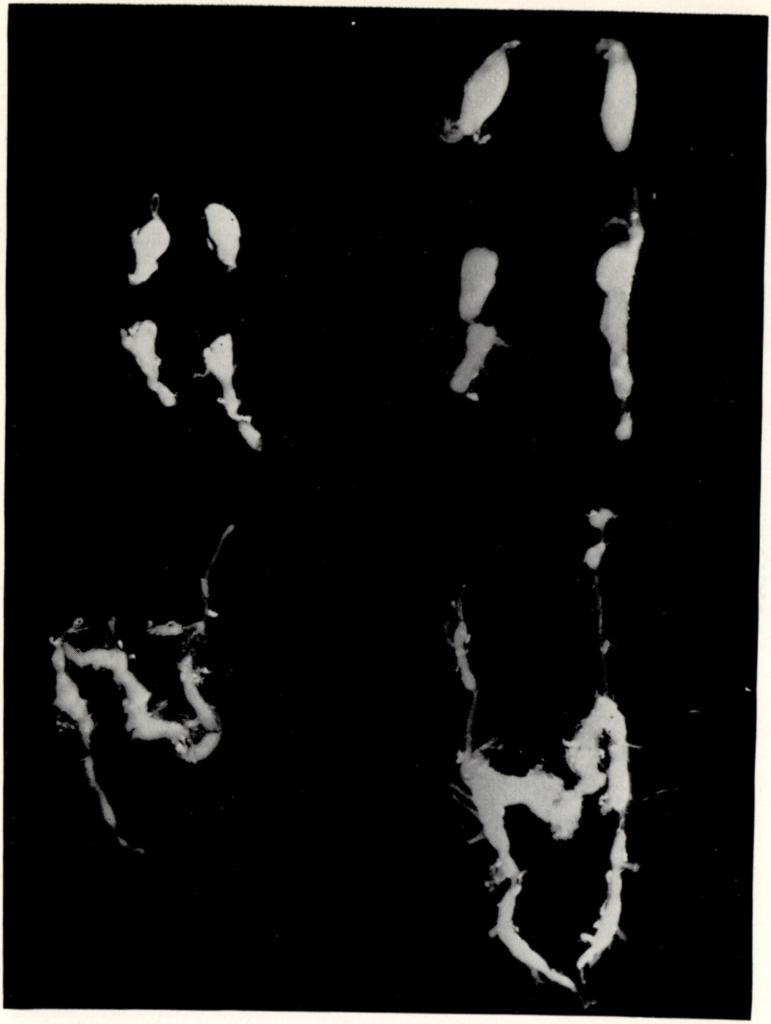

Fig. 1 Superior cervical, stellate and coeliac ganglia of ten-day-old mice. Left, ganglia from control mouse. Right, ganglia from mouse injected for nine days with 40μg NGF/g body wt/day.

Quantitative Aspects of the Effects in Mice of Nerve Growth Factor and its Antiserum

D. C. EDWARDS,* E. L. FENTON,* and I. A. HENDRY

Department of Biological Chemistry, Wellcome Research Laboratories, Beckenham, Kent, UK; Department of Pharmacology, University of Cambridge, UK*

We have made many attempts over the past several years to produce quantities of reliable nerve growth factor (NGF) and also of its antiserum. Both have proved difficult, even surprisingly difficult, to prepare, despite the fact that we have concentrated on NGF from mouse salivary gland. As a rule, it has not been too difficult to produce NGF preparations that give satisfactory haloes of fibres when used to stimulate chick embryo ganglia in tissue culture or to produce antibodies that block the stimulant action of NGF. However, a very different situation arises *in vivo*. Wide variation between batches of NGF has been found and the correlation with the *in vitro* activity is sometimes poor. Antisera in particular present problems in this respect and it is with the quantitative aspects of the effects of both the factor and its antiserum *in vivo* that we shall deal.

The production of NGF was made very much easier and more satisfactory by the work of Varon, Nomura & Shooter (1967), who isolated NGF in a high molecular weight form (7S) and then dissociated it into subunits, only one of which had the property of stimulating fibre growth *in vitro*. Using this method to isolate the 7S species, and then dissociating it into subunits on a column of CM-cellulose at pH 5 as described by Bocchini & Angeletti (1969), we have been able to produce good yields of NGF. The batches always behave quite perfectly *in vitro* in that the specific activities of the products at the various stages in the purification are highly predictable. The subunit so prepared has been used to immunize a horse. This paper will present results on the effects of these various materials on newborn mice.

Although the desirability of testing NGF *in vivo* as well as *in vitro* has been stressed in the literature (Levi-Montalcini & Angeletti, 1968), very few reports have in fact made use of studies *in vivo* and fewer still have produced quantitative data. The development of a simple and reproducible method of weighing ganglia after dissection has allowed such a study to be undertaken with respect to the effects of NGF in mice. Along with this there has been the development of a method of assessing ganglion maturation by measuring an enzyme, tyrosine hydroxylase, known to be specific to the adrenergic neurones of the sympathetic ganglia (Hendry & Iversen, 1971), which has allowed the quantitative assessment of the effectiveness of various antisera.

The experimental design adopted for testing NGF was to use two litters of eight newborn Swiss mice, each divided into four groups of two. Two groups, one from each litter, four mice in all, were injected subcutaneously with a given dose of NGF on the day of birth and for the five following days. Thus, four dose levels could be tested on the two litters. Injections were based on body weight, which was checked daily before injection and the dose adjusted accordingly. The animals were killed and the ganglia dissected on the seventh day. After dissection, each pair of superior cervical ganglia was placed in saline solution, cleaned of fat and any other debris, and finally blotted and weighed on a 5 mg torsion balance. Repeat weighings of a small object of about 1 mg showed the reproducibility of this procedure to be around ± 3 per cent. By this method it was possible to produce dose-response curves for the effect of NGF *in vivo* and to investigate various aspects of the *in vivo* effects of NGF. Potency *in vitro* was assayed by the method of Fenton (1970).

The effect of NGF in increasing the size of the ganglia of the sympathetic chain is well documented (Levi-Montalcini & Angeletti, 1968). Fig. 1 shows typical results. The increase in the size of all the ganglia is obvious, but such data, although commonly reported, provide only limited information; dose-response curves provide a much more satisfactory criterion.

Fig. 2 shows the dose-response relationship obtained using a batch of 7S NGF prepared from mouse salivary glands by the method of Varon *et al.* (1967). The average values and the range are shown in Table 1.

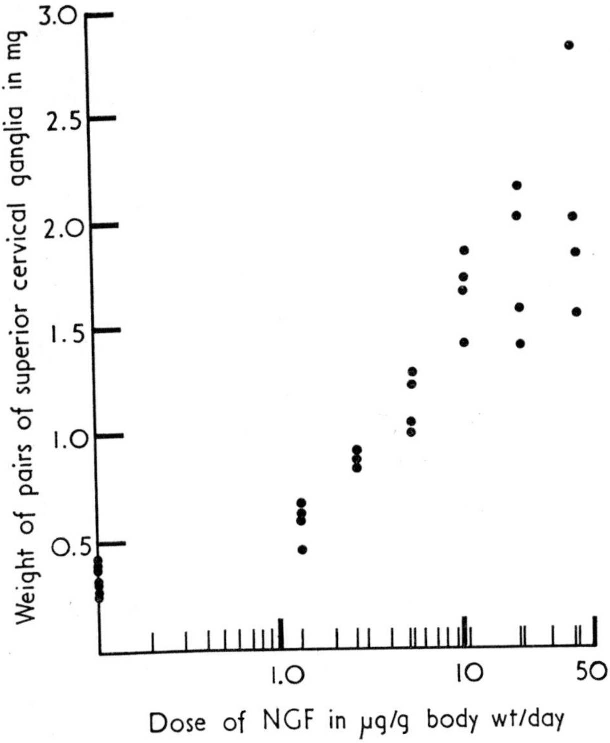

Fig. 2 Effect of NGF Batch 2470 (7S) on weight of superior cervical ganglion of the newborn mouse.

The NGF had a specific activity as measured by Fenton's method of 168 000 units/mg; and no stunting of the animals (Cohen, 1962) was found at any of the concentrations tested. It should be noted that to produce a pair of ganglia of approximately 1 mg in weight required a dose of just under 5 µg NGF/g body weight per day. The biggest average increase was around six-fold, just half of that claimed by Levi-Montalcini (1966). The increase from the smallest control to the biggest test ganglion, however, was ten-fold.

Table 1 Weights of pairs of superior cervical ganglia of mice injected with daily doses of nerve growth factor

Dose of NGF *µg/g body wt/day*	*Average weight* *mg*	*Range of weights of ganglia mg*
0	0.32	0.26–0.39
1.3	0.59	0.46–0.66
2.6	0.87	0.84–0.89
5.2	1.08	1.00–1.27
10.5	1.66	1.42–1.84
21.0	1.86	1.50–2.20
42.0	2.05	1.50–2.80

When this particular batch of 7S NGF was used to prepare the active subunit by the procedure of Bocchini & Angeletti (1969), 500 mg of 7S material yielded 50 mg of subunit, i.e. there was a 10 per cent recovery of weight. The specific activity was, however, increased to 580 000 units/mg as measured by the *in vitro* test, so the overall recovery of activity was around 35 per cent. On the basis of the considerable increase in potency *in vitro*, it was anticipated that a similar increase in activity *in vivo* would be found when the response to injected NGF was measured in the mouse. This, however, proved not to be so, as seen in Fig. 3. Because of the poor recovery of material from the column, the very high doses given in the previous experiment could not be repeated; but a dose of about 4 µg NGF/g body weight/day was required to produce pairs of ganglia weighing about 1 mg. This contrasts with the 1.4–1.5 µg dose expected from the *in vitro* titres. The average and range values included in Table 2 confirm this.

This highly unexpected and unexplained result was the first indication that the correlation between *in vitro* and *in vivo* potencies might not always be very good. This appears to be the first time that such a discrepancy has been reported. Varon *et al.* (1967) describe a loss of activity when NGF is dissociated on the CM-cellulose column, recovering between 30–40 per cent of the original activity and 10 per cent of the weight of protein. This is very much in line with our *in vitro* results. Bocchini & Angeletti (1969), on the other hand, achieved a recovery of 85–100 per cent of the original activity of the protein added to the CM-cellulose column. In neither case, however, are adequate data given on the *in vivo* effects.

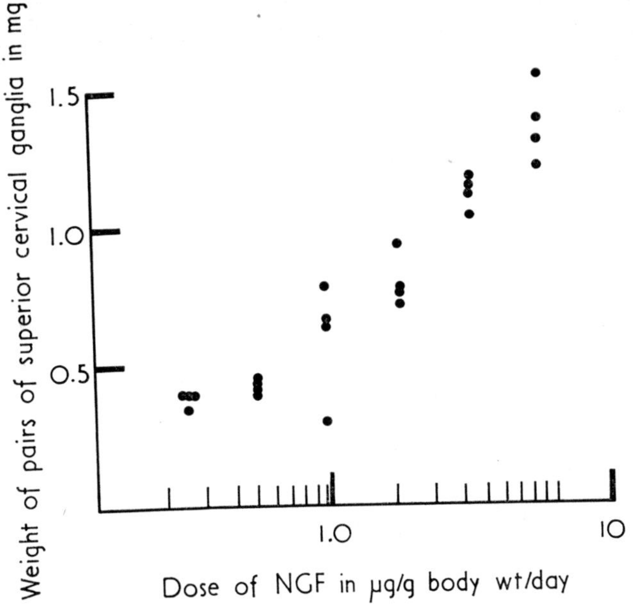

Fig. 3 Effect of NGF Batch 2470 (β-subunit) on weight of superior cervical ganglion of the newborn mouse.

Table 2 Weights of pairs of superior cervical ganglia of mice injected with daily doses of β-subunit of nerve growth factor

Dose of NGF μg/g body wt/day	*Average weight mg*	*Range of weights of ganglia mg*
0	0.28	0.22–0.32
0.25	0.38	0.35–0.39
0.5	0.43	0.40–0.44
1.0	0.70	0.65–0.79
2.1	0.79	0.72–0.93
4.1	1.11	1.04–1.16
8.6	1.31	1.12–1.54

A different phenomenon was found with another preparation. The dose-response curve for the 7S molecule is shown in Fig. 4. This material had a specific activity of 170 000 units/mg, much the same as in the previous example, but the *in vivo* activity was quite different. A considerable high-dose inhibition was seen and the material was less potent than the previous sample, doses of between 10 and 20 μg NGF/g body weight/day being required to produce pairs of ganglia in the 1 mg wet weight region.

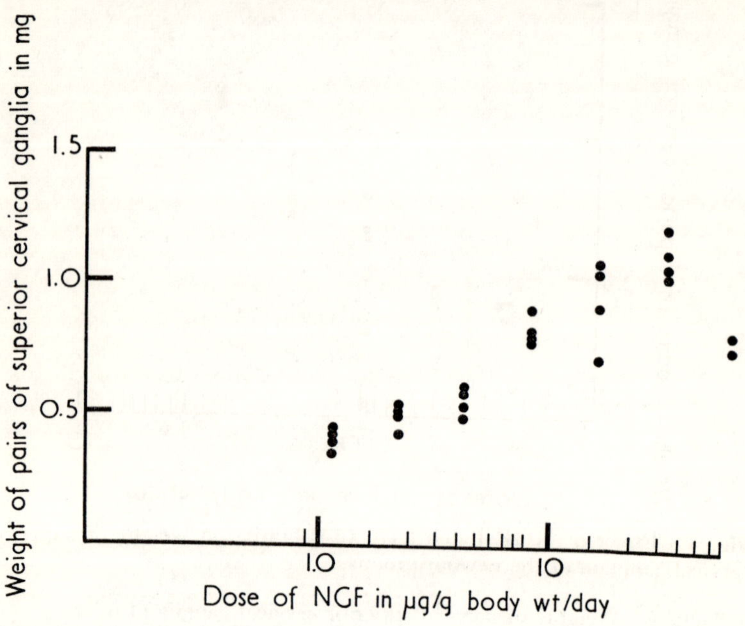

Fig. 4 Effect of NGF Batch V15 (7S) on weight of superior cervical ganglion of the newborn mouse.

This material was dissociated as before; again a recovery of 10 per cent of protein was obtained, with an increase in the *in vitro* potency to 440 000 units/mg. This subunit was injected into mice in the usual way, and the results are shown in Fig. 5. In this case, there has been an increase in activity, 5 μg/g body weight/day giving ganglia weighing 1 mg per pair, and in addition the high-dose inhibition had disappeared. The increase in activity was around four-fold and the subunit had about the same level of activity as that found in the batch previously described.

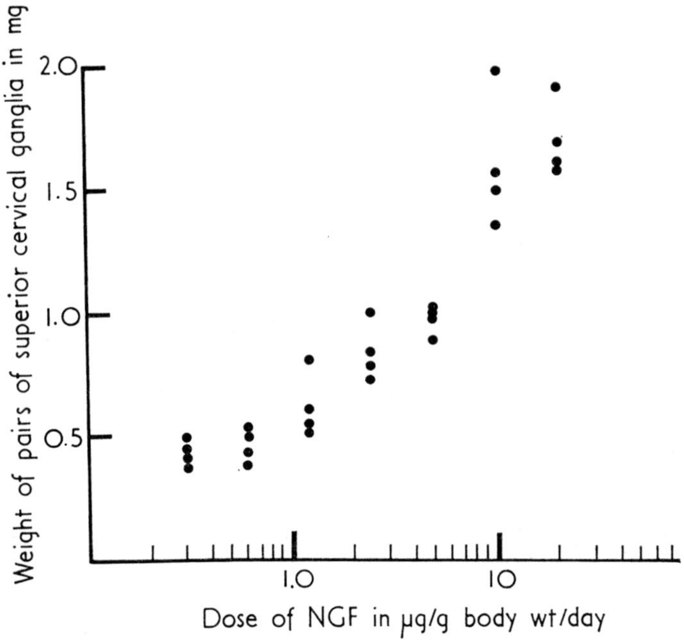

Fig. 5 Effect of NGF Batch V15 (β–subunit) on weight of superior cervical ganglion of the newborn mouse.

Since the high-dose inhibition had been removed from the 7S material by the dissociation step, it seemed reasonable to postulate the presence of an inhibitor of ganglion development. The other subunits, α and γ, resulting from the dissociation of the 7S molecule, were therefore injected into mice to examine their effect, if any, on ganglion size. The results are shown in Figs. 6 and 7; it is obvious that no marked increases or decreases of ganglion size have occurred. In other experiments with other samples of α and γ subunits from a different preparation, similar results were obtained.

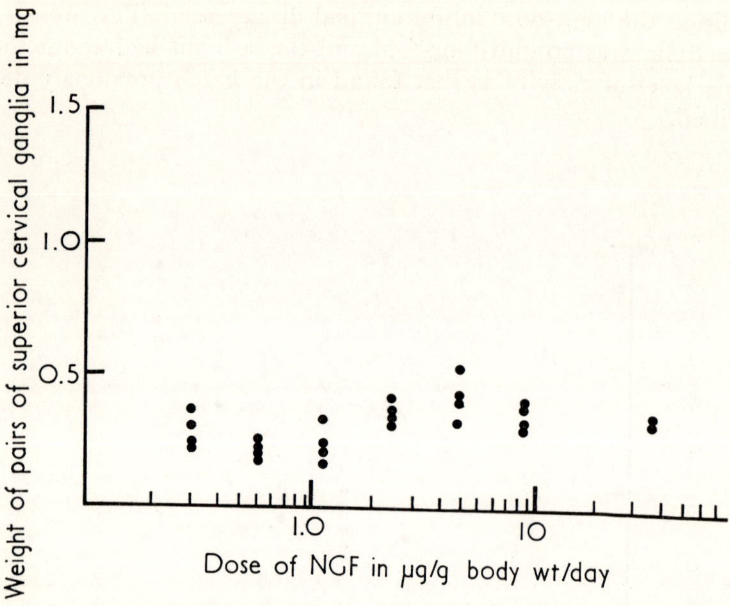

Fig. 6 Effect of α subunit from Batch V15 on weight of superior cervical ganglion of the newborn mouse.

The next experiment was obviously to recombine the fractions and test again. The recombination was done on the basis of the weight of the subunits recovered after freeze-drying the eluates from the CM-cellulose column. The proportions used were 45 per cent α, 45 per cent γ and 10 per cent β. The results obtained by injecting this mixture are shown in Fig. 8, and are quite striking. There has been a marked reduction in potency compared to the β-subunit, as might be expected, and even some reduction as compared with the result of injecting 7S NGF, to which it is very similar. The latter reduction could be expected because of the manipulations made. The most interesting feature, however, is the return of the high-dose inhibition at the same dose as seen previously; indicating that one component has an inhibitory effect in the presence of the β-subunit. Recombination studies with pairs of subunits are clearly needed and parallel studies of molecular weight and heterogeneity would be interesting.

The usefulness of the *in vivo* assay method is demonstrated in two further experiments. In the first, the reversibility of the response to NGF was investigated and in the second, two very pure preparations from different sources were compared.

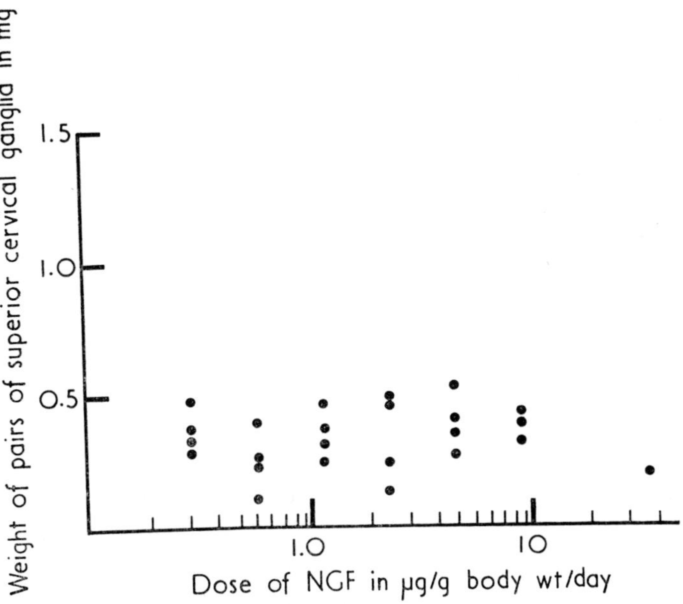

Fig. 7 Effect of γ subunit from Batch V15 on the weight of the superior cervical ganglion of the newborn mouse.

The reversibility of the effect was shown by injecting a group of mice for six days in the usual way and dissecting the ganglia of half of them on day 7. The remainder were left for a further 37 days with no further injections. Groups of control mice were also included. The results are shown in Fig. 9 and are quite clear-cut. There was a large increase in ganglion weight in animals injected for six days when compared with the ganglia of control mice of the same age. When control mice were examined after a further 37 days, a considerable increase in ganglion weight had occurred, but it was not as great as that achieved in the animals injected with NGF and dissected after seven days. Mice which had received NGF but had been left for 37 days after the injections

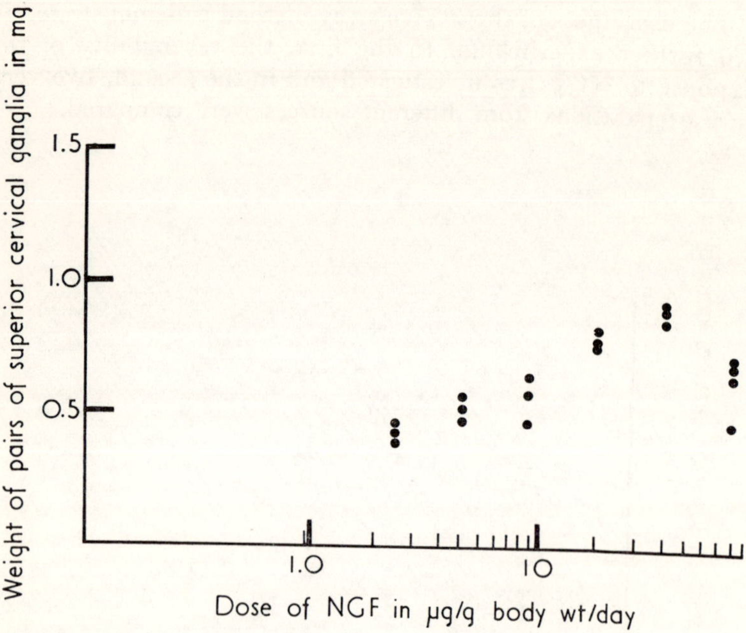

Fig. 8 Effect of α, β, and γ subunits recombined from Batch V15 on weight of superior cervical ganglion of the newborn mouse.

had been discontinued had ganglia of normal size, demonstrating that the effect of NGF is a transient one. This has not been much stressed in the literature, but it is a very important aspect of the response to NGF. Unpublished work by Katherine Charlwood of University College London has shown that the ganglia do indeed return to normal as regards both cell number and cell size. Bueker & Schenkein (1964) have demonstrated that, if injections are continued for 49 days, the increase in ganglion size is maintained. It seems clear, therefore, that NGF is required to maintain the increase and that in its absence some control process takes over and the ganglia return to normal.

In another experiment the effect of NGF isolated from mouse salivary gland was compared with that extracted from snake venom. The latter was provided by Professor C. A. Vernon and his colleagues and was a very highly purified preparation. The

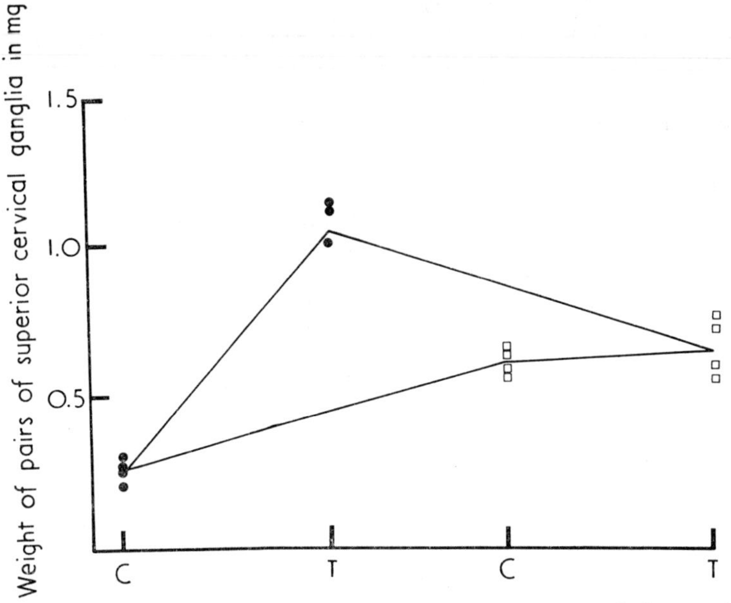

Fig. 9 Effects of injecting mice with NGF and removing their superior cervical ganglia on days 7 and 44 of life. ●, weights of ganglia from 7-day-old mice. C, controls; T, injected with NGF for six days. □, weights of ganglia from 44-day-old mice. C, controls; T, injected with NGF for first six days after birth.

results of the comparison are shown in Fig. 10. The specific activities of the two samples were 600 000 units/mg for the mouse salivary gland NGF and 300 000 units/mg for the snake venom NGF. The activities *in vivo*, however, differed by a much larger factor, of between five- and ten-fold. The sample of mouse NGF used in this experiment was certainly the most active material *in vivo* which we have found, giving pairs of ganglia of around 1 mg wet weight with a dose of only 1 μg/g body weight/day. The results, while illustrating again the discrepancy between *in vitro* and *in vivo* values, also indicate that the present technique could be applied in a classical bioassay system.

The final piece of work that we wish to describe concerns the development of antiserum to NGF. We have been trying for several years to produce a large quantity of potent antiserum;

potent in this context means a serum effective in the rat as well as in the mouse. This has proved very difficult to do. Despite many attempts and the use of various animal species, the sera remained stubbornly ineffective or only partially effective in the rat, although sera potent in mice were almost invariably obtained.

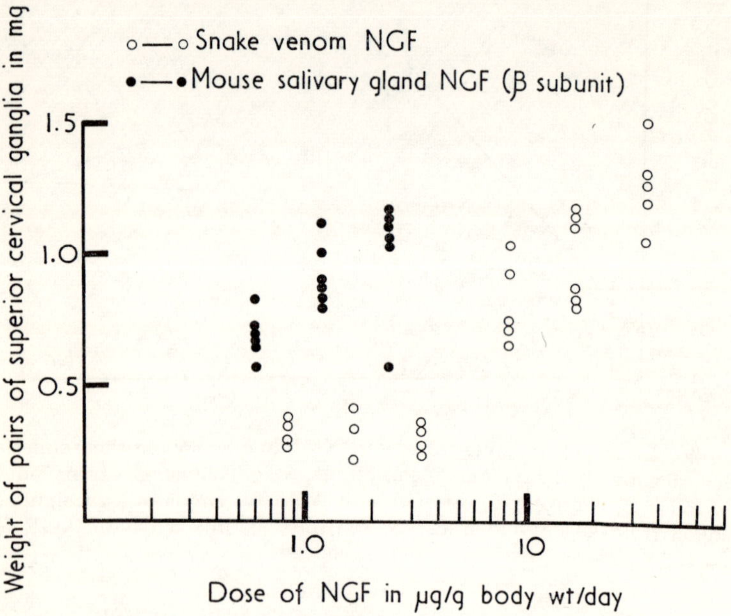

Fig. 10 Comparison of effect of snake venom NGF and mouse salivary gland NGF (β-subunit) on weight of superior cervical ganglion of the newborn mouse.

When we started to use β-subunit to immunize rabbits the situation appeared to change. The animals responded with very high titres, as judged by the ability of the antiserum to block the effect of NGF *in vitro* in the Fenton (1970) assay system. The results of a typical experiment are shown in Fig. 11. The maximum titres found in this work were much greater than any we had seen before and the value of the Abbott serum was exceeded by six-fold. Further, these sera were found by Professor E. Zaimis to give a very satisfactory degree of immunosympathectomy in rats.

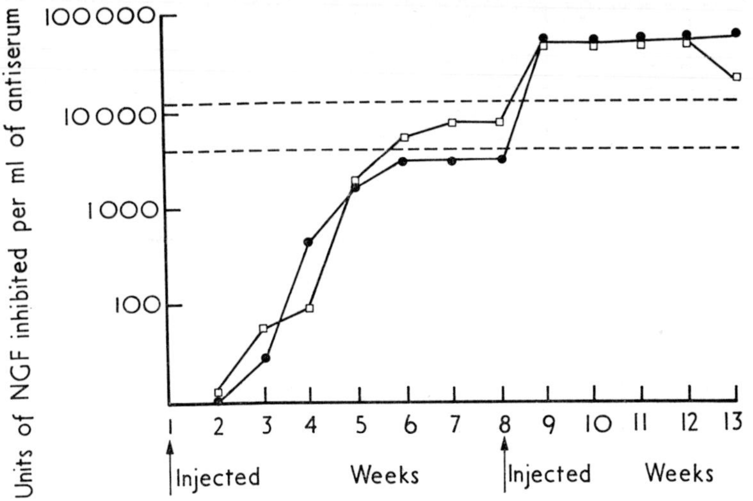

Fig. 11 Two rabbits (●, □) immunized with 1 mg β-subunit in Freund's complete adjuvant. For comparison, the value of Abbott antiserum (upper broken line) and an early horse serum (lower broken line) are shown.

Encouraged by these results, we proceeded to immunize a horse. The animal was given 1 mg of β-subunit NGF in Freund's complete adjuvant in multiple subcutaneous sites. Eight weeks later a second similar dose was given. The animal was bled weekly and the sera were analysed. The results show a clear primary response followed, after boosting, by a massive secondary response (Fig. 12). The titre at the peak value was six times higher than that of Abbott antiserum in a directly comparable test.

A study was then made of the effects of these various antisera *in vivo*. Litters of eight mice were divided into two groups of four mice. Each group was injected subcutaneously with a single dose of antiserum. Doses of 0.5, 1.0, 2.0, 5.0, 10.0, and 20.0 μl were given. The animals were injected once only, on the day of birth. The ganglia were dissected out on day 7, placed into 10 μl distilled water, allowed to stand for 30 minutes and then the droplet was frozen and analysed for tyrosine hydroxylase. From the results, the dose necessary to reduce the enzyme level by 50 per cent from the control value was calculated, and the result

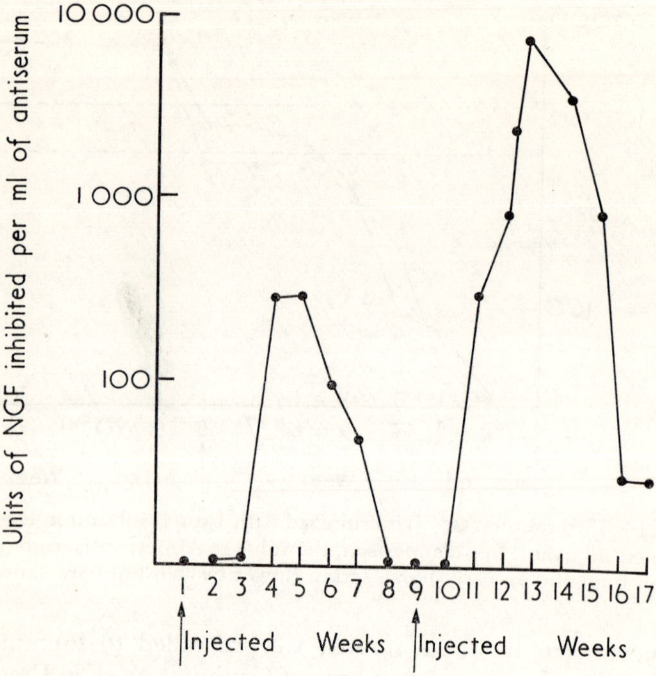

Fig. 12 Immunization of a horse with two doses of β-subunit NGF in Freund's complete adjuvant.

obtained was expressed as a reciprocal in order to give values that increased with increasing potency. Fig. 13 shows the results obtained, together with the *in vitro* results for comparison. The most striking point is that serum 10 appears to be just about as effective *in vivo* as any other of the sera, despite its low value *in vitro*. It should also be noted that the result for Bleed 13 is not included in the curve. This is because we believe it to be wrong and that it should be repeated. The reason for thinking that the result for Bleed 10 is correct, while that for Bleed 13 is wrong, is that we have fractionated all the sera into IgM and IgG by gel filtration on Sephadex G-200. The results show that the activity resides in the 7S group of molecules; but, more importantly, that the IgG from Bleed 10 is just as active as that from Bleeds 11 or 12, although its *in vitro* titre is still extremely low. On the other hand, the titre for the IgG from Bleed 13 is actually higher than that of the unfractionated serum. A comparison of the *in vitro* and *in vivo* values is shown in Table 3. Even if we ignore the result with Bleed 10, the discrepancy between the *in vivo* and *in vitro* values of the sera is great, but if we include it, and we feel we must, the difference is greater than three orders of magnitude, and it can be said with some confidence that the effect *in vivo* is not a reflection of the ability of the antiserum to neutralize NGF in tissue culture.

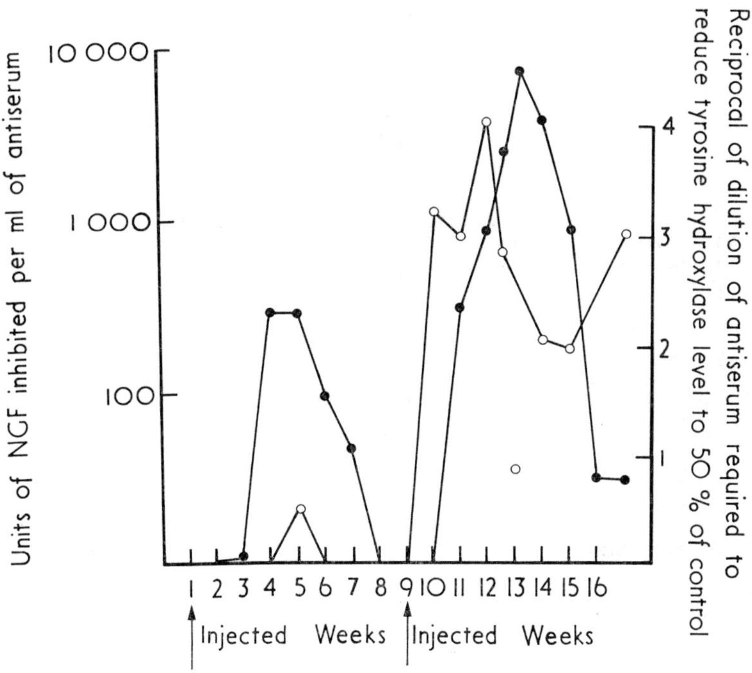

Fig. 13 Comparison of *in vitro* and *in vivo* properties of antisera to NGF. ●, *in vitro* titres; ○, *in vivo* titres.

The experimental approach of applying a quantitative *in vivo* measurement to NGF and its antiserum has produced results that create more problems than the use of the method has solved. The fact that discrepancies exist between the biological activities of these agents in different test systems, however, emphasizes the need for such an approach; and it also underlines the dangers inherent in a too ready extrapolation from *in vitro* to *in vivo* situations.

Table 3 Comparison of *in vitro* and *in vivo* titres of horse anti-NGF sera

Bleed no.	*'In vitro' titre*[1]	*'In vivo' titre*[2]
9	36	<0.5
10	36	3.2
11	3 000	3.0
12	9 000	4.2
13	26 000	2.9
14	78 000	0.9
15	39 000	2.1
16	9 000	2.1
17	300	3.0
18	300	2.7

[1] Units of NGF inhibited per ml of antiserum.
[2] Reciprocal of volume of antiserum required to reduce tyrosine hydroxylase level of superior cervical ganglion by 50 per cent.

Acknowledgements

We wish to express our thanks to Mrs I. Bushby for her highly skilled technical assistance. The Abbott antiserum was kindly supplied by Dr K. R. Richards.

References

Bocchini, V. & Angeletti, P. U. (1969). *Proc. natn. Acad. Sci. U.S.A.* **64**, 787.
Bueker, E. D. & Schenkein, I. (1964). *Ann. N.Y. Acad. Sci.* **118**, 183.
Cohen, S. (1962). *J. biol. Chem.* **237**, 1555.
Fenton, E. L. (1970). *Expl Cell Res.* **59**, 383.
Hendry, I. A. & Iversen, L. (1971). *Brain Res.* (in the Press).
Levi-Montalcini, R. (1966). *Harvey Lectures*, Ser. **60**, 217.
Levi-Montalcini, R. & Angeletti, P. U. (1968). *Physiol. Rev.* **48**, 534.
Varon, S., Nomura, J. & Shooter, E. M. (1967). *Biochemistry, N.Y.* **6**, 2202.

Problems in the Assay of Nerve Growth Factor

F. L. PEARCE

Department of Chemistry, University College London, UK

The standard method for assaying nerve growth factor (NGF) was developed by Levi-Montalcini and her co-workers (Levi-Montalcini, Meyer & Hamburger, 1954; Cohen, Levi-Montalcini & Hamburger, 1954; Cohen & Levi-Montalcini, 1957), and it involves examination of the outgrowths of nerve fibres from the sensory ganglia of chick embryos, when these fibres are grown in tissue culture in the presence of the active protein. How many nerve fibres are produced by an individual ganglion depends upon the concentration of NGF in the culture medium; and, although the outgrowths cannot be measured quantitatively they can as a rule be assessed subjectively and graded on some arbitrary scale, usually between 0 and 4 or between 0 and 5. The activity of a given sample of NGF may then be expressed in terms of the minimum concentration of protein required to produce some standard response. To facilitate this determination, the outgrowths produced by a range of concentrations of the test material are examined and the dose-response relationship is then plotted. The nature of this relationship for purified NGF has by now become well established: as the concentration of the active protein is increased, the response rises to a maximum value; but thereafter, it appears to fall, as the outgrowth of nerve fibres becomes progressively shorter and denser. This apparent decrease in response at high concentrations of NGF was originally attributed to an unspecified inhibitory effect. However, later histological examinations showed that the affected nerve fibres did not grow in a radial direction from the explant but formed a dense fibrillar capsule around the ganglion (Levi-Montalcini, 1966). The thickness of this capsule increased with the concentration of NGF, indicating that the production of neurofibrillar material was in fact stimulated, and not inhibited, by high concentrations of the factor. The reason for the abnormal type of outgrowth produced under these conditions is not known. Examples of the various responses produced by different concentrations of NGF have been illustrated by Cohen *et al.* (1954).

In view of the apparent simplicity of the above procedure, it is rather surprising to find that individual workers (Angeletti, 1969; Levy, Schenkein, Boesman, Tokarsky & Bueker, 1969) have had considerable difficulty in obtaining reliable and reproducible results for the assay of given samples of NGF; and also that there are widely conflicting reports on the activities of different batches of active material. Levels of activity vary between 10^{-1} and 10^{-8} μg/ml for the NGF from snake venoms (Cohen, 1959; Banks *et al.*, 1968) and between 10^{-1} and 10^{-10} μg/ml for the NGF from mouse salivary gland (Schenkein & Bueker, 1964; Schenkein, Levy, Bueker & Tokarsky, 1968). These variations are too large to reflect any real differences in the purity of the samples in question. In view of this confusion a thorough investigation of the problems involved in assaying NGF was made in our laboratories, and the procedure used for diluting the sample to concentrations appropriate for the assay was found to be of critical importance in determining the apparent biological activity of the test material. In particular, the level of activity of NGF from the venom of the Russell's viper (Pearce *et al.*, p. 3) varied between 10^{-1} and 10^{-10} μg/ml according to the dilution procedure adopted. The true level of activity of this material is believed to be between 10^{-2} and 10^{-3} μg/ml. It is considered that these effects are produced by the reversible adsorption of NGF on to the walls of the pipettes used in making the dilutions and that this phenomenon may explain both the irreproducible results obtained by many workers and the anomalously high activities reported in the literature. Some of the experiments which led to these conclusions are described below.

The range of concentrations required for the assay of NGF may be simply prepared by making a series of ten-fold dropwise dilutions from a starting solution of known concentration. Dropwise dilutions of this type, while not being particularly accurate, are very convenient for routine purposes. The serial dilution may be made in one of two ways: either a single pipette may be used throughout the procedure, or a separate pipette may be used for each successive dilution step.

Dose-response curves were obtained by both these methods, from a starting solution of concentration 300 μg/ml, for a sample of NGF from Russell's viper venom. The two curves were found to be remarkably different (Fig. 1). The curve obtained by dilution with a single pipette showed a broad region of strong activity which persisted until very low concentrations were reached. The response also decreased at high concentrations of NGF. In contrast, the curve obtained by diluting with a series of pipettes had a well-defined maximum of activity; and the response decreased sharply on either side of this optimum concentration. The levels of activity of the sample, defined for convenience as the minimum concentration required to produce the mid-response of 2.5 on the scale 0 to 5, were between 10^{-10} and 10^{-11} μg/ml won the dilution was made with a single pipette and between 10^{-1} and 10^{-2} μg/ml when it was made with a series of pipettes.

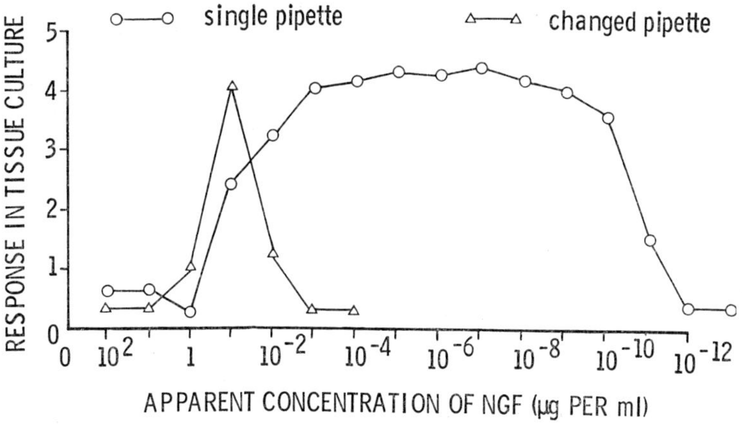

Fig. 1 Dose-response curves obtained by dropwise dilution methods using glass apparatus.

The only obvious explanation of these results is that the NGF is reversibly adsorbed on to the pipettes used in the dilution of the sample. When a single pipette is used for dilution, active material is adsorbed on to the pipette at the highest concentrations of NGF, and is progressively released from the pipette at the lower concentrations. In this way activity is spread over the entire range of dilutions. When a series of pipettes is used there is a continuous loss of NGF as the active material is adsorbed on to the walls of the pipettes and discarded after each successive dilution step. A dropwise method of dilution using a single pipette will thus overestimate the activity of a given sample of NGF, whereas the corresponding method using a series of different pipettes will underestimate this activity. Neither method will give the correct activity.

The effects of changing the diluent, and the materials of which the pipettes were made, were then examined. Samples of NGF were diluted in various sera, in solutions containing inert proteins and amino acids, and in buffers at different pH values. The dilutions were made from Pasteur pipettes constructed of glass, polypropylene, polystyrene, Teflon and glass that had been coated with silicone. All the results obtained, with the exception of those given by pipettes made of polystyrene and Teflon, were essentially identical with those already described. The same large difference in the dose-response curves for the two methods of dilution was observed in each case. The differences between the curves for pipettes made of polystyrene and Teflon were, however, much smaller. The adsorption of NGF is therefore apparently independent of the nature of the diluent, and the protein is adsorbed not only on to glass surfaces but also onto surfaces of polypropylene and silicone. The adsorption onto polystyrene and Teflon is considerably less.

The effects of changes in the starting concentration of the test solution of NGF were then examined. Solutions of different concentration were prepared by direct weighing and were diluted using glass pipettes by the two dropwise methods previously described. The regions of the dose-response curves of interest in determining the levels of activity of the samples are shown in Figs. 2 and 3. When the dilution was made with a single pipette (Fig. 2) the apparent activity of the test material fell rapidly as

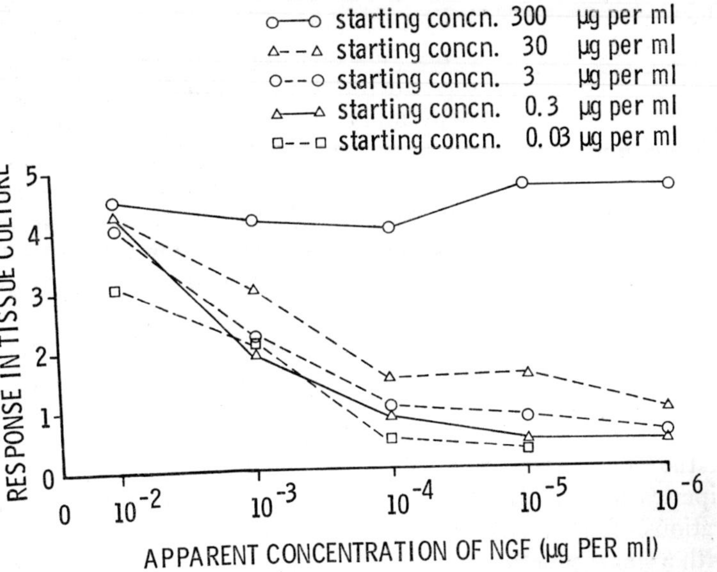

Fig. 2 Dose-response curves obtained from starting solutions of different concentrations by dropwise dilution using a single glass pipette.

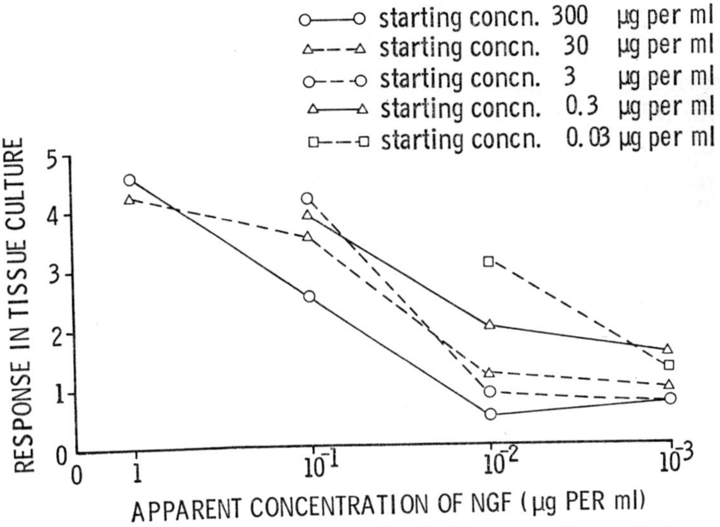

Fig. 3 Dose-response curves obtained from starting solutions of different concentrations by dropwise dilution using a series of glass pipettes.

the concentration of the starting solution was lowered. The level of activity corresponding to a starting solution of 300 μg/ml was 10^{-10}–10^{-11} μg/ml; the level corresponding to a starting concentration of 0.03 μg/ml was 10^{-2}–10^{-3} μg/ml. When the sample was diluted with a series of pipettes (Fig. 3), the apparent activity of the test material gradually rose as the concentration of the starting solution was lowered. The level of activity corresponding to a starting solution of 300 μg/ml was 10^{-1}–10^{-2} μg/ml whereas that corresponding to a starting concentration of 0.03 μg/ml was 10^{-2}–10^{-3} μg/ml.

These results are consistent with the hypothesis that NGF is reversibly adsorbed onto the pipettes used in the dilution procedures. This effect will predominate at high concentrations of NGF and will be minimized by lowering the concentration of the starting solution of the test material. In this way, the pipettes are not brought into contact with very high concentrations of the factor. The apparent activity of a sample diluted with a single pipette will therefore fall as the concentration of the starting solution is lowered and as the adsorption of NGF onto the pipette is reduced. Conversely, the apparent activity of a sample diluted with a series of pipettes will rise under these conditions, the losses of material being diminished. In addition to providing impressive confirmation of the hypothesis of adsorption, this experiment also confines the level of activity of the sample to within relatively narrow limits. The level of activity given by both methods of dilution from a starting concentration of 0.03 μg/ml was 10^{-2}–10^{-3} μg/ml. Since one method will overestimate this level and the other will underestimate it, the true level of activity must lie between these limits.

In the experiments described above, the ranges of concentrations required for the assay of NGF were prepared by making a series of ten-fold dropwise dilutions from a standard starting solution. The adsorption of NGF will, however, be maximized in dropwise dilutions of this type, since the active solution is drawn into a capillary region of each pipette where the ratio of the surface area to the volume is relatively high. The adsorption should then be minimized by diluting larger volumes of the sample from pipettes of wider bore in which this ratio is reduced. A ten-fold dilution of this type may conveniently be made by pipetting 1 ml of the test solution into 9 ml of the diluent. The dose-response curves obtained in this way, and by dropwise dilutions, using glass and polystyrene apparatus, are shown in Figs. 4 and 5.

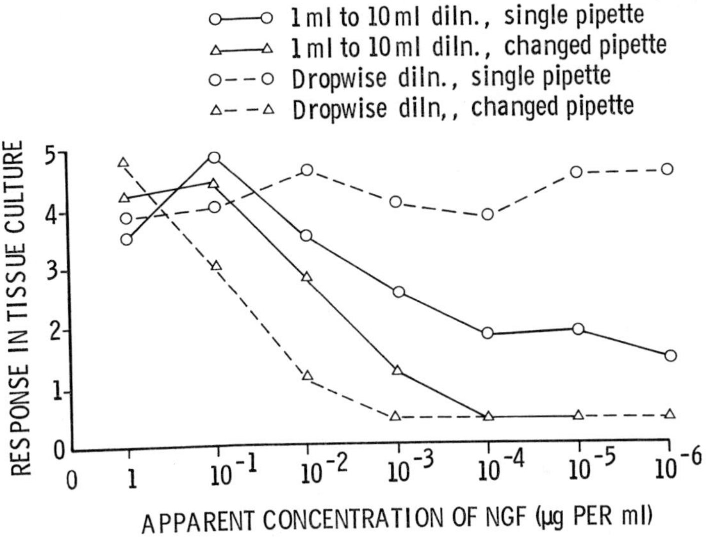

Fig. 4 Dose-response curves obtained by various dilution methods using glass apparatus.

As expected, when the dilution was made by means of a single pipette, the apparent activity of the test material was decreased by changing from a dropwise method of dilution to a volumetric method in which 1 ml is diluted to 10 ml. Conversely, when the dilution was made by means of a series of different pipettes, the activity measured was increased by changing the method of dilution in this way. The most marked displacements in the dose-response curves occurred when the sample was diluted with pipettes made of glass (Fig. 4), and the displacements were considerably smaller when the sample was diluted with pipettes made of polystyrene (Fig. 5). Furthermore, while the dose-response curves obtained by the two methods of volumetric dilution were not exactly superimposable, the level of activity of the sample was again confined within acceptably narrow limits between 10^{-2} and 10^{-3} μg/ml.

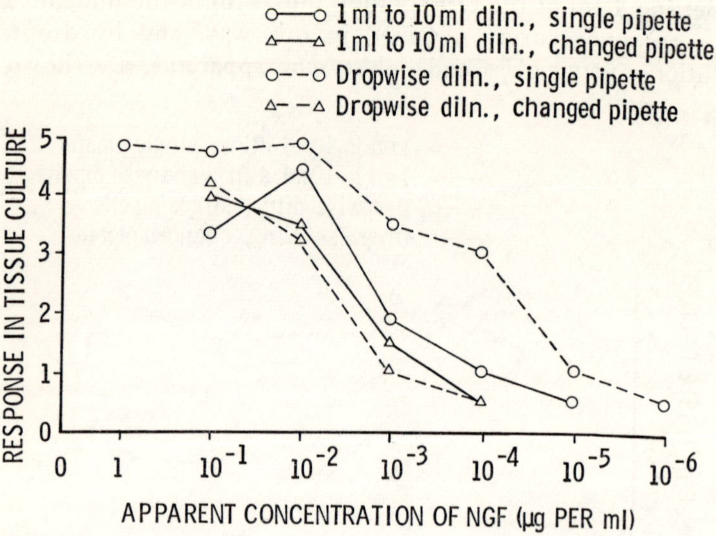

Fig. 5 Dose-response curves obtained by various dilution methods using polystyrene apparatus.

In conclusion, the observation that NGF may be reversibly adsorbed onto a variety of solid surfaces probably accounts for the considerable difficulty that has been experienced by many workers in obtaining meaningful results for the assay of given samples of active material. The adsorption is, however, minimized for surfaces of polystyrene and the most accurate and convenient method for the dilution of samples of NGF consists of making a series of 1 ml to 10 ml dilutions, using polystyrene apparatus. The dose-response curves obtained by this method are reproducible and do not vary appreciably with changes in the starting concentration of the test solution. Finally, it should be emphasized that the experiments described were done with samples of NGF from Russell's viper venom. The same effects are observed for the NGF from the venom of the common European viper; but the adsorption on to solid surfaces of the high molecular weight aggregate from mouse salivary gland is much less. The extent to which NGF from other sources exhibits this behaviour is therefore of interest.

References

Angeletti, R. (1969). *Brain Res.* **12**, 234.
Banks, B. E. C., Banthorpe, D. V., Berry, A. R., Davies, H. ff. S., Doonan, S., Lamont, D. M., Shipolini, R. & Vernon, C. A. (1968). *Biochem. J.* **108**, 157.
Cohen, S. (1959). *J. biol. Chem.* **234**, 1129.
Cohen, S. & Levi-Montalcini, R. (1957). *Cancer Res.* **17**, 15.
Cohen, S., Levi-Montalcini, R. & Hamburger, V. (1954). *Proc. natn. Acad. Sci. U.S.A.* **40**, 1014.
Levi-Montalcini, R. (1966). *Harvey Lectures*, Ser. **60**, 217.
Levi-Montalcini, R., Meyer, H. & Hamburger, V. (1954). *Cancer Res.* **14**, 49.
Levy, M., Schenkein, I., Boesman, M., Tokarsky, E. and Bueker, E. D. (1969). *Fedn. Proc. Fedn. Am. Socs exp. Biol.* **28**, 872.
Schenkein, I. & Bueker, E. D. (1964). *Ann. N.Y. Acad. Sci.* **118**, 171.
Schenkein, I., Levy, M., Bueker, E. D. & Tokarsky, E. (1968). *Science* **159**, 640.

Radioimmunoassay of Nerve Growth Factor from Mouse Salivary Gland

I. A. HENDRY, G. M. ADDISON and L. L. IVERSEN

Departments of Pharmacology and Biochemistry, University of Cambridge, UK

For the routine assay of protein hormones, the technique of radioimmunoassay has several advantages over biological assays. The existing assay for the nerve growth factor (NGF) (Levi-Montalcini, Meyer & Hamburger, 1954; Cohen, 1959; Fenton, 1970) requires the growth of 8-day-old chick embryo sensory ganglia in tissue cultures containing serial dilutions of NGF. Subjective estimates are then made to determine the concentration which produces a maximum fibre outgrowth (the 4+ response): this concentration is defined as one Biological Unit (B.U.)/ml. Accurate determination of this concentration requires a large number of dilutions, thus limiting the number of samples that can conveniently be assayed, as well as reducing the practical sensitivity of this method. Subjective estimates of concentrations of less than 1 B.U./ml can be made, using the 1+, 2+ and 3+ responses, but such estimates are not quantitatively accurate.

We have developed a radioimmunoassay procedure for NGF isolated from mouse salivary gland. Because of the tendency of the 7S species of NGF to dissociate into subunits, the active β-subunit was chosen for the development of this assay. The assay is thus specific for the biologically active component of the 7S protein, and is effective whether this component is present in free or aggregated form. For convenience we shall refer to the β-subunit as 'β-NGF'. This assay shares with other radio-immunoassays the advantages of sensitivity and precision in comparison with the biological methods. We are able to measure accurately amounts of less than 0.05 B.U., giving a twenty-fold improvement over the previous maximum sensitivity of the biological assay.

The form that our assay takes follows the principle of the two-site assay procedure of Addison & Hales (1971) which has been shown to be valid for insulin, growth hormone and parathyroid hormone. The protocol is shown in Fig. 1, which illustrates the two stages of the procedure. The NGF to be assayed is first bound to a solid-phase antibody and this complex is then reacted with radioactively labelled specific anti-β-NGF antibodies which bind to the β-NGF already fixed. This has the advantage of yielding a low zero value, and since there is a proportionate increase in bound radioactivity with increasing amounts of β-NGF, the assay has a high sensitivity. It also has the advantage of increased selectivity, as two antigenic sites are required for the complete reaction.

The solid-phase antibody is the base on which all subsequent reactions take place. Whatman No. 1 filter paper was converted to aminocellulose by a modification of the method of Gurvich, Kuzovleva & Tumanova (1961) using *m*-nitrobenzylomethyl-pyridinium chloride. Semi-purified IgG was prepared from β-NGF rabbit antiserum* by sodium sulphate precipitation at 18 per cent w/v. The precipitated IgG was dissolved in 5 mM-potassium phosphate buffer, pH 8.0, dialysed against this buffer and then linked to the filter paper by the method of Addison & Hales (1971). The paper was finally washed in a buffer pH 8.6, containing 0.5 M-veronal, 0.9 per cent sodium chloride, 0.5 per cent bovine serum albumin and 0.1 per cent sodium azide ('veronal buffer'). It was finally cut into 0.5 cm squares for use in the assay, and stored in this buffer at 4°C. The paper retained its immunological reactivity for at least six months under these storage conditions.

The second stage of the reaction involves the use of labelled specific anti-β-NGF antibodies. The preparation of these is

* β-NGF and β-NGF rabbit antiserum were generously donated by Dr D. C. Edwards of the Wellcome Research Laboratories, Beckenham, Kent. The preparation of β-NGF used was electrophoretically homogeneous, and yielded only one precipitin band on immunodiffusion against anti-β-NGF rabbit antiserum. In the tissue culture bioassay method of Fenton (1970), this preparation of β-NGF had an activity of 1 B.U. per 2 ng of protein.

shown in outline in Fig. 2. An immunoadsorbent containing β-NGF was prepared by fixing β-NGF to cellulose powder, as described above. Diazo-cellulose powder (10 mg/ml) was suspended in 0.2 M-borate buffer, pH 8.0. To 1 ml of this suspension 0.25 ml of borate buffer containing 2.5 mg of β-NGF was added, giving a final protein concentration of 2 mg/ml. After 72 hours

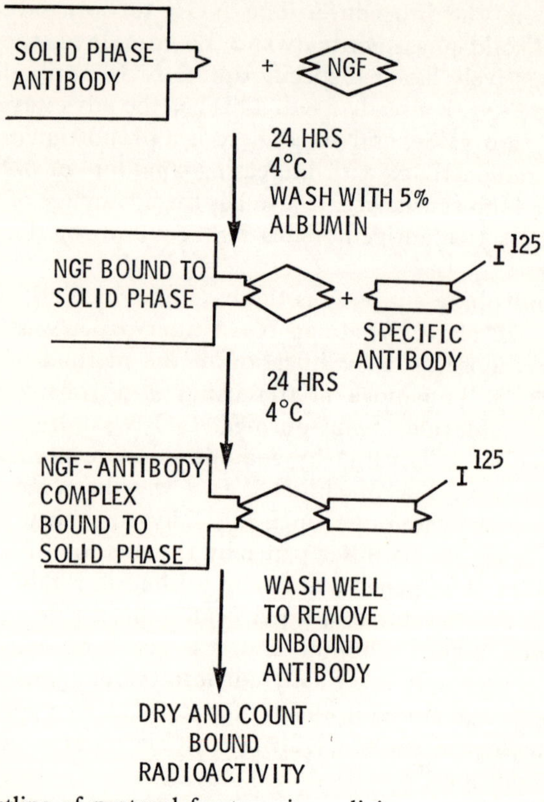

Fig. 1 Outline of protocol for two-site radioimmunoassay of β-NGF.

the unchanged diazo groups were inactivated by the addition of 1 ml of a saturated solution of glycine and mixing for 24 hours. The suspension was centrifuged and the supernatant sampled and assayed for protein content. The amount of β-NGF fixed to the cellulose was 160 mg/g of matrix, or 64 per cent of the added protein. This immunoadsorbent was washed six times with water and then suspended in veronal buffer. Specific anti-β NGF-antibodies were isolated from rabbit antiserum by use of this immunoadsorbent and were labelled with ^{125}I while bound to the immunoadsorbent. This procedure ensures the protection of at least one antigen-binding site during the iodination reaction. The β-NGF immunoadsorbent (1 mg) was saturated with anti-β-NGF antibody by mixing for 24 hours at 4°C with 1 ml of antiserum. The immunoadsorbent was

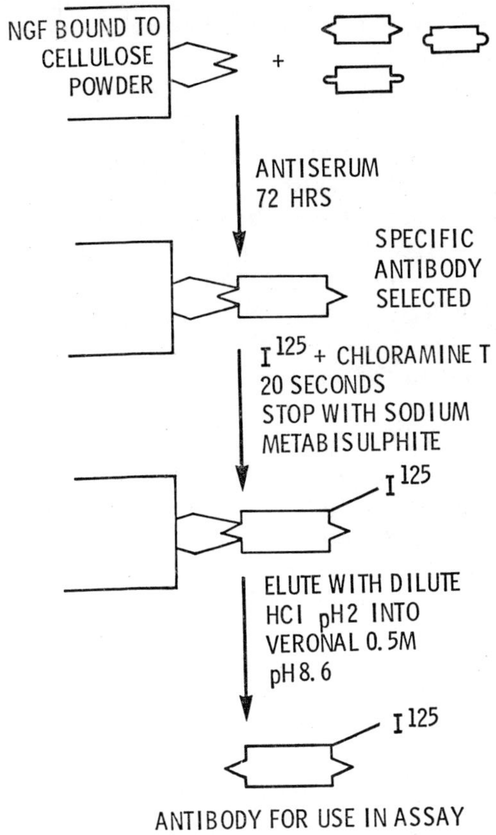

Fig. 2 Summary of procedure used to prepare radioactively labelled specific anti-β-NGF antibodies.

recovered by centrifugation, and was resuspended in a further 1 ml of antiserum before being left for 24 hours at 4°C. This procedure was repeated once more, and the complex was then washed thoroughly with a potassium phosphate buffer, 0.4 M, pH 7.6 (five times). Approximately 100 μg of antibody protein was bound per 1 mg of immunoadsorbent. An amount of immunoadsorbent containing 25 μg of antibody protein was centrifuged and the supernatant was discarded. The bound antibody was then iodinated by the method of Greenwood, Hunter & Glover (1963); 25 μg chloramine-T dissolved in 0.1 M-phosphate buffer at pH 7.4 in a volume of 10 μl and 1 μCi of ^{125}I were added. After 20 seconds the reaction was stopped with 60 μg of sodium metabisulphite in 10 μl of the phosphate buffer. The suspension was rapidly washed through a filter-funnel lined by two Whatman No. 1 papers with 200 ml of veronal buffer pH 8.6. After successive washes with 100 ml each of water and 0.001 N-hydrochloric acid the antibodies were eluted with three 4 ml washes of 0.01 N-hydrochloric acid into 4 ml of veronal buffer. About 10–15 per cent of the original quantity of ^{125}I was recovered by this elution, yielding approximately one iodine atom per antibody molecule. The iodination yielded sufficient amounts of labelled antibodies for several thousand assays and these were stored, rebound to the immunoadsorbent, at 4°C. The length of storage is limited only by the half-life of ^{125}I, which is 60 days. The antibodies were washed on the immunoadsorbent and eluted before each assay, thus ensuring the removal of any molecules damaged by radiochemical decomposition.

In the first stage of the assay (Fig. 1), solid-phase antibody is incubated with the solution to be assayed, after which it is washed well with veronal buffer containing a high protein (albumin) concentration (1 per cent). The washed paper containing the bound NGF is then incubated with 100 μl of the specific ^{125}I-labelled antibodies. The labelled antibodies were diluted with the high-protein veronal buffer to give approximately 20 000 d.p.m. in each incubation tube. The high protein concentrations were required to reduce the non-specific binding of the labelled antibodies to the paper. After this incubation the paper was again washed thoroughly with the high-protein veronal buffer to remove any unbound radioactivity. The paper was then dried and immersed in scintillant solution (0.4 per cent butyl PBD*, CIBA Ltd, in toluene) for counting. There was an increase in the sensitivity of the assay with duration of incubation for at least 40 hours in both stages of the reaction (Fig. 3). Incubation periods of 24 hours were chosen for each stage of the assay for convenience: these were a compromise between the time taken to perform the assay and its sensitivity. If an increase

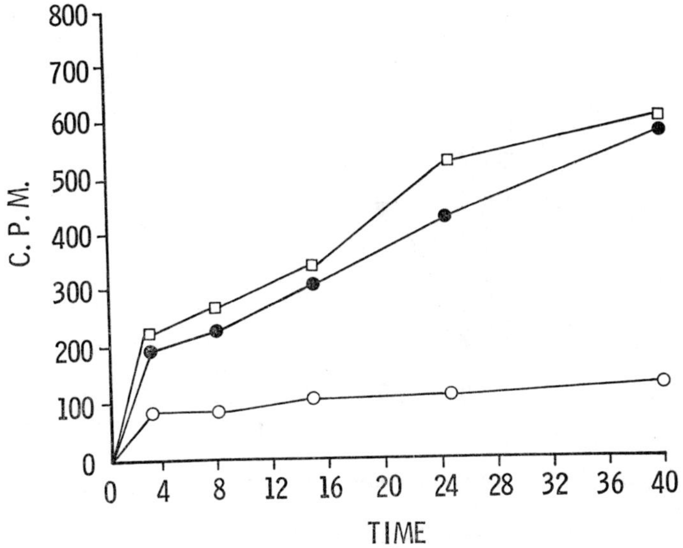

Fig. 3 Effect of incubation time on NGF radioimmunoassay results. Amount of bound radioactivity is shown after various incubation times (in hours) using 10 ng β-NGF in the first incubation:
□—□ first incubation, varying times. Second incubation 16 hours.
●—● first incubation 16 hours. Second incubation, varying times.
○—○ results after varying times of second incubation with no NGF in first incubation.

in sensitivity is required, longer incubation times can be used. However, in most of the work involved in the purification of NGF, such sensitivity is not required. In situations where many fractions have to be assayed from column eluates, a fast assay is required. By sacrificing sensitivity, incubation times can be

* 2-(4′-t-butylphenyl)-5-(4″-biphenyl)-1,3,4-oxdiazole.

very much reduced. For example, if incubation periods of three hours for each stage are used, the sensitivity of the assay is reduced by ten-fold, to about 10 ng/ml. The results, however, may be obtained in one day.

A typical standard curve is shown in Fig. 4. The β-NGF we used had an activity of 1 B.U./2 ng; 100 pg on quadruplicate

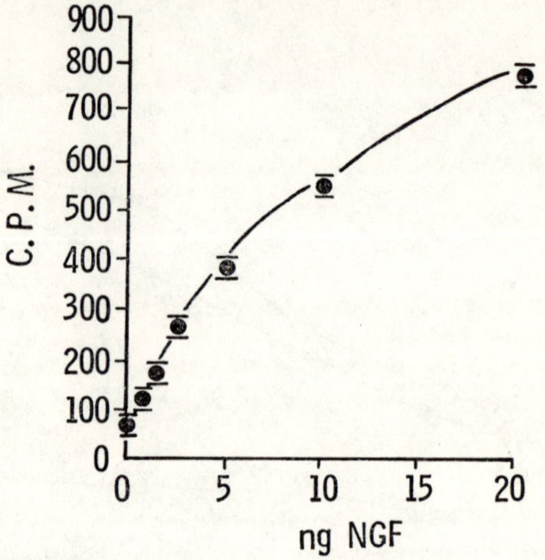

Fig. 4 Standard curve for radioimmunoassay of β-NGF. Each point is the mean ± S.E.M. for quadruplicate determinations; incubation periods of 24 hours were used for both stages of the assay.

assays gave values significantly higher than the background radioactivity. Thus this assay has a sensitivity of 0.05 B.U. We also obtained samples of NGF at various stages during the purification of the '7S' species (supplied by S. Walters and C. A. Vernon of the Department of Chemistry, University College London). There was a good correlation between the bioassay results obtained on these samples and the results of the immunoassay (Table 1). This result confirmed that the immunoassay was applicable to the assay of NGF in its aggregated '7S' form. In this case, the number of assays that could be performed in the bioassay system permitted only a ten-fold series of dilutions, and hence it was only possible to obtain approximate estimates

Table 1 Comparison of bioassay with radioimmunoassay of NGF in partially purified preparations from mouse salivary glands

	Amount of protein (μg) *equivalent to 1 B.U. of NGF*	
Fraction no.	*Bioassay*	*Radioimmunoassay*
1	0.3	0.1
2	10–100	20
3	1–10	1.7
4	0.3	0.05
5	10–100	30
6	10–100	25

One B.U. is the amount of NGF yielding a 4+ response in tissue culture (bioassay) or equivalent to 2 ng of β-NGF (radioimmunoassay). Bioassays were performed by S. Walters (Department of Chemistry, University College London). Radioimmunoassay results are from duplicate determinations.

of NGF concentration. The immunoassay, however, always gives a definite value for NGF concentration. We have also assayed mouse submaxillary glands using this method. These results (Table 2) agree well with those found previously using Cohen's

Table 2 Radioimmunoassay of NGF content of mouse salivary glands

Source of tissue	β-*NGF concentration* μ*g/g wet weight*
Prepubertal male and female mice	0.6 ± 0.02
Adult female mice	60.0 ± 3.0
Adult male mice	170.0 ± 24.0

Submaxillary glands were dissected from Swiss Albino mice and homogenized in 10 volumes of veronal buffer and serial dilutions prepared in this buffer; aliquots of the diluted homogenates were used for radioimmunoassay of β-NGF content (duplicate assay). Results are mean values ± S.E.M. for groups of four animals.

bioassay method (1960). The salivary glands from male mice contained higher concentrations of β-NGF than had those from females, and the tissue from prepubertal animals contained very much lower concentrations of β-NGF than did that from adults.

The present assay has the advantage over existing bioassay

methods of increased sensitivity and ease of performance. The subjective role of the experimenter is removed and a precise value for NGF concentration is obtained. For NGF from species other than the mouse, comparison with a bioassay will be required, as the antigenicity of the protein from other species will probably vary.

Acknowledgements

I.A.H. holds a Fellowship from the Postgraduate Medical Foundation of Sydney. G.M.A. is a Junior Research Fellow of the Medical Research Council. These studies were supported by a grant to L.L.I. from the Medical Research Council. We are very grateful to Dr D. C. Edwards of the Wellcome Research Laboratories for his advice and for generous supplies of the materials used in this study.

References

Addison, G. M. & Hales, C. N. (1971). *Horm. Metab. Res.* **3**, 59.
Cohen, S. (1959). *J. biol. Chem.* **234**, 1129.
Cohen, S. (1960). *Proc. natn. Acad. Sci. U.S.A.* **46**, 302.
Fenton, E. L. (1970). *Expl Cell Res.* **59**, 383.
Gurvich, A. E., Kuzovleva, O. B. & Tumanova, A. E. (1961). *Biokhimiya* **26**, 803.
Greenwood, F. C., Hunter, W. M. & Glover, J. S. (1963). *Biochem. J.* **89**, 114.
Levi-Montalcini, R., Meyer, H. & Hamburger, V. (1954). *Cancer Res.* **14**, 49.

Index

X19.90
N
+1.40 prl

WITHDRAWN

QP
363
N47

A10202 846110